PENGUIN BOOKS

jamie's dinners

'If you're sick of sticking a TV dinner in the microwave and fancy trying
something a little more creative, then call on the ever-pukka Jamie for
a little bit of nosh advice'
OK!

'Thank God for Jamie Oliver'
Fiona Phillips, *Daily Mirror*

'When it comes to getting our nation of young people eating healthily,
there are no limits to the lengths Jamie will go to'
Heat

'Jamie is a national asset'
Daily Mail

'Jamie – every parent's best friend'
Sunday Times

'Jamie is encouraging parents to look at what they give their own
children and provides easy, interesting recipes'
The Times

'I have become obsessed with the wondrous goodness of Jamie
Oliver... the country's most deserving candidate for canonization'
Sunday Times

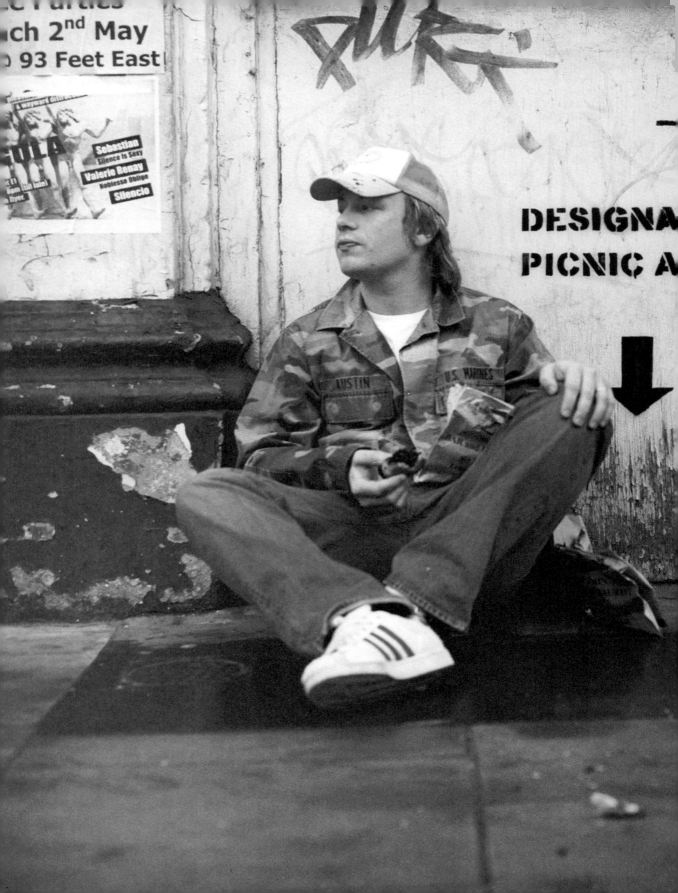

LOVE
TANYA
ROBINSON

JAMIE OLIVER

jamie's dinners

with photographs by david loftus and chris terry
and illustrations by marion deuchars

PENGUIN BOOKS

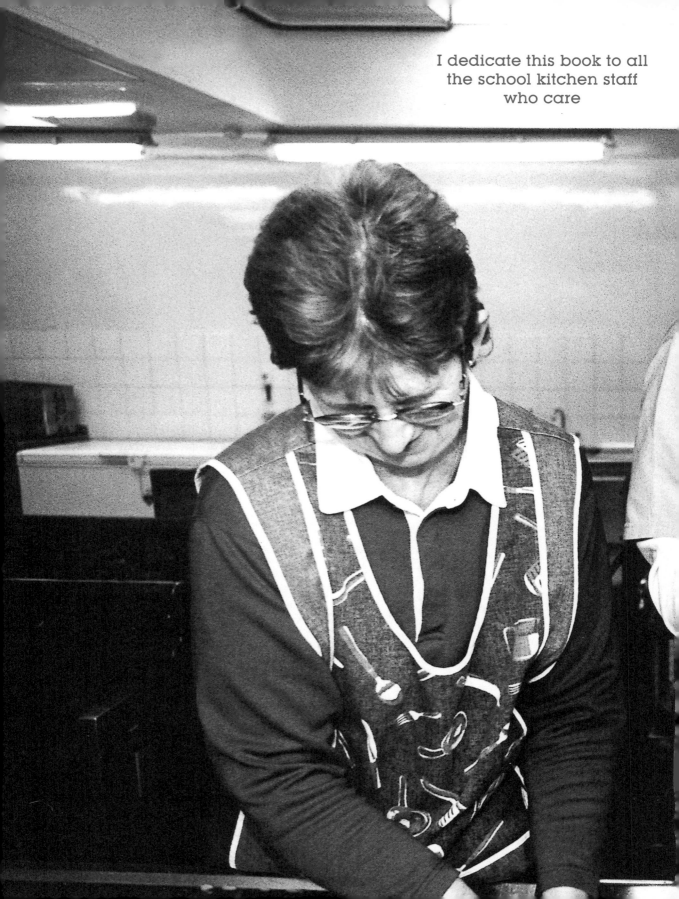

I dedicate this book to all
the school kitchen staff
who care

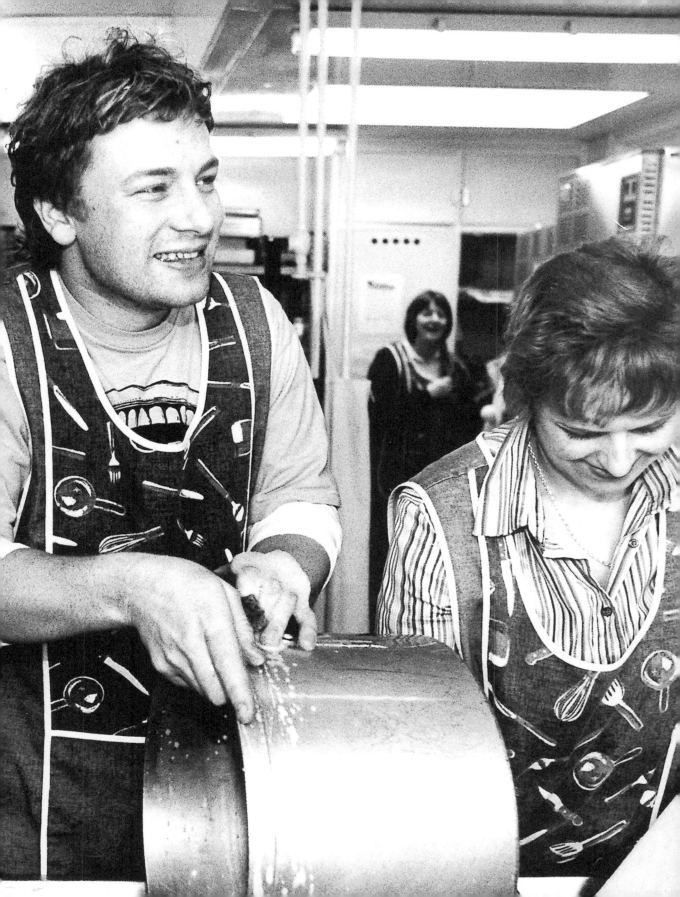

PENGUIN BOOKS

Published by the Penguin Group
Penguin Books Ltd, 80 Strand, London WC2R 0RL, England
Penguin Group (USA) Inc., 375 Hudson Street, New York, New York 10014, USA
Penguin Group (Canada), 90 Eglinton Avenue East, Suite 700, Toronto, Ontario,
Canada M4P 2Y3 (a division of Pearson Penguin Canada Inc.)
Penguin Ireland, 25 St Stephen's Green, Dublin 2, Ireland (a division of Penguin Books Ltd)
Penguin Group (Australia), 250 Camberwell Road, Camberwell, Victoria 3124, Australia
(a division of Pearson Australia Group Pty Ltd)
Penguin Books India Pvt Ltd, 11 Community Centre,
Panchsheel Park, New Delhi – 110 017, India
Penguin Group (NZ), 67 Apollo Drive, Rosedale, North Shore 0632, New Zealand
(a division of Pearson New Zealand Ltd)
Penguin Books (South Africa) (Pty) Ltd, 24 Sturdee Avenue, Rosebank,
Johannesburg 2196, South Africa

Penguin Books Ltd, Registered Offices: 80 Strand, London WC2R 0RL, England

www.penguin.com

First published by Michael Joseph 2004
Published in Penguin Books 2006
Reissued in Penguin Books 2010
1

Copyright © Jamie Oliver, 2004
Photographs copyright © David Loftus and Chris Terry, 2004
Illustrations copyright © Marion Deuchars, 2004
All rights reserved

The moral right of the author has been asserted

Set in Helvetica and Lubalin Graph
Typeset by Rowland Phototypesetting Ltd, Bury St Edmonds, Suffolk
Printed in China

Except in the United States of America, this book is sold subject
to the condition that it shall not, by way of trade or otherwise, be lent,
re-sold, hired out, or otherwise circulated without the publisher's
prior consent in any form of binding or cover other than that in
which it is published and without a similar condition including this
condition being imposed on the subsequent purchaser

ISBN: 978–0–141–04300–5

jamieoliver.com

contents

INTRODUCTION

I'm really proud of this book because it's full of recipes for great family dinners, and what I want is to get you all cooking and enjoying them together at home. I've noticed, as I continue to work as a chef and grow as a parent, that there are a whole bunch of people who just don't cook at all, or do so very rarely. But I truly believe that anyone can cook and love it – and that everyone has it in them to hold great dinner parties, family occasions or everyday meals that are remembered for a long time. What I hope this book will do is show that anyone can have a go at cooking. It's totally aimed at families and at those who have an interest in good food, no matter what your budget is. Probably someone like you!

Over the last two and a half years I've been researching and filming a documentary series looking at the food being served in British schools, to see if we can at last cook tasty and nutritious meals for school kids. I decided to use the same idea in my approach to this book, which means the food is cheap, economical, accessible, easy and time-efficient to make. We all want the same things when making dinner at home for our families.

All the major factors that are needed to make a good affordable school dinner also apply to a mindful, clever cook at home. Availability, accessibility, regionality, affordability, simplicity and a tasty product are the key, with not too much washing-up if you're lucky! Just taking all these words has provided me with a great brief for this cookbook. It's not concerned with fillet steak and lobster and posh stuff. Most of the recipes use pretty standard ingredients that you can buy from street markets or supermarkets all over the country, if not the world.

I think you'll get a lot out of these chapters. They concern themselves with the types of food that most of us are eating every day. For instance, there is a lovely little chapter called Five Minute Wonders, which gives you eight fantastically quick recipes. Perfect for busy lives as each one only takes five minutes or so. I hope a chapter like The Top Ten is really going to inspire you. It's like Top of the Pops, but for food, and it gives you ten crowd-pleasers that everyone loves to eat. The Family Tree chapter takes recipes like a simple tomato sauce or pesto and shows you how to take them further by changing and tweaking here and there, so you can make a whole handful of dishes from just one recipe. I've also included a chapter on sandwiches – you might think this sounds a bit naff, but it's great because it acknowledges that sandwiches are the most widely eaten food product in most western countries. I've tried to show you how you can make really good portable meals to make your work colleagues or friends jealous at lunchtime! Have a look at the picture of the lunchbox on page 76. Then all your normal chapters follow, like Pasta, Meat and Fish. With Vegetables I've kept things really chatty and shown you that veggies can be a real highlight to your dinner, not just an extra. I've given you various different ways of cooking each vegetable so you can widen your repertoire even more.

I was brought up around food, around chefs and cooks, and I also love nature, agriculture and farming, the changing seasons and the produce that comes with them. You may feel the same way as I do about these things – however, I do think a lot of people just don't understand the importance of where their food comes from or what might have been done to it before they buy it. It's good to question these things.

First, good-quality food and produce – and yes, this may involve organics – is always considered to be middle-class or rich people's food. Wrong. I've worked with students and people on the dole who eat better than some city boys earning hundreds of thousands of pounds a year, and the reason is that they use their heads when buying. Why is this important? Why should you have standards when buying? Because you're going to put this food in your mouth and swallow it and you'll do this two or three times every single day of your life. Everything you eat contributes to you being happy, or fit, or lethargic, or full of energy, or susceptible to colds and flu, or being able to think better and hold your concentration. Your hair, your fingernails, your height, your skin, everything you are is made from the food you eat.

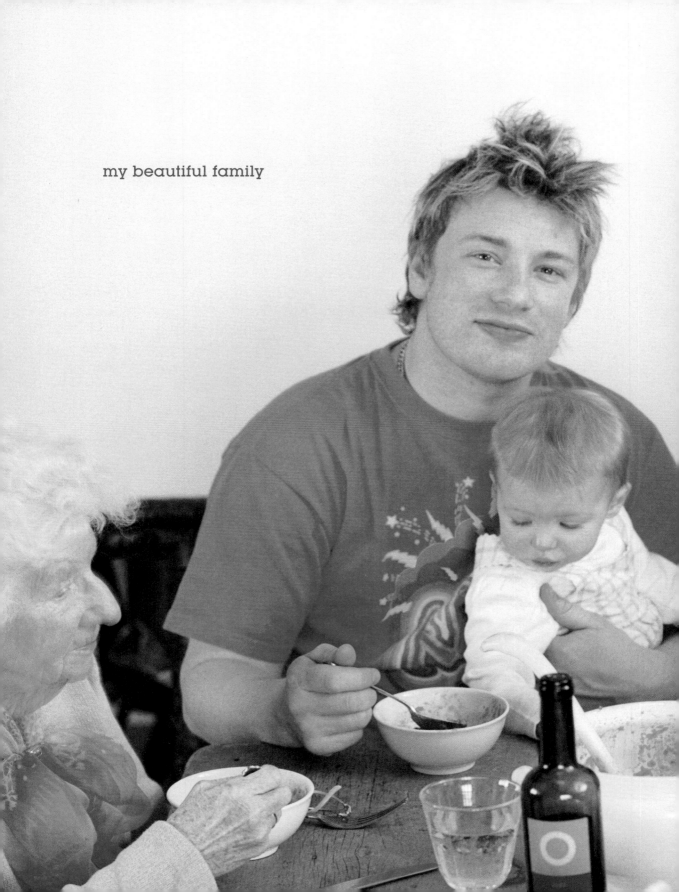

my beautiful family

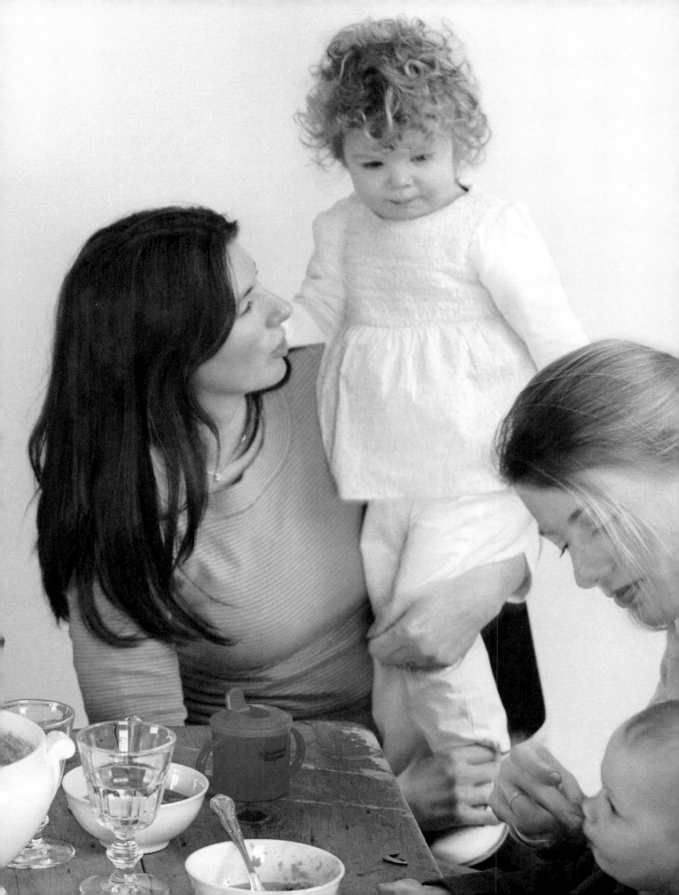

Very rarely does anyone go into a garage, phone shop or shoe shop and ask for 'the cheapest, most rubbish one'. So why do we walk into super-markets and support those companies that are producing cheap products? As a general rule, when food is cheap the quality is not going to be so good. I'm happy to say that the supermarket I work with sells the largest amount of British organic products compared to the others, but we should all try to steer them in the right direction. All supermarkets have got to push forward, try harder to support regional, or at least British, produce and strive for more integrity.

It all comes down to your perception of value – is it about buying the cheapest thing you can get, or is it about spending a little more and getting something that tastes nicer, smells better and makes you feel good in return? People in Britain spend the smallest percentage of their weekly wage on food compared to most of the rest of Europe. Europeans tend to spend more on better produce. I think it's a matter of priorities. For instance, before I got married, if I'd suggested that we go out to a half decent restaurant to spend £25 to £30 on a meal, with a few bottles of wine to get tiddly, my friends would not have been interested in the slightest, but if I'd said, 'Why don't we go to the local nightclub?' where we'd have ended up spending £50 on drinks, even my friends who were unemployed or on the dole would have found the money somehow. I don't think it always comes down to money, I think it's a priority thing.

I'd never try to persuade you to necessarily spend more money, but I'd really like you to spend the money you've got more wisely when shopping for food. I've got friends who are unemployed and have time on their hands, yet they fill their shopping trolleys with packets of processed food and soft drinks, with no veggies in sight. And yet this is the most expensive way to feed your family. It is much cheaper to buy fresh produce and cook it than to heat up pre-packaged, processed food. There really isn't much excuse for not giving cooking a go.

Whether I'm at home with my family, or at work with my surrogate family at the restaurant, I enjoy sitting down to eat and chat with them. So what I hope will happen with this book is that you'll get stuck in and enjoy some of these recipes with your friends and family.

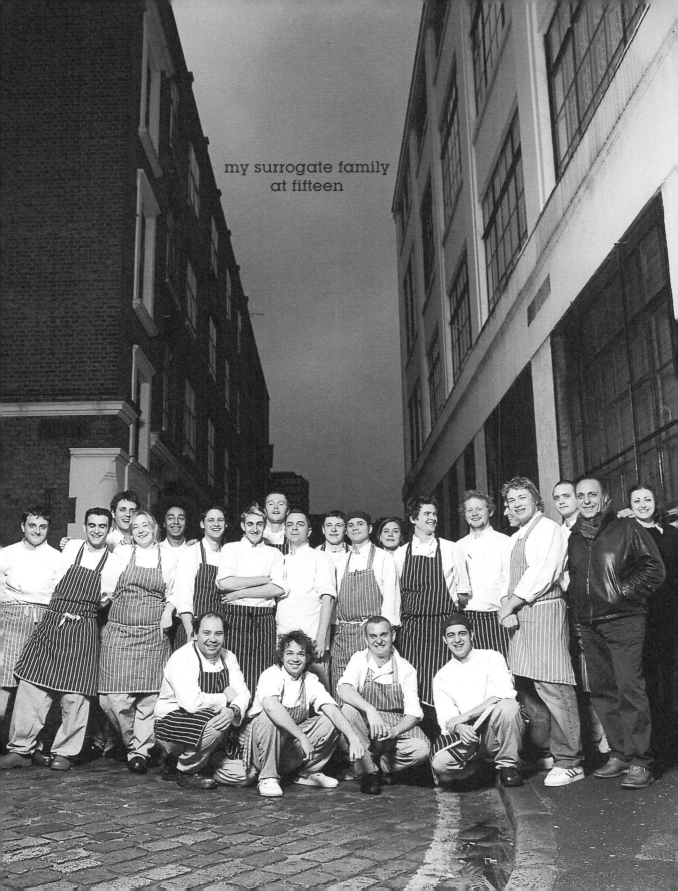

my surrogate family
at fifteen

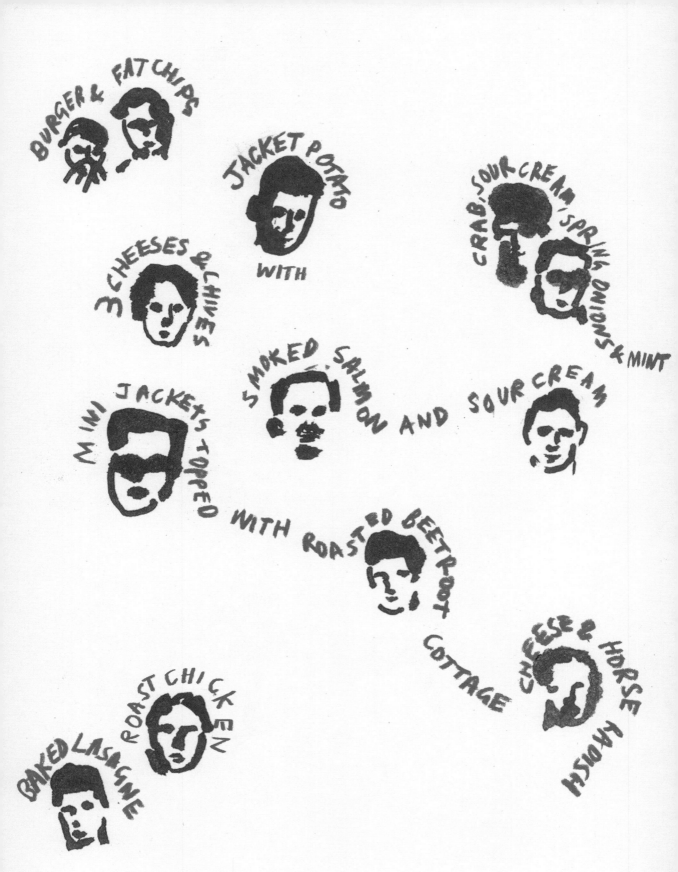

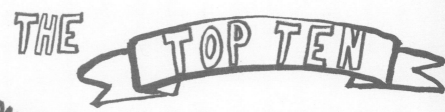
THE TOP TEN

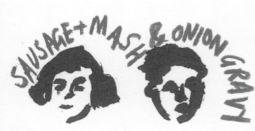
SAUSAGE + MASH & ONION GRAVY

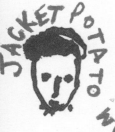
JACKET POTATO

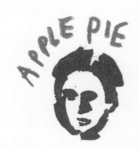
WITH PRAWNS & MARIE ROSE SAUCE

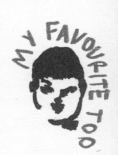
MY FAVOURITE TOO

APPLE PIE

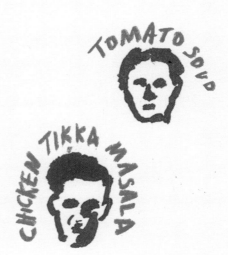
TOMATO SOUP

CHICKEN TIKKA MASALA

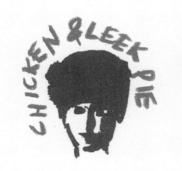
CHICKEN & LEEK PIE

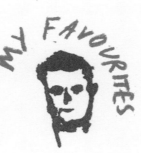
MY FAVOURITES

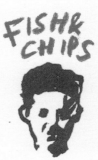
FISH & CHIPS

As this is a friendly book about everyday dinners for all of us, I thought I'd hit you with a collection of favourite dishes early on and not muck about! But I don't just want to give you my own thoughts (although, if you're interested, I've listed my personal favourites below!). We're always hearing about Top Tens for music, films and books, so, knowing that every one of you will have your own Top Ten dinners, I asked people who visit my website to write in and tell me about their favourite food. Over the course of about six months I had thousands of ideas coming in from all over the world and, although they differed from country to country, it was interesting to see that we all have favourites in common. So this chapter is based on ten dishes that I love to cook and eat with my family, but that are also your favourites.

MY FAVOURITE DINNERS ...

Mum's superb roasted chicken; spaghetti arrabiatta; a spicy noodle laksa soup; a fantastic bacon sandwich; the ultimate steak and chips; simply poached salmon with asparagus, new potatoes and homemade mayonnaise; Peking roasted duck and pancakes; shepherd's pie; fish pie; fruit pie (apple or cherry); rhubarb crumble ...

... and now we're over ten, you see! And that's without even mentioning roast leg of lamb, spaghetti bolognaise or meatballs, all of which I love ... It's very hard to narrow it down to ten!

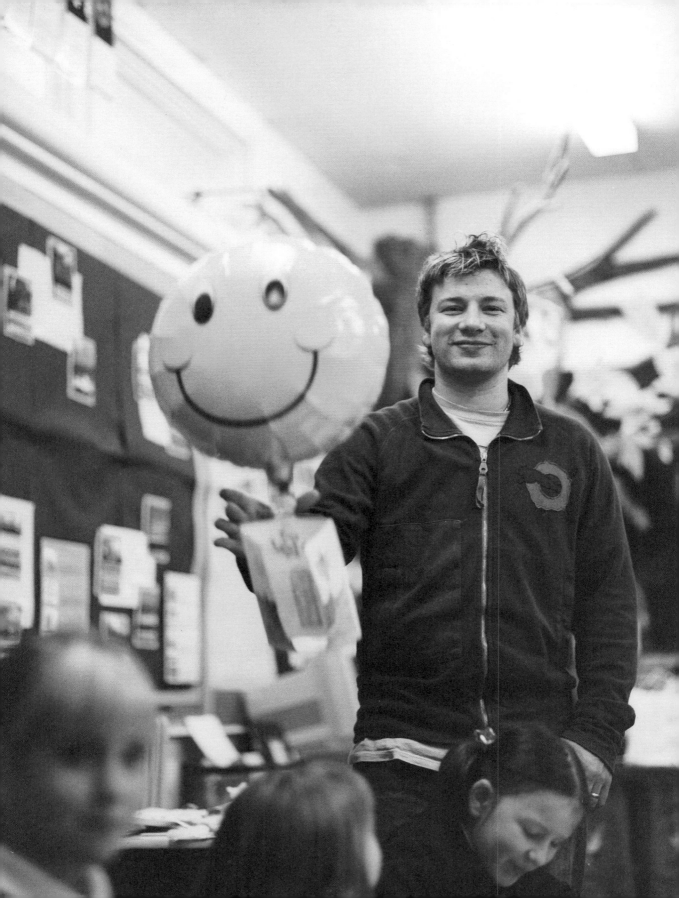

THE BEST SAUSAGE AND SUPER MASH WITH ONION GRAVY

I really love this recipe for sausage and mash – you must have a go at it! I made it on Bonfire Night last year, inspired by my mate Peter Gott's award-winning Cumberland sausages. If you can't get hold of the traditional curled sausage, just roll up a string of about eight normal ones to give you a similar shape. You will need some wooden skewers or long, sharpened rosemary sticks.

SERVES 4

2 long, curled Cumberland
    sausages
2 cloves of garlic, peeled and
    finely sliced
a bunch of fresh sage,
    leaves picked
olive oil
a bunch of fresh rosemary,
    leaves picked
2kg/4½lb potatoes, peeled

sea salt and freshly ground
    black pepper
300ml/just over ½ pint milk
115g/4oz butter
4 tablespoons freshly grated horseradish,
    or use jarred
4 medium red onions, peeled and
    finely sliced
5 tablespoons balsamic or red
    wine vinegar
2 beef or chicken stock cubes

Preheat your oven to 200°C/400°F/gas 6. If you're using the traditional round Cumberland sausage, tuck the garlic and most of the sage leaves between the layers of sausage. If you're using normal sausages, untwist the links and squeeze the meat through, rolling them into a tight circle and pushing in the garlic and sage as you go. (This will give the sausages a terrific flavour.) Secure the sausages with a couple of skewers or some sharp rosemary stalks. Place them on an oiled baking tray, drizzle them with olive oil and sprinkle them with the rosemary leaves. Cook in the preheated oven for 20 minutes, or until crisp and golden. Five minutes before the sausages are ready, remove the baking tray from the oven, place the rest of the sage leaves next to the sausages, drizzle with olive oil, then return the tray to the oven. The leaves will go lovely and crispy.

While the sausages are cooking, chop your potatoes into rough chunks and boil them in salted water until cooked. Drain well, using a colander, then return them to the pan. Mash until smooth, adding the milk, 70g/2½oz of the butter and the horseradish (use more if needed). Season well to taste, then put the lid on the pan and keep warm at the back of the stove.

Making the onion gravy is simple. Fry the onions – really slowly – in a little oil, covered, for about 15 minutes until soft. Remove the lid, turn the heat up, and as soon as the onions become golden brown, pour in the vinegar and boil until it almost disappears. Turn the heat down again, add the rest of the butter, crumble in your stock cubes and 565ml/1 pint of water and stir well. Let this simmer until you have a nice gravy consistency. To serve, dollop some oozy potatoes on the plate, chop up the sausages (discarding the skewers), put them alongside the mash, and spoon over the onion gravy. Scatter with the crispy sage leaves. Proper comfort food!

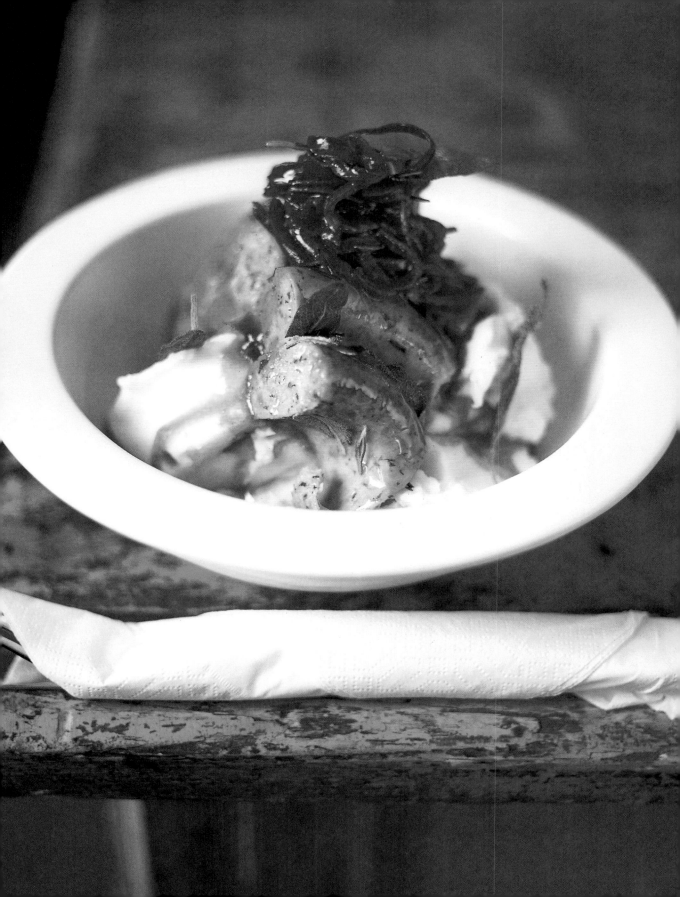

THE ULTIMATE BURGER AND CHIPS

One of the best meals in the world is burger and chips, and this burger is fantastic. A useful tip when it comes to mince is to buy some good chuck steak, either pulse it in a food processor or ask your butcher to mince it up for you – that way you always know what's in it. And the chips are so fantastic, far healthier than the deep-fried variety. The rosemary salt can be kept for months in a little airtight jar and has a fantastic, intense flavour that is great with chicken or pork chops, too.

MAKES APPROX. 8 BURGERS
1kg/2lb 3oz chuck steak, or
    good minced steak
1 onion, peeled and
    finely chopped
olive oil
a pinch of cumin seeds
1 tablespoon coriander seeds
sea salt and freshly ground
    black pepper
a handful of freshly grated
    Parmesan cheese
1 heaped tablespoon
    English mustard

1 large free-range egg
115g/4oz breadcrumbs
8 burger buns

FOR THE CHIPS
2kg/4½lb large potatoes, skins left on,
    cut into chips 1cm/½ inch thick
olive oil
1 whole bulb of garlic
freshly ground black pepper
3 sprigs of fresh rosemary
zest of 1 lemon
85g/3oz sea salt

If you're using chuck steak to make your burgers, slice it up and pulse it in a food processor. Transfer the meat to a bowl. In a big frying pan, slowly cook the onion in a little olive oil for about 5 minutes until softened but not coloured. Add the onion to the meat – it will give sweetness to the burger. Using a pestle and mortar, bash up the cumin and coriander seeds with a pinch of salt and freshly ground black pepper until fine and add to the meat. Then add the Parmesan, mustard, egg and half the breadcrumbs and mix well. If the mixture is too sticky, add a few more breadcrumbs.

Lay some greaseproof paper on a tray or large plate and sprinkle over some of the remaining breadcrumbs. Shape the meat into 8 fat burgers and place these on top of the crumbs on the tray. Sprinkle more crumbs on top and press down gently. The burgers are better if they are chilled before cooking, so put them in the fridge for an hour or so.

Half an hour before you want to cook the burgers, put a large flat baking tray in the oven and turn the heat to 230°C/450°F/gas 8. Parboil your chips (still with their skins on) for about 10 minutes in salted boiling water and drain in a colander. Heat some olive oil in a frying pan, smash the garlic bulb up and chuck in the cloves, then add the chips. Toss in the oil and season with freshly ground black pepper. Transfer the contents of the pan to the preheated tray and cook for 20 to 25 minutes until crisp and golden. Now make your rosemary salt. Remove the leaves from the rosemary and put them in a pestle and mortar with the lemon zest and salt. Bash up to make a green paste, adding more salt if the mixture is too wet. Push this paste through a sieve, and keep to one side until you're ready to serve.

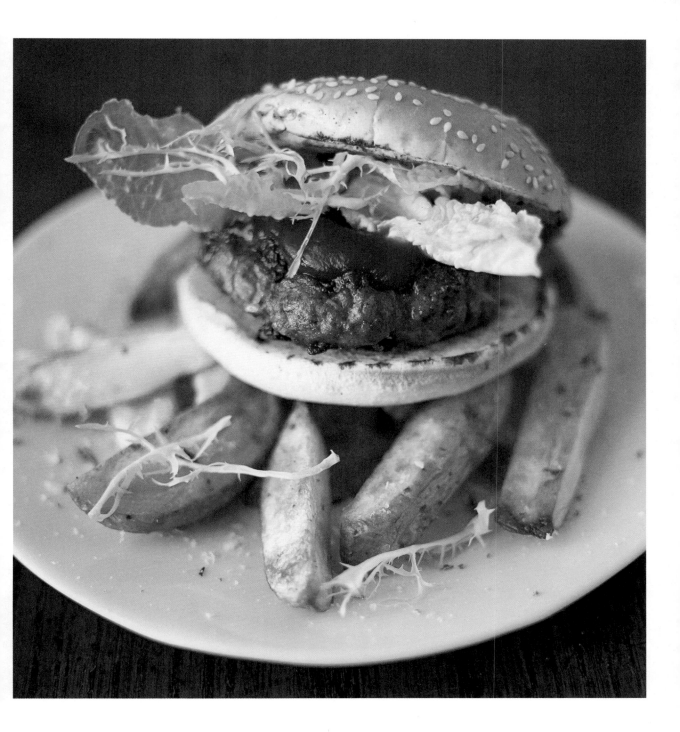

Take your burgers out of the fridge and fry them in a little oil on a medium to high heat for about 8 to 10 minutes, depending on the thickness of the burgers and how you like them, turning occasionally. Serve them on toasted burger buns, with tomato ketchup, and your fat chips sprinkled with the rosemary salt. Other great things to top your burger with are layers of sliced beef tomatoes, thinly sliced cheese, raw onion rings, lettuce, a grating of fresh horseradish – even a fried egg!

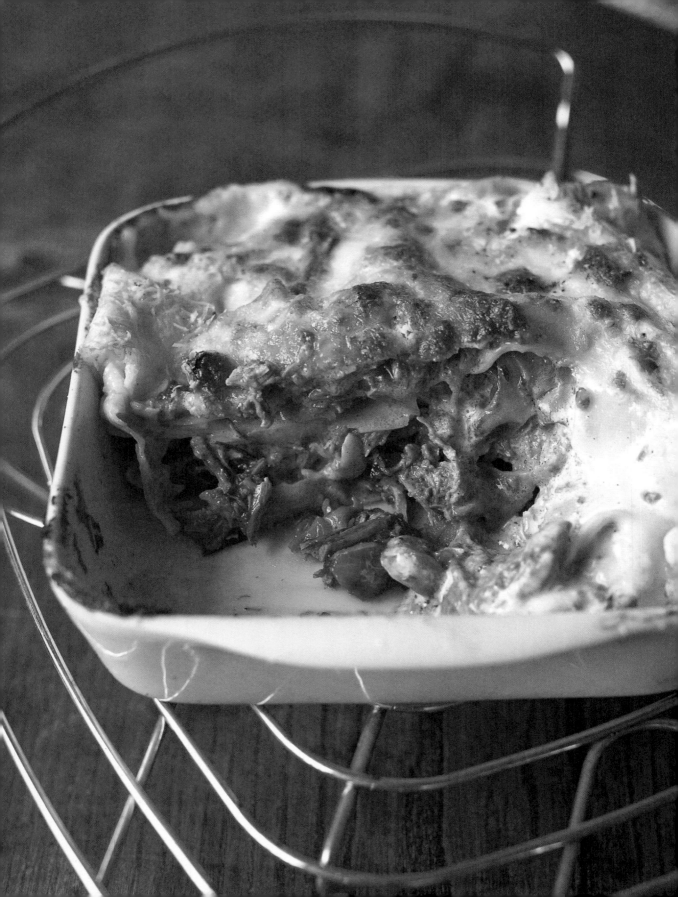

SIMPLE BAKED LASAGNE

Lasagne is always best when made with fresh sheets of pasta, and these are now available in packets in all good supermarkets. Dried lasagne is fine as well, but it will need to be simmered gently to soften it before using. I haven't used a béchamel sauce because it takes too long – I've used a crème fraîche mixture that does a great job. A mixture of beef and pork is really tasty – it's just a brilliant sauce which can also be used for making spaghetti bolognaise, stuffing cannelloni, mixing with sautéd mushrooms and pappardelle.

SERVES 6
4 rashers pancetta or smoked
   bacon, finely sliced
a pinch of cinnamon
1 onion, finely chopped
1 carrot, finely chopped
2 cloves of garlic, peeled and
   finely chopped
2 handfuls of fresh herbs (sage,
   oregano, rosemary, thyme)
olive oil
400g/14oz shin of beef or stewing
   beef, minced coarsely
200g/7oz pork belly, skin
   removed, minced
2 x 400g tins of good-quality
   plum tomatoes

2 glasses of red wine or water
2 bay leaves
1 butternut squash, halved, deseeded
   and roughly chopped
1 tablespoon coriander seeds, bashed
1 dried red chilli, bashed
sea salt and freshly ground
   black pepper
400g/14oz fresh lasagne sheets
400g/14oz mozzarella, torn up

FOR THE WHITE SAUCE
1 x 500ml tub of crème fraîche
3 anchovies, finely chopped
2 handfuls of freshly grated
   Parmesan cheese
optional: a little milk

Preheat the oven to 180°C/350°F/gas 4. In a large casserole-type pan slowly fry the pancetta and cinnamon until golden, then add the onion, carrot, garlic and herbs and about 4 tablespoons of olive oil. Mix together, then add the beef and pork. Cook for about 5 minutes, then add the tinned tomatoes and the wine or water. Add the bay leaves and bring to the boil. Then get some grease-proof paper, wet it and place it on top of the pan with a lid placed on top as well. Then place in the preheated oven for 2 hours or simmer on the hob over a gentle heat for around an hour and a half. Rub your butternut squash slices with olive oil, and sprinkle with salt, pepper and the bashed-up coriander seeds and chilli. Place on a baking tray and roast in the oven for the last 45 minutes of cooking the sauce. When the sauce is done, season to taste and put to one side. Mix together your crème fraîche, anchovies, and a handful of Parmesan, and season with salt and pepper. You may need to loosen the mixture with a little milk.

Turn the oven to 200°C/400°F/gas 6. To assemble the lasagne, rub an earthenware lasagne dish with olive oil, lay some sheets of lasagne over the bottom and drape them over the sides (see pages 10–11). Add a layer of meat, a little white sauce and a sprinkling of Parmesan. Break the butternut squash into pieces and use this as one layer, then repeat the layers, finishing with a layer of pasta covered in white sauce. Tear over the mozzarella and sprinkle with some extra Parmesan. Cook in the preheated oven for 30–35 minutes until golden.

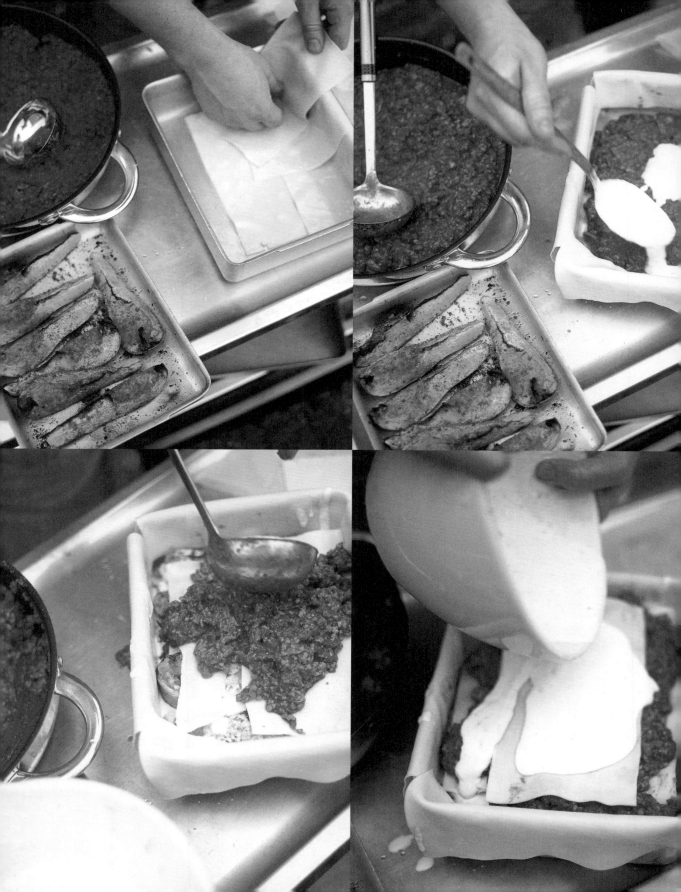

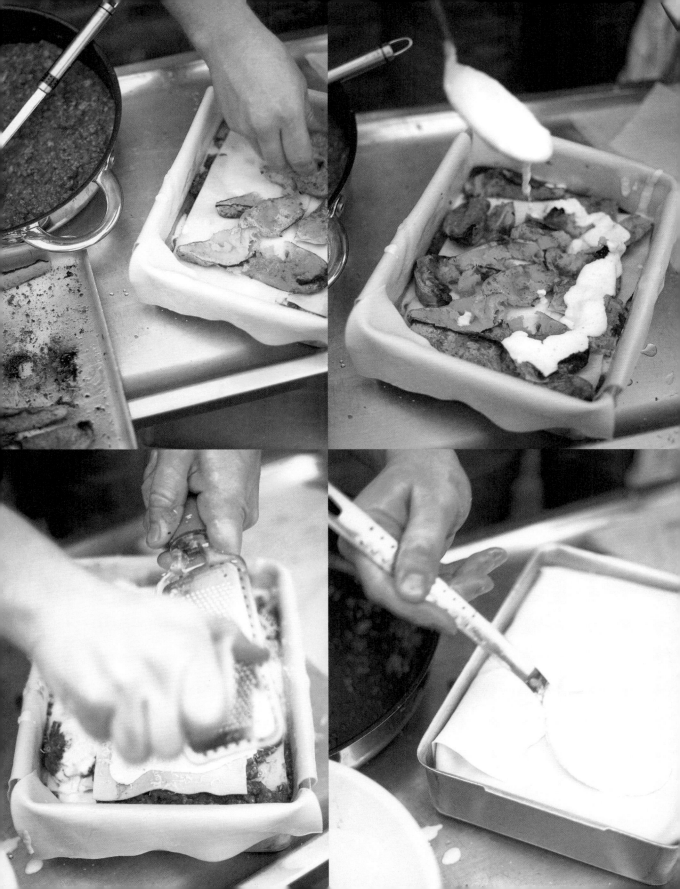

THE FAMOUS JACKET POTATO

There is nothing better when you're hungry than a hot, steaming, fluffy jacket potato. Even simply served with a knob of butter, or a drizzle of olive oil, or maybe a dollop of sour cream, and some salt and pepper, it is one of the most comforting things to eat. The trouble is, most people think of jacket potatoes as nothing more than boring old high street or canteen food, but they can actually be the basis of a really memorable, luxurious dinner. It just depends how you think about it. But the beauty of them is that they can be topped with some amazing combinations. I've decided to give you my favourite ways, including a recipe for making mini jackets by roasting some new potatoes in oil, garlic and rosemary – yum! – and one for sweet potatoes which I think you will love.

To bake your potatoes, simply wash them, prick them with a fork so they don't explode in the oven, rub them with olive oil and sea salt and then place in the oven at 190°C/375°F/gas 5 for between an hour and an hour and 20 minutes. The cooking time will depend on how large your spuds are. Split open your potatoes and add a knob of butter to the centre of each one before adding your chosen topping.

THREE CHEESES WITH CHIVES

Grate over some lovely red Leicester followed by some Cheddar. Crumble up a little Roquefort or other blue cheese and sprinkle over the top. The heat from the potato will melt the cheeses together into a lovely oozy topping. Sprinkle over some finely chopped chives.

CRAB, CRÈME FRAÎCHE, SPRING ONIONS, CHILLI AND MINT

For 4 people, you will need 6 tablespoons of lovely freshly picked white crabmeat. Dress this with the juice of 1 lemon, twice as much olive oil, salt and freshly ground black pepper, 4 finely chopped spring onions, a small handful of finely chopped mint and 1 chilli, deseeded and finely chopped. Add a tablespoon of crème fraîche to the crab mixture and divide between your 4 potatoes.

PRAWNS AND MARIE ROSE SAUCE

For 4 people you will need 4 handfuls of prawns. To make your Marie Rose sauce, get 2 heaped tablespoons of mayonnaise, 1 tablespoon of ketchup, 1 teaspoon of brandy to give it a nice buzz and a pinch of cayenne pepper. Season with salt and pepper and mix it all together. Squeeze over the juice from one lemon – enough to give it a twang – then dress your prawns with the Marie Rose sauce and spoon over your 4 buttered potatoes. Sprinkle with cress and a little parsley.

SMOKED SALMON AND SOUR CREAM

When you split your potatoes open, make quite a large well in the centre and add your knob of butter. Then take 2 handfuls of the small inner leaves of a cos lettuce and mix them with a handful of roughly chopped fresh flat-leaf parsley. Dress the leaves with 1 tablespoon of soured cream, 2 tablespoons of extra virgin olive oil and the juice of 1 lemon. Finish with a pinch of salt and freshly ground black pepper and mix together well. Divide into 4 portions, then get 1 or 2 nice slices of smoked salmon and wrap them round a portion before lifting it carefully on to one of your waiting buttered and seasoned jacket potatoes. Repeat with the other 3 portions. Serve with lemon wedges and extra black pepper. Lovely.

MINI JACKETS TOPPED WITH BEETROOT, COTTAGE CHEESE AND HORSERADISH

If you don't fancy a big baked potato, then try baking some new potatoes instead – lovely as a veg dish to go with meat or fish and perfect for a barbecue. For 4 people you'll need about 1kg/2lb 3oz. Wash and prick them, then roll them in some sea salt, olive oil and rosemary leaves. This will give them incredible flavour. Add them to a roasting tray. Take a whole bulb of garlic and break it up into cloves then scatter these, unpeeled, all over the potatoes. Place in the oven to roast for 45–50 minutes until soft in the middle and crispy outside. When your potatoes are cooked, serve them topped with a little cottage cheese or soured cream and some diced vinegary beetroot. You can also grate over some fresh horseradish to give them a kick. Sprinkle over some chopped fresh herbs such as basil, parsley or chervil. These make great little canapés to munch before dinner!

SWEET POTATO TOPPED WITH CHILLIES, BUFFALO MOZZARELLA AND BASIL

Sweet potatoes are lovely roasted, as the juices caramelize slightly where you prick the skin. They won't look much from the outside, but when you split them open the flesh will be a vibrant orange and so tasty. I love to top them with some torn-up pieces of buffalo mozzarella, some finely chopped fresh red and green chillies, a little squeeze of lemon juice and some fresh whole basil leaves, a drizzle of olive oil and some salt and pepper. You'll love it!

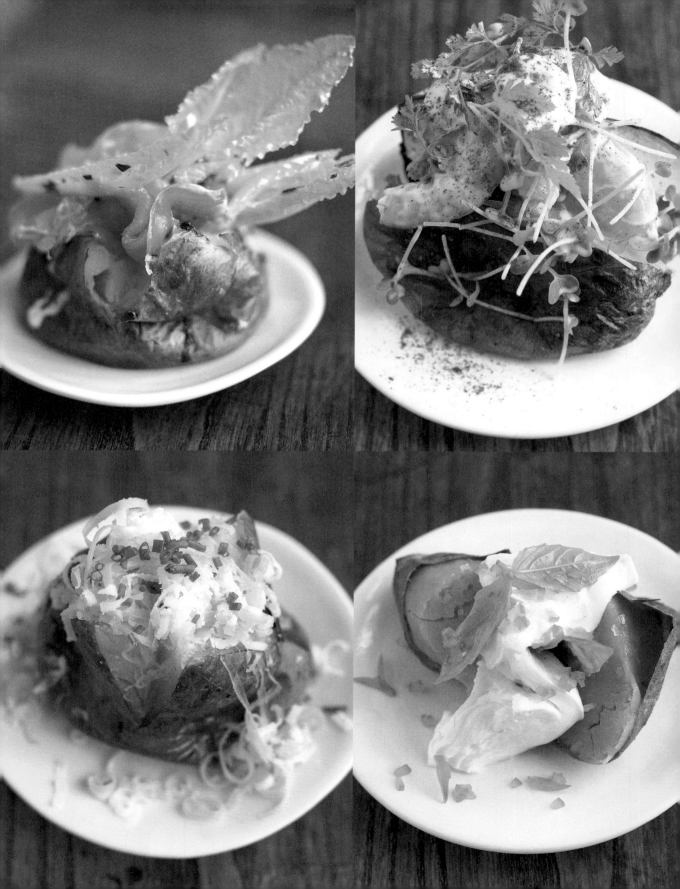

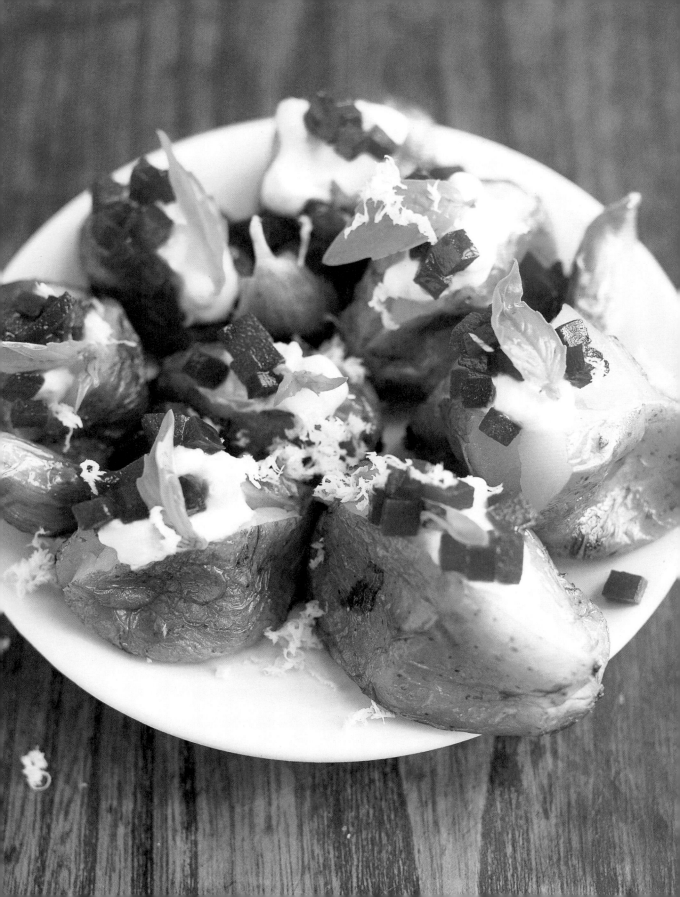

APPLE PIE

Obviously apple pie is one of the classic all-time desserts. I can't even imagine how good they must have tasted in the old days when England used to have hundreds and hundreds of different varieties of apples – they would have tasted like heaven. My tip to you is to use both cooking and eating apples in the filling. The best apple pies I've ever made are from apples bought at farmers' markets. As the year progresses it's also a treat to substitute some of the apples with beautiful pears and then wonderful blackberries.

SERVES 6

FOR THE PASTRY
225g/8oz plain flour
140g/5oz butter
85g/3oz caster sugar
finely grated rind of 1 lemon
2 egg yolks
salt

FOR THE FILLING
a small knob of butter
flour, for dusting

1 large Bramley cooking apple
4 eating apples (try Cox's or Braeburn)
3 tablespoons Demerara or
   muscovado sugar
zest of ½ a lemon
½ teaspoon ground ginger
a handful of raisins or sultanas
1 egg yolk mixed with a splash of milk

Preheat the oven to 180°C/350°F/gas 4. To make the pastry, in a Magimix or food processor, pulse up the flour, butter, caster sugar and lemon rind with a pinch of salt, then add the egg yolk and a tiny drop of water to bind the mix together. Butter a 20cm/8 inch metal pie dish – the reason for using a metal one is because it will conduct heat better so the bottom of the pie will cook at the same time as the top.

Divide your pastry dough into two and roll half of it out on a flour-dusted surface until 0.5cm/¼ inch thick. Lay the pastry in the metal dish and gently push it down into the sides. Don't worry if it tears or breaks – just patch it up – as it will look nice and rustic! Pop the pie dish and the remaining half of your pastry into the fridge while you peel your apples. Quarter the Bramley apple and cut the eating apples into eighths. Toss the apples in a small pan with the sugar, lemon zest, ginger, sultanas or raisins, and a tablespoon of water. Simmer gently for 5 minutes or until the apples are just tender. Remove from the heat and allow to cool completely.

Remove the pie dish and pastry from the fridge and pack the apple mix tightly into the pie dish. Egg-wash the pastry rim and then roll out the other half of the dough. Drape this over the top of the pie and roughly pinch the edges together using your finger and thumb and trim any excess pastry. Egg-wash the top, make a couple of small incisions and bake in the bottom of the oven for 45 to 50 minutes. Spoon out the portions of apple pie and serve with some custard!

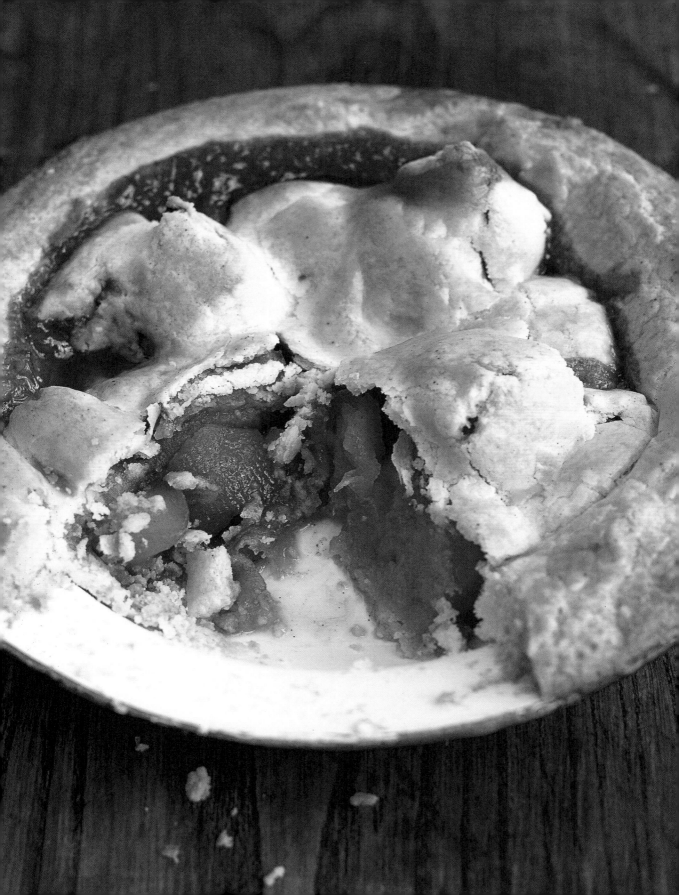

ROAST CHICKEN WITH LEMON AND ROSEMARY ROAST POTATOES

Roast chicken remains one of our favourite dishes at home, so that's why I've included it in The Top Ten. I recently discovered a way to make the chicken taste even better, by putting a lemon in with my potatoes when I was parboiling them. It smelt fantastic and flavoured the potatoes. Then when I was draining them I decided to stab the lemon, which hissed out juice and steam, and quickly jammed it inside the chicken! The benefits of the hot steaming lemon going into the chicken are very obvious as the meat tastes amazing, and the chicken cooks slightly quicker because of it.

SERVES 4
1 x 2kg/4½lb free-range organic chicken
sea salt and freshly ground black pepper
2kg/4½lb potatoes, peeled
1 large, preferably unwaxed, lemon
1 whole bulb of garlic, broken into cloves
a handful of fresh thyme
olive oil
a handful of fresh rosemary sprigs, leaves picked
optional: 8 rashers of smoked streaky bacon

Rub the chicken inside and out with a generous amount of salt and freshly ground black pepper. Do this in the morning if possible, then cover the chicken and leave in the fridge until you're ready to start cooking it for lunch or dinner. By doing this, you'll make the meat really tasty when cooked. Preheat your oven to 190°C/375°F/gas 5. Bring a large pan of salted water to the boil. Cut the potatoes into golf-ball-sized pieces, put them into the water with the whole lemon and the garlic cloves, and cook for 12 minutes. Drain and allow to steam dry for 1 minute (this will give you crispier potatoes), then remove the lemon and garlic. Toss the potatoes in the pan while still hot so their outsides get chuffed up and fluffy – this will make them lovely and crispy when they roast.

While the lemon is still hot, carefully stab it about 10 times. Take the chicken out of the fridge, pat it with kitchen paper and rub it all over with olive oil. Push the garlic cloves, the whole lemon and the thyme into the cavity, then put the chicken into a roasting tray and cook in the preheated oven for around 45 minutes. Remove the chicken to a plate. Some lovely fat should have cooked out of it into the roasting tray, so toss the potatoes into this with the rosemary leaves. Shake the tray around, then make a gap in the centre of the potatoes and put the chicken back in. If using the bacon, lay the rashers over the chicken breast and cook for a further 45 minutes, or until the chicken is cooked and the potatoes are nice and golden. (You can tell the chicken is cooked when the thigh meat pulls easily away from the bone and the juices run clear.)

I like to remove the bacon from the chicken and crumble it up over the potatoes. Then I remove the lemon and garlic from inside the chicken, squeeze all the garlic flesh out of the skin, mush it up and smear it all over the chicken, discard the lemon and rosemary and carve the chicken at the table. Heaven!

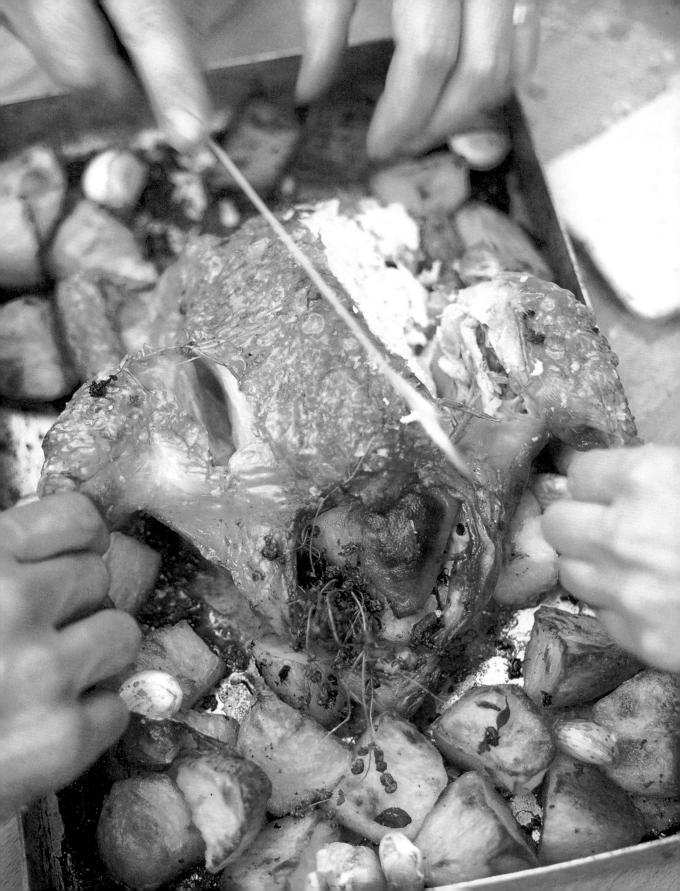

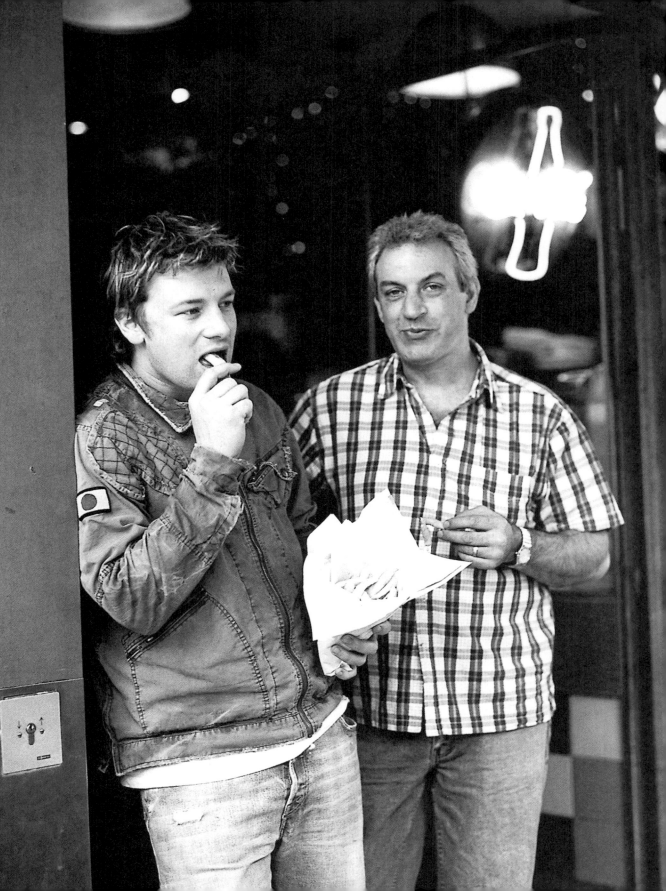

FISH, CHIPS AND MUSHY PEAS

Good fish and chips are becoming harder to find these days, but there are still some good boys out there making the real deal. However, if you want to make your own at home, here's the recipe I use. Unless you've got a really big fryer I'd say it's not really worth trying to make fish and chips at home for more than 4 people – otherwise it becomes a struggle. Other things to have on the table are some crunchy sweet pickled gherkins, some pickled onions (if your other half isn't around!) – and pickled chillies are good too. Then you want to douse it all with some cheap malt vinegar and nothing other than Heinz tomato ketchup.

SERVES 4
sunflower oil for deep-frying
½ teaspoon sea salt
1 teaspoon freshly ground
    black pepper
225g/8oz nice white fish fillets,
    pinboned
225g/8oz flour, plus extra for
    dusting
285ml/½ pint good cold beer
3 heaped teaspoons baking
    powder

900g/2lb potatoes, peeled and
    sliced into chips

FOR THE MUSHY PEAS
a knob of butter
4 handfuls of podded peas
a small handful of fresh mint, leaves
    picked and chopped
a squeeze of lemon juice
sea salt and freshly ground
    black pepper

To make your mushy peas, put the butter in a pan with the peas and the chopped mint. Put a lid on top and simmer for about 10 minutes. Add a squeeze of lemon juice and season with salt and pepper. You can either mush the peas up in a food processor, or you can mash them by hand until they are stodgy, thick and perfect for dipping your fish into. Keep them warm while you cook your fish and chips.

Pour the sunflower oil into your deep fat fryer or a large frying pan and heat it to 190°C/375°F. Mix the salt and pepper together and season the fish fillets on both sides. This will help to remove any excess water, making the fish really meaty. Whisk the flour, beer and baking powder together until nice and shiny. The texture should be like semi-whipped double cream (i.e. it should stick to whatever you're coating). Dust each fish fillet in a little of the extra flour, then dip into the batter and allow any excess to drip off. Holding one end, lower the fish into the oil one by one, carefully so you don't get splashed – it will depend on the size of your fryer how many fish you can do at once. Cook for 4 minutes or so, until the batter is golden and crisp.

Meanwhile, parboil your chips in salted boiling water for about 4 or 5 minutes until softened but still retaining their shape, then drain them in a colander and leave to steam completely dry. When all the moisture has disappeared, fry them in the oil that the fish were cooked in at 180°C/350°F until golden and crisp. While the chips are frying, you can place the fish on a baking tray and put them in the oven for a few minutes at 180°C/350°F/gas 4 to finish cooking. This way they will stay crisp while you finish off the chips. When they are done, drain them on kitchen paper, season with salt, and serve with the fish and mushy peas.

opposite: george's portobello
fish bar, portobello road, london

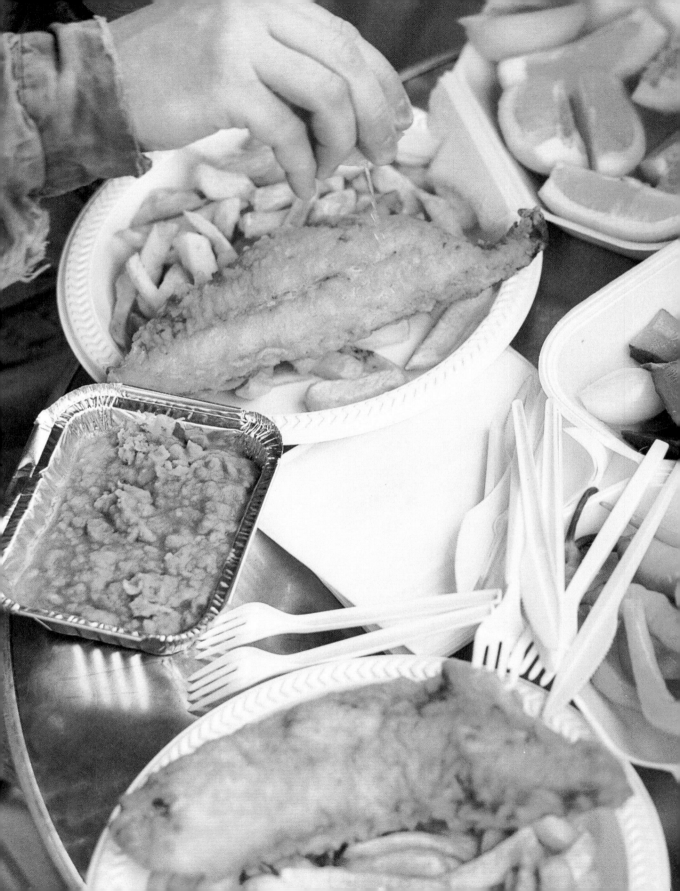

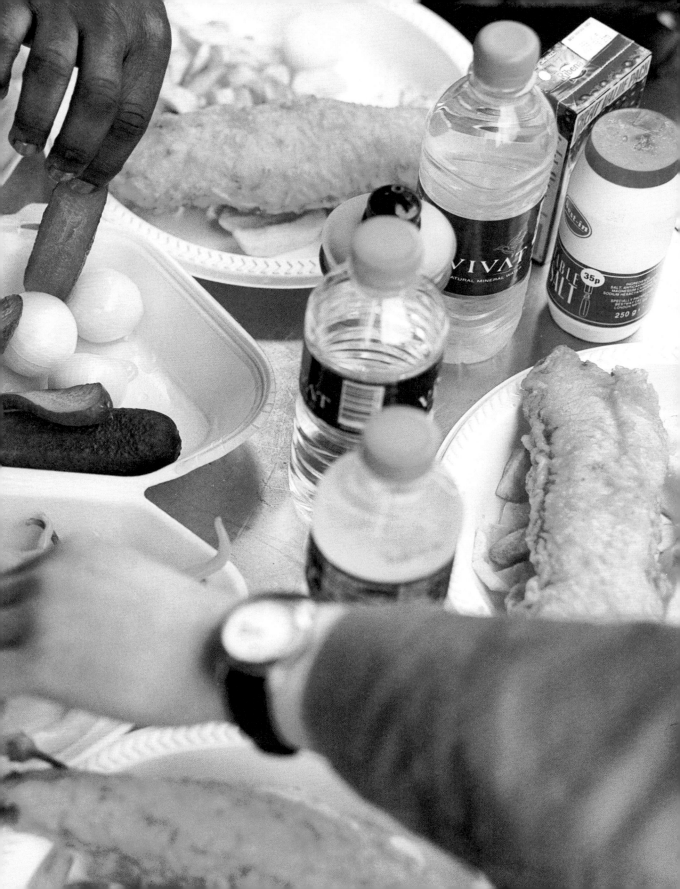

THE BEST CHICKEN AND SWEET LEEK PIE WITH FLAKY PASTRY

I've always loved chicken pie. Apart from being quick, simple and scrumptious, puff pastry gives you a really flaky, crispy top, which I can never get enough of. I was invited to dinner at the food critic Fay Maschler's home a while back and she made me a wonderful chicken pie. Her tip was to put some sausagemeat balls in the stew and they tasted fantastic. Three stars!

SERVES 4
olive oil
2 knobs of butter
1kg/2lb 3oz boned and skinned
 chicken thighs, cut into pieces
2 medium leeks, trimmed, washed
 and sliced into 1cm/½ inch
 pieces
2 carrots, peeled and roughly
 chopped

3 sticks of celery, finely sliced
a small handful of thyme, leaves picked
2 tablespoons flour
1 wineglass of white wine
285ml/½ pint milk
sea salt and freshly ground
 black pepper
255g/9oz good pork sausages
1 x 500g pack of all-butter puff pastry
1 egg

Preheat the oven to 220°C/425°F/gas 7. Take a large casserole pot and add a lug of olive oil and your butter. Add the chicken, leeks, carrots, celery and thyme and cook slowly on the hob for 15 minutes. Turn the heat right up, add the flour, and keep stirring for a couple of minutes before adding the wine, a wineglass of water and the milk. Season with a little salt and freshly ground black pepper, then cover with a tight-fitting lid and simmer very slowly on the hob for 30–40 minutes until the chicken is tender. Stir it every so often so it doesn't catch on the bottom of the pan. The sauce should be loose but quite thick. If it's a little too liquid, just continue to simmer it with the lid off until it thickens slightly. (At this point you could let it cool and keep it in the fridge for a couple of days if you want to – it can also be eaten as a stew.)

Pour the chicken mixture into an appropriately sized pie dish. Squeeze the meat out of the sausage skins, roll it into little balls, brown them in a little oil and sprinkle them over the stew. Roll out your pastry to about 0.5cm/¼ inch thick. Egg-wash the rim of the dish and drape over the pastry, using a knife to trim the edge of the dish. Egg-wash the top of the pastry to make it go golden while cooking, then pinch it to crimp it round the edges (there's no need to do this, but I like to as my mum always does it and it makes it look pretty). I use the back of a knife to lightly criss-cross the top – this allows the pastry to go crisp and flaky. Cook the pie in the centre of the oven for about 30 to 40 minutes, until golden on top. I like to serve this with sweetcorn and mashed potato.

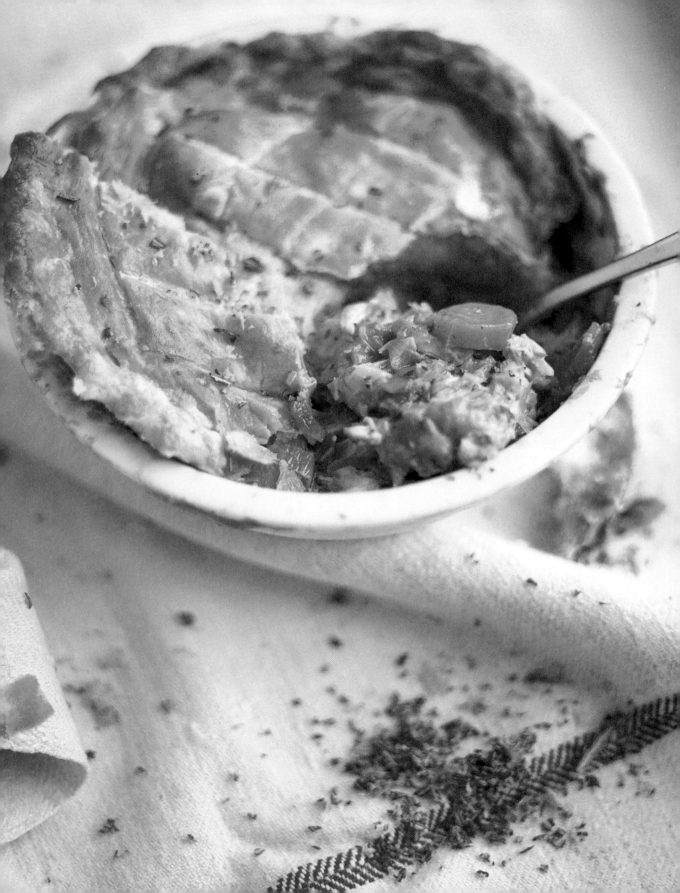

TOMATO SOUP

I've made all sorts of different tomato soups over the years, and this is probably one of the simplest and tastiest. Here's the trick ... if you go down to your local market at the end of the day you may find they are selling off tomatoes cheap. More than likely the seller thinks they are over-ripe, but they are more probably just perfect and will make great soup. If you can't get these, buy tomatoes two or three days before you need them, but don't keep them in the fridge as they won't ripen. Leave them on a windowsill to get ripe. If there's a choice then have a taste – you'll be amazed how different they can be, so choose the ones that taste the best. The second trick is the slow cooking, which makes them very sweet. Best served in warm bowls or mugs at the table with some really fresh bread.

SERVES 4
1 onion, peeled and finely chopped
1 clove of garlic, peeled and finely chopped
1 carrot, peeled and coarsely grated
a handful of fresh basil, leaves picked, stalks finely chopped
olive oil
6 tablespoons double cream
1 teaspoon red wine vinegar
2 egg yolks
1kg/2lb 3oz super-ripe tomatoes
1.1 litres/2 pints chicken or vegetable stock
sea salt and freshly ground black pepper

Put your onion, garlic, carrot and basil stalks into a large pot with a couple of lugs of olive oil. Cover the pan, and simmer gently without colouring for 20 minutes, stirring every couple of minutes. Whisk together the cream, vinegar and egg yolks in a small bowl and put to one side. While the veg are simmering, drop the tomatoes into boiling water for 30 seconds, then remove the skins and roughly chop the flesh. Add these to the veg, then pour in the stock and simmer for a further 20 minutes with the lid on. At this point it's nice to purée the soup using either a food processor, a liquidizer or a hand-held blender, but be careful as it will be hot. Once you've puréed the soup, put it back into the pan, bring it back to a simmer, and season very carefully with salt and freshly ground black pepper.

Just before serving, to enrich the soup and give it a shine and silky texture, whisk in the cream mixture (don't reboil it after adding the egg yolks or it will scramble) and serve straight away, sprinkled with a few torn-up basil leaves, if you like.

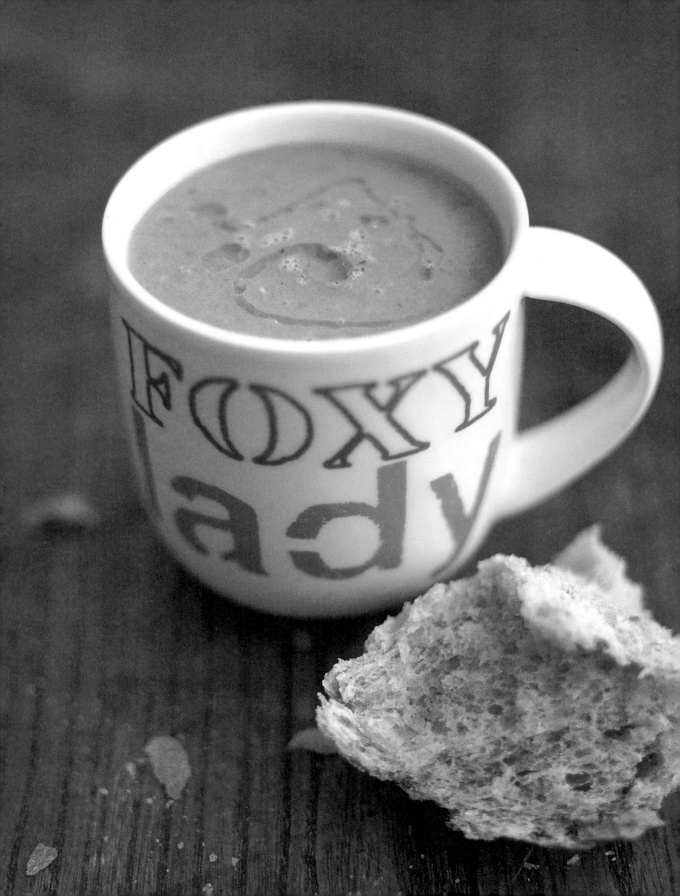

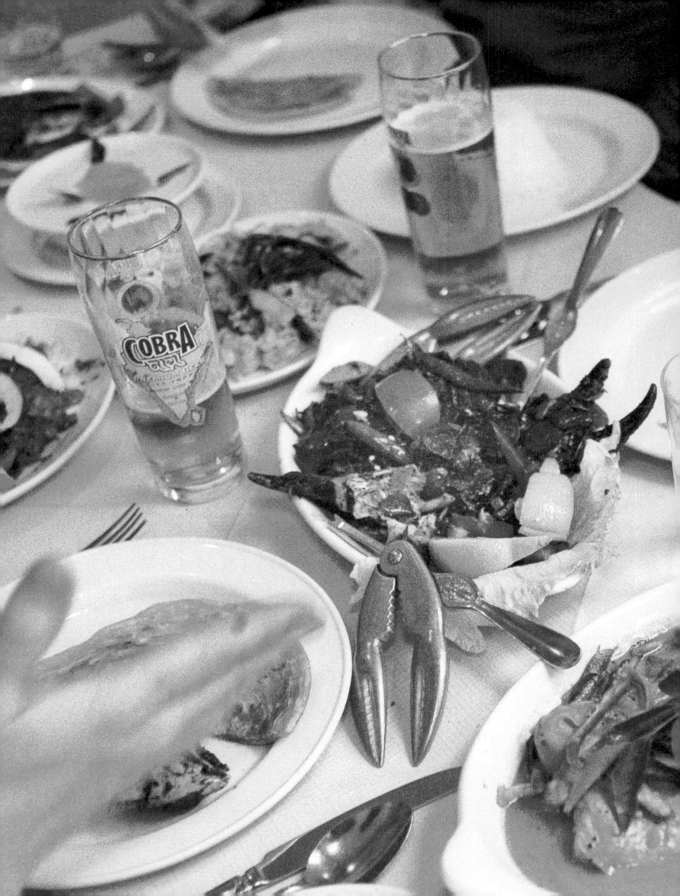

CHICKEN TIKKA MASALA

This is a really popular curry dish which loads of people order from their local curry houses at the weekend. If you've ever thought of making it at home you may have been slightly mystified about how to make it taste so good, but have a go at this recipe and I'm sure you won't be disappointed. The great thing about it is that if you don't fancy chicken you can try using lamb instead, because it's cooked separately from the sauce.

SERVES 4
6 cloves of garlic, peeled
7.5cm/3 inches of fresh
   ginger, peeled
2–3 fresh red chillies, deseeded
olive oil
1 tablespoon mustard seeds
1 tablespoon paprika
2 teaspoons ground cumin
2 teaspoons ground coriander
3 tablespoons garam masala
200g/7oz natural yoghurt

4 medium chicken breasts, skinned and
   cut into large chunks
1 tablespoon butter
2 medium onions, peeled and
   finely sliced
2 tablespoons tomato purée
a small handful of ground cashew nuts
   or almonds
sea salt
115ml/4fl oz double cream
a handful of fresh coriander, chopped
juice of 1–2 limes

Grate the garlic and ginger on the finest side of a cheese grater and put to one side in a bowl. Chop the chillies as finely as you can and mix them in with the ginger and garlic. Heat a good splash of oil in a pan and add the mustard seeds. When they start to pop, add them to the ginger and garlic mixture along with the paprika, cumin, ground coriander and 2 tablespoons of the garam masala. Put half of this mix in a bowl, add the yoghurt and the chicken pieces to it, stir and leave to marinate for half an hour or so.

Melt the butter in the saucepan the mustard seeds were in and add the sliced onions and the remaining half of the spice mix. Cook gently for 15 minutes or so without browning too much – it should start to smell fantastic! Add the tomato purée, the ground nuts, half a litre/1 pint of water and ½ a teaspoon of salt. Stir well and simmer gently for a few minutes. Let this sauce reduce until it thickens slightly and then place to one side.

Put the marinaded chicken on a hot griddle pan or barbecue and sear until cooked through – you can also do this under a preheated grill if you like.

Warm the sauce and add the cream and the other tablespoon of garam masala. Taste and correct the seasoning if necessary. As soon as it boils, take off the heat and add the grilled chicken. Check the seasoning once more and serve sprinkled with the chopped coriander, and the lime juice. Then all you need is a huge bowl of steaming basmati rice, some poppadums and lots of cold beer!

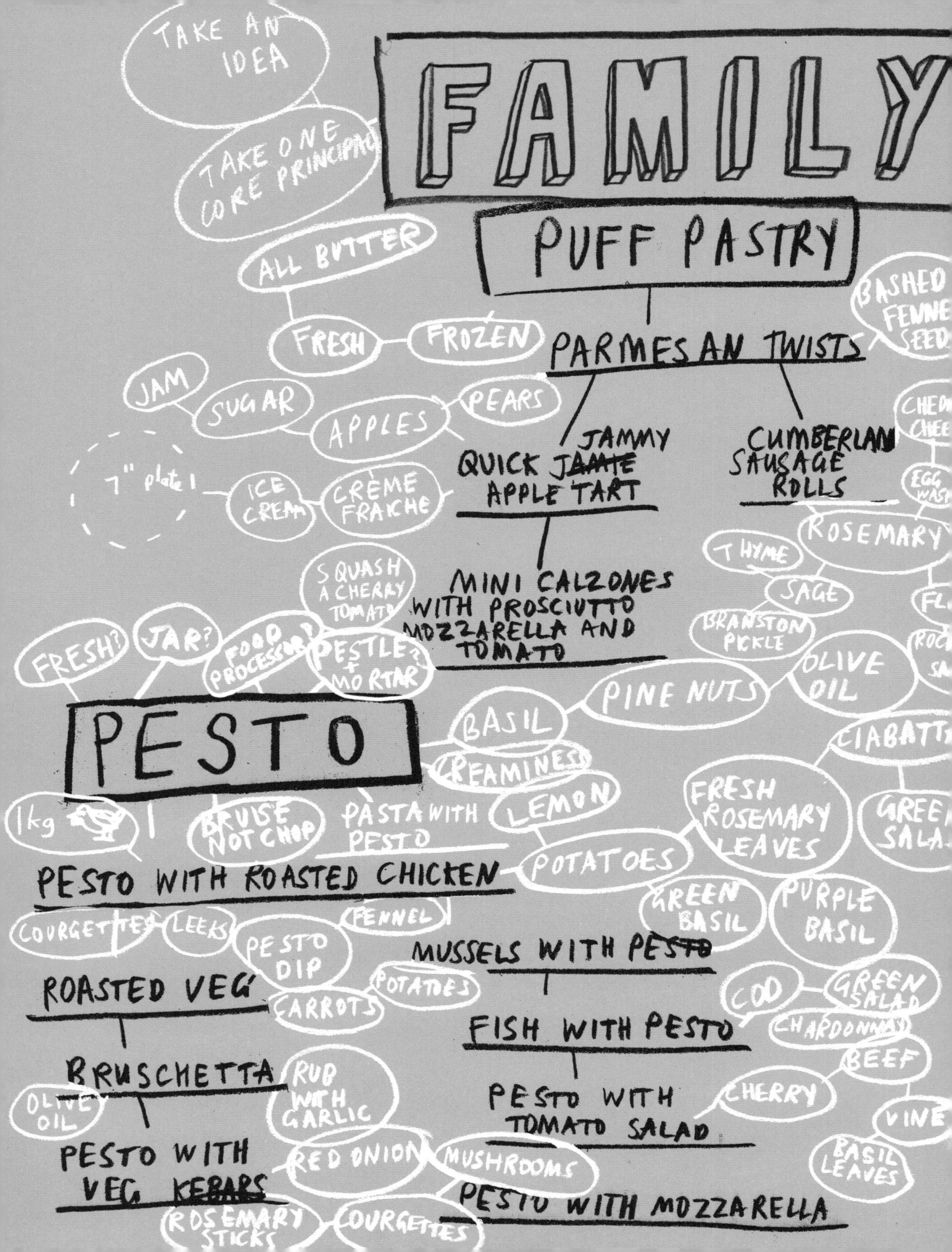

TAKE AN IDEA

TAKE ONE CORE PRINCIPLE

FAMILY

PUFF PASTRY

ALL BUTTER

FRESH — FROZEN

PARMESAN TWISTS

BASHED FENNEL SEEDS

JAM

SUGAR

APPLES

PEARS

JAMMY

QUICK JAMIE APPLE TART

CUMBERLAND SAUSAGE ROLLS

CHEDDAR CHEESE

7" plate!

ICE CREAM

CRÈME FRAICHE

EGG WASH

ROSEMARY

SQUASH A CHERRY TOMATO

THYME

SAGE

FL...

MINI CALZONES WITH PROSCIUTTO MOZZARELLA AND TOMATO

BRANSTON PICKLE

ROC... SA...

FRESH?

JAR?

FOOD PROCESSOR

PESTLE + MORTAR

OLIVE OIL

PINE NUTS

PESTO

BASIL

CREAMINESS

LEMON

CIABATTA

1kg

BRUISE NOT CHOP

PASTA WITH PESTO

FRESH ROSEMARY LEAVES

GREEN SALAD

POTATOES

PESTO WITH ROASTED CHICKEN

COURGETTES LEEKS

FENNEL

GREEN BASIL

PURPLE BASIL

PESTO DIP

MUSSELS WITH PESTO

ROASTED VEG

POTATOES

COD

GREEN SALAD

CARROTS

FISH WITH PESTO

CHARDONNAY

BRUSCHETTA

RUB WITH GARLIC

BEEF

OLIVE OIL

PESTO WITH TOMATO SALAD

CHERRY

VINE

PESTO WITH VEG KEBABS

RED ONION

MUSHROOMS

BASIL LEAVES

ROSEMARY STICKS

COURGETTES

PESTO WITH MOZZARELLA

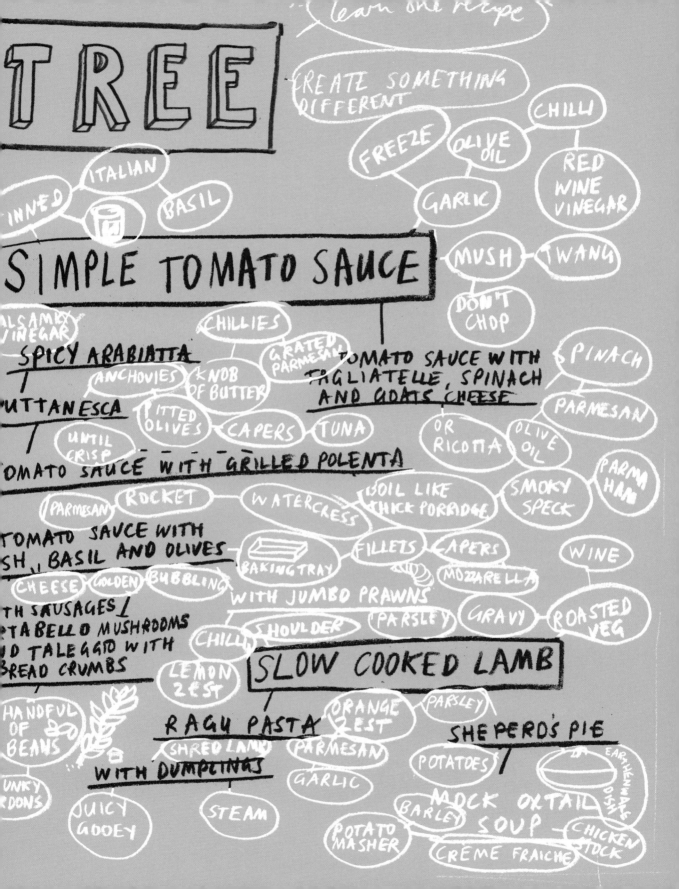

I've called this chapter 'Family Tree' because once you've perfected one really good 'parent' recipe, you can make lots of 'offspring' recipes. It's a chapter for nervous or novice cooks, and it should give you the confidence to think, 'I'm the boss, I'm in control and I'm going to cook an amazing meal tonight, and the next night, and the next . . . !'

Many years ago I worked with a waiter called Angus who never cooked. Between services one day he was helping out by picking the basil for me to make fresh pesto. He'd seen me make it a few times and wanted to have a go himself, so I taught him how to do it. 'Unbelievable!' he said. 'That's so easy, even an idiot could do it!'

This was around the time of the World Cup, so he had all the boys round to his house for a few bevvies and some food. He told me afterwards that he put a pound of pasta on to boil, bashed up the basil, then added the pine nuts and cheese to make the pesto. He made it with complete ease, and plonked it down in front of his (very!) impressed mates, who wasted no time tucking in with gusto. For weeks after that they were all saying what a great cook Angus was. Then he came over to me one day and told me he'd had his girlfriend and family over. He'd roasted a chicken, served a green salad out of a packet, dressed with a little bit of oil and vinegar, and then made the pesto at the table and served it with the chicken – his parents were amazed! They couldn't believe how independent their son had become and how tasty the food was!

So this chapter is all about showing you how you can learn one recipe and then use it to champion a whole set of different meals while fooling everyone into believing you're the best cook in the world! Being a cook is about ducking and diving your way around dishes. I just love the fact that I can take an idea and move it on in some small way to create my own customized recipes. After you've had a look through this chapter, have a go at coming up with your own ideas or ways of doing things.

Some of the recipes in this chapter haven't got lists of ingredients because I wanted them to be chatty. I also feel that sometimes it's important to read the whole recipe through before you start, to get more of an understanding of how the whole thing works. Instead I have high-lighted the ingredients in the method so you can see, at a glance, what you'll need.

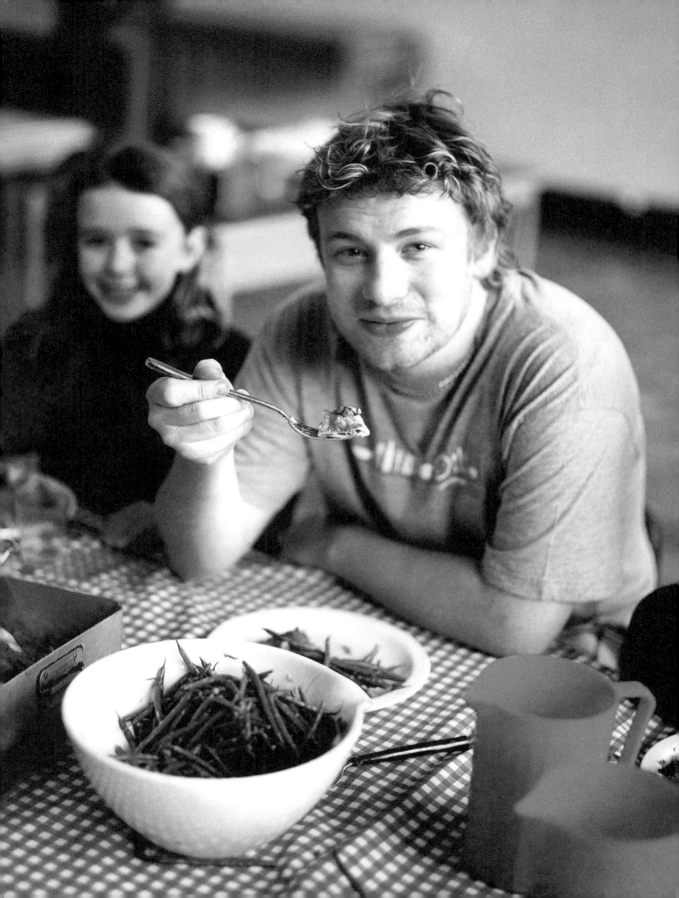

PESTO

First I'm going to show you an easy recipe for making pesto and then I'll give you some ideas on how best to use it, instead of just having it with pasta all the time. When it comes to making pesto, you can invest in a good processor if you like, but you can also make it using a pestle and mortar. If you have a blunt blade from your processor then don't chuck it, but keep it specially for making pesto or marinades where you need to bruise out the flavour, instead of chopping. You may think it's nice to toast the pine nuts until they're coloured, to give them a nutty taste, but the really good pestos I've tasted in Italy just have them very lightly toasted, to give a creaminess rather than a nuttiness. Pesto is normally made with green basil, but purple basil looks good if you can get hold of some. Another way, slightly more American, uses rocket instead of basil – it's fragrant and interesting with roasted meats, but I prefer this classic pesto recipe.

SERVES 4
½ a clove of garlic, chopped
sea salt and freshly ground black pepper
3 good handfuls of fresh basil, leaves picked and chopped
a handful of pine nuts, very lightly toasted
a good handful of freshly grated Parmesan cheese
extra virgin olive oil
optional: a small squeeze of lemon juice

Pound the garlic with a little pinch of salt and the basil leaves in a pestle and mortar, or pulse in a food processor. Add a bit more garlic if you like, but I usually stick to ½ a clove. Add the pine nuts to the mixture and pound again. Turn out into a bowl and add half the Parmesan. Stir gently and add olive oil – you need just enough to bind the sauce and get it to an oozy consistency.

Season to taste, then add most of the remaining cheese. Pour in some more oil and taste again. Keep adding a bit more cheese or oil until you are happy with the taste and consistency. You may like to add a squeeze of lemon juice at the end to give it a little twang, but it's not essential. Try it with and without and see which you prefer.

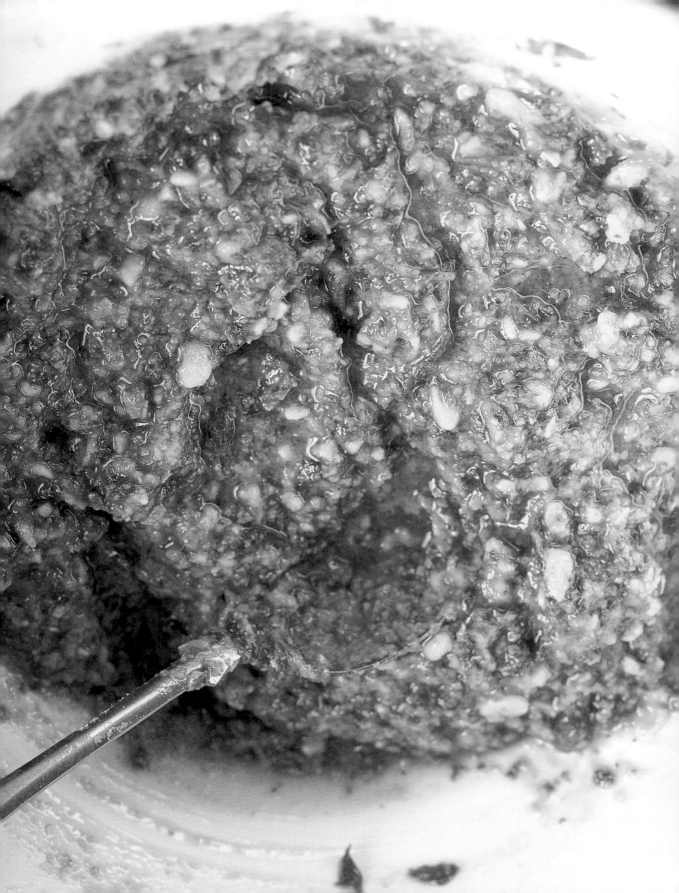

PESTO

with Roasted Chicken

For 4 people, get yourself a 2kg/4½lb chicken. Parboil 2kg/4½lb of potatoes with a whole lemon in the water to give some flavour. Drain the spuds, then remove the lemon and prick it with a knife a few times before pushing it inside the chicken. Bash up a handful of fresh rosemary leaves, drizzle them with olive oil and stuff them into the chicken as well. Roast the chicken for 30 minutes at 220°C/425°F/gas 7, then throw the parboiled potatoes into the tray and put it back into the oven for an hour, until the chicken is cooked and the potatoes are browned. Then what I really like to do is make the pesto at the table – it only takes 4 minutes if you've got everything ready on a tray. But if you prefer, you can make it while the chicken is cooking. Serve the pesto with the chicken and the lovely roast potatoes, and maybe with some ciabatta bread, a big green salad and some beers.

with Mussels

This is a creamy mussel dish which is a little bit like the French way of serving mussels with a garlicky sauce. When you put pesto with garlic into a broth or soup it really makes the room smell amazing as it hits the warmth. For 4 people get 2kg/4½lb of nice mussels, chuck away any open shells and debeard the rest if they need it. By this I mean pull off the little scruffy 'beards' which hang out of the shells. Get yourself an appropriately sized pan, heat it up, add a couple of lugs of olive oil and fry a peeled and finely chopped onion, 3 or 4 peeled and chopped cloves of garlic and a little deseeded and finely chopped fresh chilli. Throw the mussels in with one glass of white wine and one glass of cream. Put a lid on top and simmer for about 10 minutes until the shells have opened. Discard any that remain closed. Add a knob of butter and give the pan a little shake. The mussels should be really soft and tender. Correct the seasoning with a little salt and freshly ground black pepper – though you might not need salt – and a squeeze of lemon juice. Serve in a big bowl with all the juices and a handful of chopped fresh flat-leaf parsley or basil sprinkled over. Serve the pesto spooned over the top. Really nice with a warm baguette.

with Bruschetta

When your mates turn up for a barbecue and are having a few beers while they wait for their food, just toast some slices of ciabatta, rub with the cut side of a garlic clove and then spoon over some pesto and finish with a drizzle of olive oil.

with Fish

A simple meal. Get yourself a fillet of nice white fish, such as cod, and rub it with olive oil. Season it with salt and freshly ground black pepper, then either grill or pan-fry and serve with a nice big spoonful of pesto over the top. On the side, have a green salad and a nice glass of white wine.

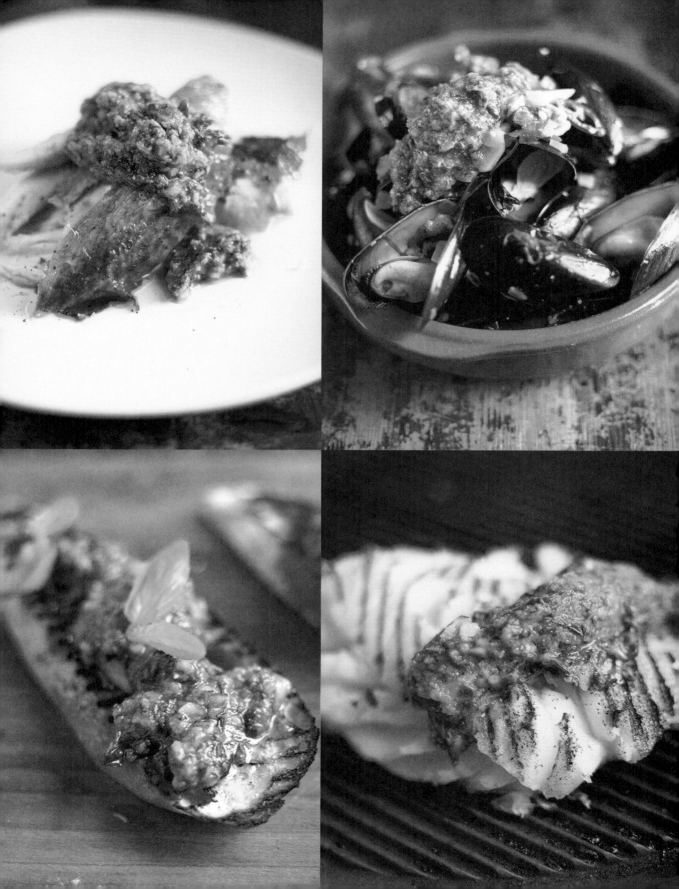

PESTO

with Mixed Tomato Salad

Get yourself some different varieties of tomato – little cherry ones, big beef ones or ones on the vine – and slice them all up. Lay them on a plate with some basil leaves torn over, a drizzle of peppery olive oil, some sea salt and freshly ground black pepper and a big dollop of pesto. You could even stir this tomato salad through some hot, drained pasta – lovely.

with Roasted Vegetables

There are so many combinations of vegetables that can be roasted well together: carrots, squash, parsnips, turnips, potatoes, celeriac, swede, fennel and red onions. All you need to do is cut them into similar sized chunks and roast them all together, in the same roasting tray, in a little olive oil with some sea salt and freshly ground black pepper at 190°C/375°F/gas 5 for about 45 minutes until golden and soft. Mix all the veg together and serve with a little bowl of pesto – lovely. If you want to make these part of a more substantial dinner, you can roast a leg of lamb to go with them, but either way these veggies are fantastic served as a starter, a vegetable dish or an accompaniment to meat or fish.

with Vegetable Kebabs

These kebabs are lovely cooked on the barbecue, but are just as easily done under the grill. Get yourself a selection of veggies – try aubergine, mushrooms, peppers, red onion and courgettes. Dice them into pieces roughly the same size and spear them on to some rosemary sticks or skewers. Drizzle over some olive oil, season with sea salt and freshly ground black pepper, and grill or barbecue for 5 to 10 minutes until soft and nicely cooked. Serve with your pesto.

with Mozzarella

Get yourself a nice ball of buffalo mozzarella, tear it up, and eat it with pesto as a great starter. Lovely served with some roasted peppers, ciabatta and basil or wild rocket.

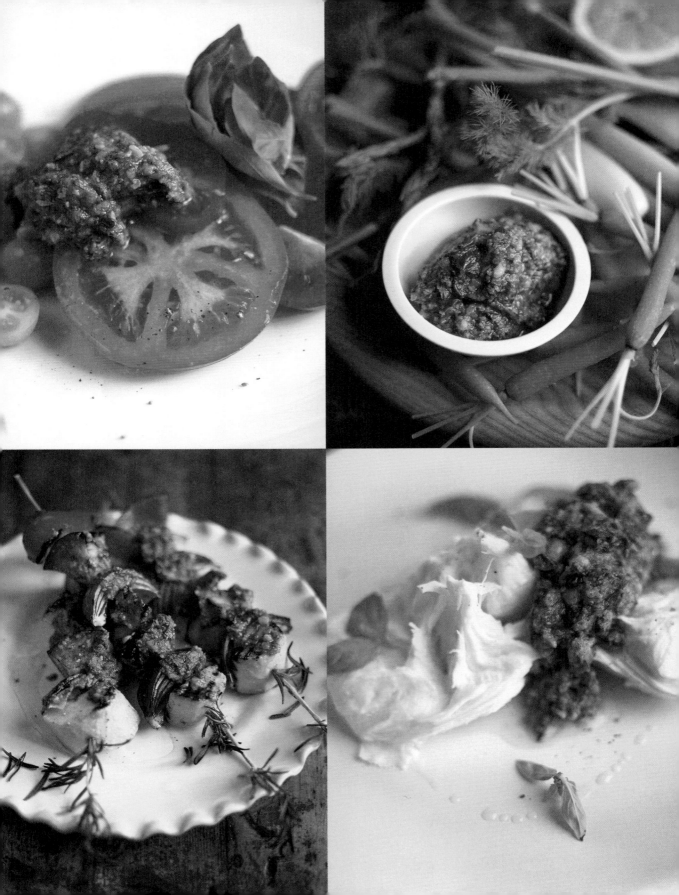

SIMPLE TOMATO SAUCE

I'm a great believer in a simple tomato sauce, but it has to be made properly. The quality of the tinned tomatoes is important, and the only way to tell the difference between good ones and great ones is to try out a few varieties. I've recently come across an Italian brand called La Fiammante. Each tin contains one basil leaf to flavour the tomatoes and they taste superb. I find it's more economical to make one big batch of tomato sauce every so often – I divide it up into sandwich bags and pop them into the freezer (where they will keep for a couple of months) or into the fridge for a week.

First of all, chop 2 or 3 cloves of garlic and fry them gently in olive oil with either some chopped basil stalks or a good pinch of dried oregano, and a whole fresh red chilli. Pierce the chilli once with a knife so it doesn't explode when frying. It will give a subtle heat to the sauce. Add a couple of tins of plum tomatoes – try to get hold of the best Italian ones you can – and leave the tomatoes whole. The seeds can be a little bitter, so if you chop the tomatoes up straight away the sauce won't be as sweet as it should be. Lightly season with sea salt and freshly ground black pepper, then gently simmer for 30 minutes. Remove the chilli.

Break and mush the tomatoes up with a spoon, season the sauce really carefully with more salt and pepper, and add a tiny swig of red wine vinegar to give it a little twang. It should now be perfect! There are so many different ways you can take this sauce forward . . .

PASTA SAUCES

- For a spicy arrabiatta, start the tomato sauce off by adding a few more whole fresh chillies. After the sauce has simmered for 15 to 20 minutes, remove the chillies, chop them up and add back as much as you need to give your arrabiatta the desired heat. One of my favourites.

- A real crowd-pleaser can be made by taking the tomato sauce off the heat when it's ready and adding a big handful of torn fresh basil, a nice swig of balsamic vinegar, a good knob of butter and a handful of grated Parmesan. This is fantastic with pasta like rigatoni or tagliatelle, or with grilled meats and fish.

- To make a puttanesca, simmer the sauce gently with a handful of good pitted and squashed olives, a couple of anchovies and a handful of capers. You can take this in a different direction by flaking in a tin of tuna when the sauce is ready.

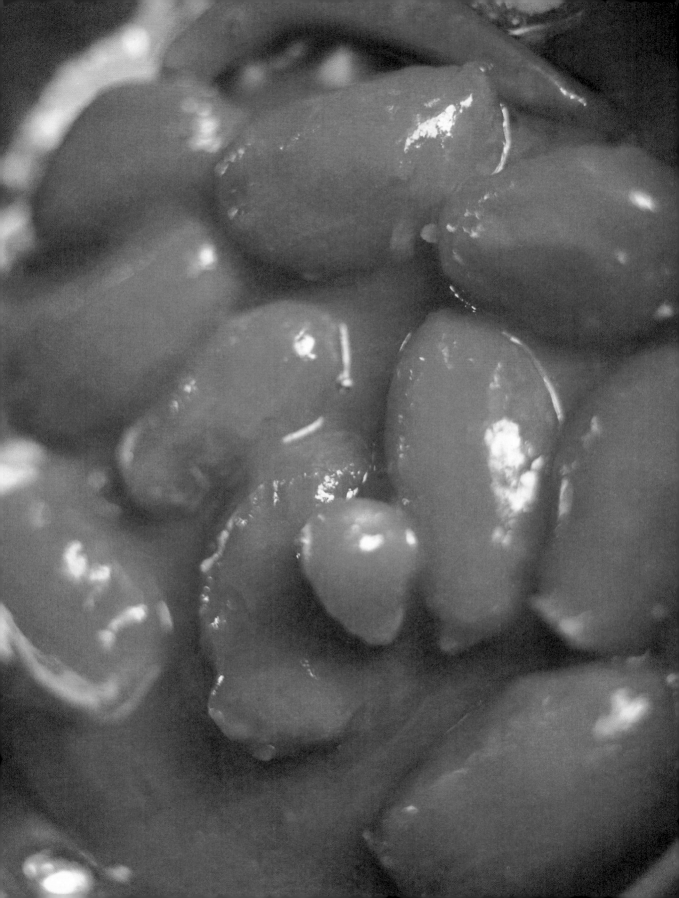

TOMATO SAUCE

with Tagliatelle, Spinach and Goat's Cheese

Once I've made my basic tomato sauce, this is one of my favourite ways to turn it into a desirable pasta dish. Simmer it in a large pan while you cook some tagliatelle in salted, boiling water according to the packet instructions. Just before the pasta is ready, add a large handful of spinach to the tomato sauce and check the seasoning. Drain the pasta in a colander, saving a little of the cooking water. Then toss the pasta with a little olive oil and some of the reserved water to loosen it, and pour your tomato and spinach sauce over the top. Toss again. Divide on to plates, sprinkle over some grated Parmesan and crumble over some goat's cheese. You can also try using crumbled feta or ricotta – you'll love it.

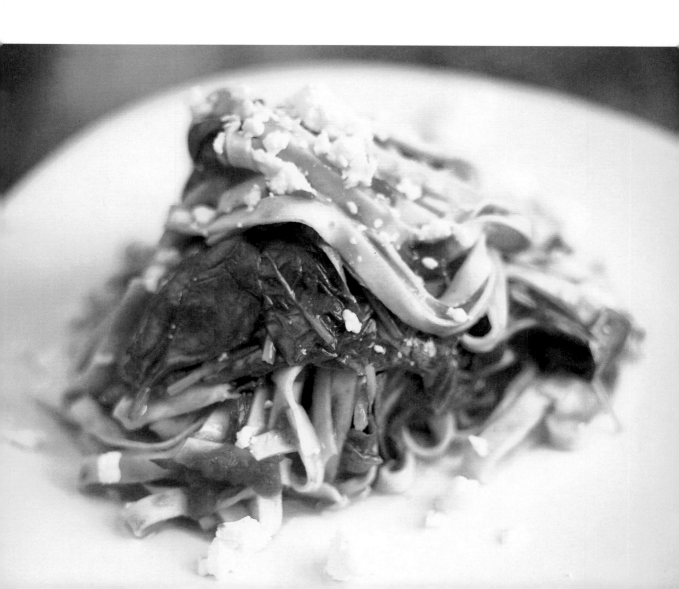

with Grilled Polenta   You can use your tomato sauce as a posh version of ketchup to serve with grilled chicken or white fish. Or even with polenta – here's an easy recipe. Boil your polenta grains according to the packet instructions, stirring all the time, until you have a stodgy consistency like thick porridge. Season with sea salt and freshly ground black pepper, add a little knob of butter and some grated Parmesan, then pour the polenta out on to an oiled baking tray so that it's about 2.5cm/1 inch thick. Leave it to cool and set – anything between 1 and 2 hours – then grill it till it's crisp. Serve with some tomato sauce spooned over the top, and a little bunch of dressed watercress or rocket wrapped up in some smoky speck or Parma ham. Shave over some Parmesan, using a speed peeler, and finish with a drizzle of olive oil.

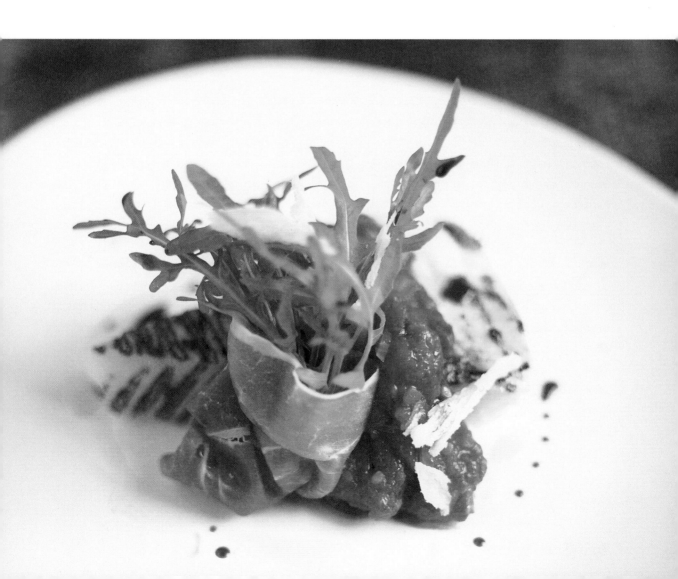

TOMATO SAUCE

with Fish, Olives and Basil
Pour your warmed tomato sauce into a small baking tray and put a couple of fish fillets on top. If you prefer to use chicken breasts, brown them first in a little oil before placing on top. Sprinkle with some pitted olives, capers and basil leaves and, if you have any to hand, a little torn mozzarella, and place in the oven at about 220°C/425°F/gas 7 for around 15 minutes until the fish is cooked. If using chicken breasts they will need 20 minutes.

with Portabello Mushrooms and Taleggio
Pour your warmed tomato sauce into a small baking tray and place some nice Portabello or field mushrooms, with the stalks facing up, on top. Slice over some taleggio – this is a lovely melting cheese and it's beautiful with these mushrooms – and sprinkle over some picked thyme leaves. You could even scatter over some torn-up breadcrumbs, drizzled with olive oil. Bake in the oven at 220°C/425°F/gas 7 for 15 to 20 minutes.

with Sausages
Pour your warmed tomato sauce into a baking tray or ovenproof dish. Get yourself some nice sausages and toss them in a little olive oil, then place them on top of the sauce and cook at 220°C/425°F/gas 7 for about 30 minutes, or until the sausages are golden and crisp on top. It will be almost like a cassoulet – the sausages will be soft and juicy on the bottom from the sauce, and lovely and crisp on top. On the cassoulet vibe, a tin of beans such as cannellini, flageolet, haricot or chickpeas, or chunky lardons of smoked bacon added to this would be fantastic.

with Marinated Jumbo Prawns
Ask your fishmonger to remove the shells from a couple of handfuls of large raw prawns, then when you get home all you have to do is run a knife down the back of each one to remove the little black vein. Once you've done this, squeeze over some lemon juice, olive oil, chopped fresh flat-leaf parsley and chopped fresh chilli and let the prawns marinate for at least 5 minutes and up to an hour. Put your tomato sauce into a pan and sprinkle in the prawns and their marinating juices. Put the lid on and either slowly simmer on the hob or pop the pan in the oven for just 5 minutes at 220°C/425°F/gas 7. Serve with a big pile of grilled ciabatta and a nice chilled bottle of white wine – makes a great starter. You could even chuck a handful of mussels or clams in with the prawns, or try having the sauce with a whole lobster cut in half. All good.

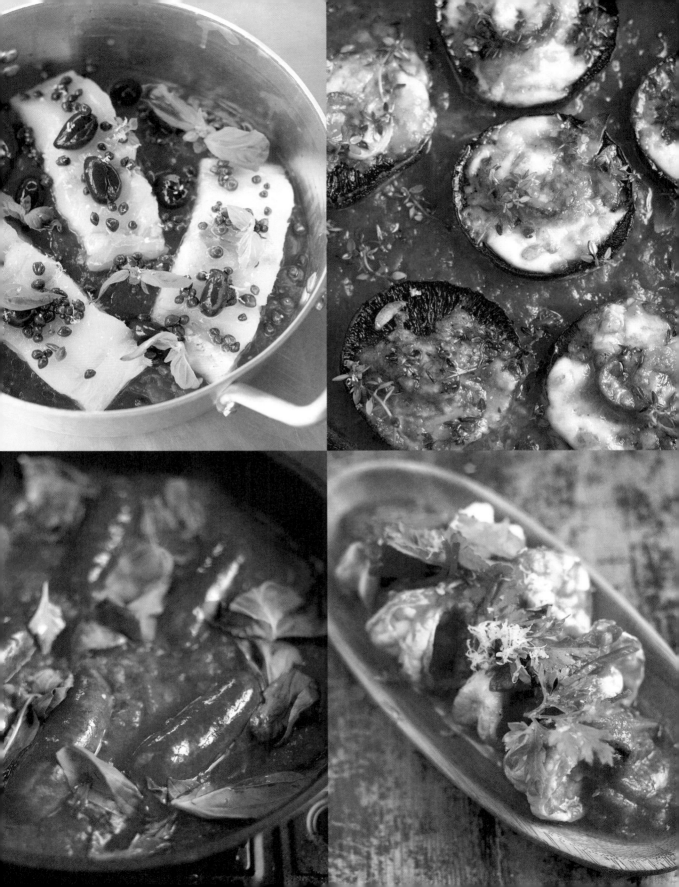

SLOW-COOKED SHOULDER OF LAMB WITH ROASTED VEGETABLES

This is a recipe that I first made as an alternative to roasting a leg of lamb. I wanted to save time and make my own gravy, so I turned it into a pot roast by adding vegetables and wine. I think shoulder of lamb is one of the best cuts by far – it's tastier than leg and much more economical. I've taken it in various different directions and have come up with some fantastic Family Tree ideas . . .

SERVES 6–8
1 x 2.25kg/5½lb shoulder of lamb, bone in
olive oil
sea salt and freshly ground black pepper
1 whole bulb of garlic, broken into cloves
a handful of fresh rosemary sprigs
2 red onions, peeled and quartered
3 carrots, peeled and roughly chopped
2 sticks of celery, cut into pieces
1 large leek or 2–3 baby leeks, trimmed and cut into pieces
a handful of ripe tomatoes, halved
2 bay leaves
a handful of fresh thyme sprigs
2 x 400g tins of good-quality plum tomatoes
1 bottle of red wine

Preheat your oven to 200°C/400°F/gas 6. Rub the lamb with oil, sea salt and freshly ground black pepper and put it into a roasting tray. Using a sharp knife, make small incisions all over the lamb and poke rosemary leaves and some quartered cloves of garlic into each one. This will give great flavour to the meat. Add the rest of the garlic cloves, the onions, carrots, celery, leeks and fresh tomatoes to the tray, then tuck the remaining herbs under the meat. Pour the tinned tomatoes over the top, followed by the wine. Cover the tray tightly with a double layer of foil and put it into the oven. Turn down the oven temperature to 170°C/325°F/gas 3 and cook for 3½ to 4 hours, or until the lamb is soft, melting and sticky and you can pull it apart with a fork. Gently break up the meat, pull out the bones, and extract any herb stalks. Squeeze the garlic out of the skins and mush it in. Shred the lamb, and check the seasoning.

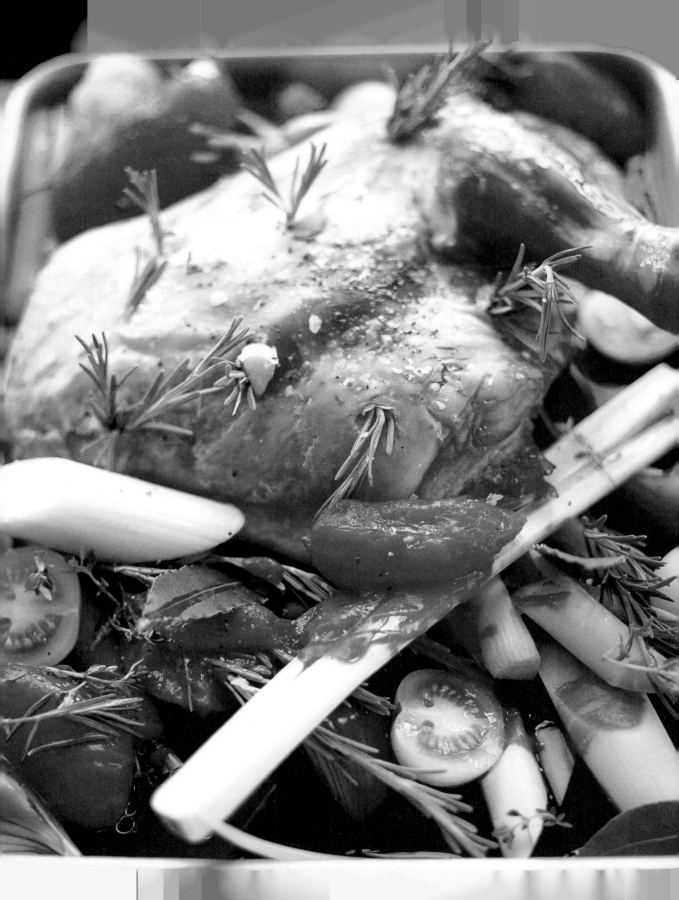

SLOW-COOKED LAMB

Ragù Pasta Using the slow-cooked lamb for this recipe makes it far closer to an original ragù dish than if you use mince. I think you'll really love it. If you happen to have the zest from an orange, some chopped fresh flat-leaf parsley and a peeled and chopped clove of garlic, mix them together and try sprinkling over the top of the pasta just before serving – it will give an incredible flavour. Cook your spaghetti or tagliatelle – 455g/1lb for 4 people – in salted boiling water according to the packet instructions, then drain it in a colander, reserving a little of the cooking water. Stir your shredded lamb through your pasta and add a good handful of grated Parmesan. Serve in large bowls.

with My Mum's Dumplings This recipe is really simple because all you have to do is stir the following ingredients together in a bowl: 225g/8oz of self-raising flour, 115g/4oz of suet or butter, a handful of chopped fresh rosemary, thyme or flat-leaf parsley, 30g/1oz of grated Cheddar or Gruyère cheese and ½ a level teaspoon of salt. Slowly add 140ml/¼ pint cold water and mix until the dough binds together. Then divide it into 8 pieces and roll them into golf-ball-sized dumplings. Once your lamb is cooked and shredded, put it into a pan and warm gently – you may need to add a little water to thin the sauce out. Lay your dumplings on top of the stew (or dunk them under if you prefer – this will make them glossy and dark when cooked) and then, if your pan is ovenproof, put it into the oven for 40 minutes at 190°C/375°F/gas 5, covering the pan for the first 25 minutes. Or put a tight-fitting lid on the pan and finish it on top of the stove so the dumplings can steam, for an hour. Either way, the dumplings will suck up loads of the fantastic cooking juices, leaving you with nice, firm, tasty meat and juicy, gooey dumplings.

Shepherd's Pie Once your lamb is cooked and shredded, transfer it to a casserole pan or earthenware-type dish that will allow the meat to sit about 2.5cm/1 inch deep. Cover with mashed potato, add a sprig of rosemary and bake in the oven at 200°C/400°F/gas 6 for 35 minutes until golden.

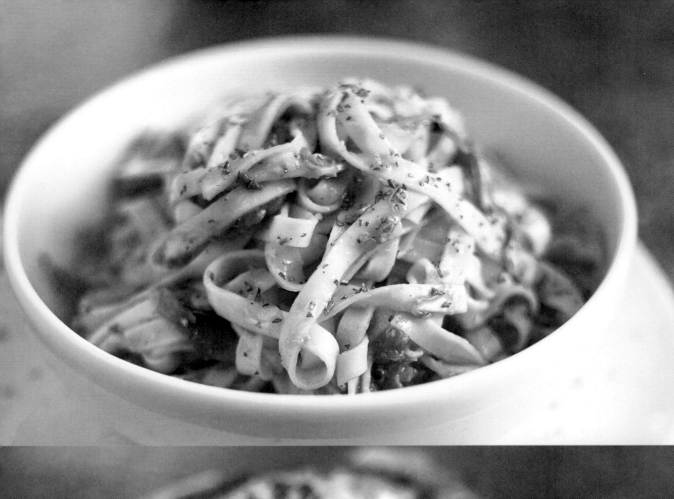
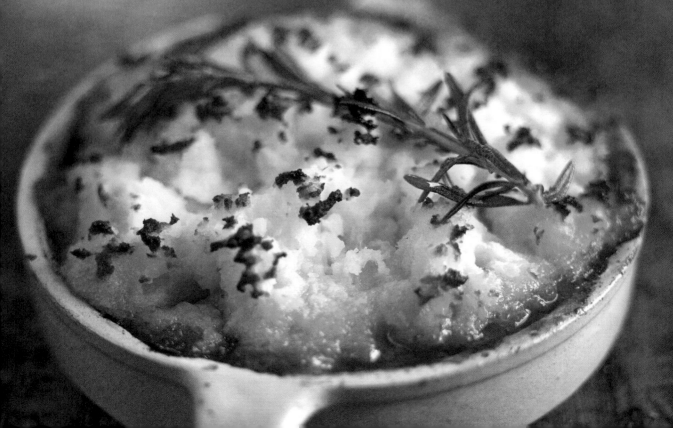

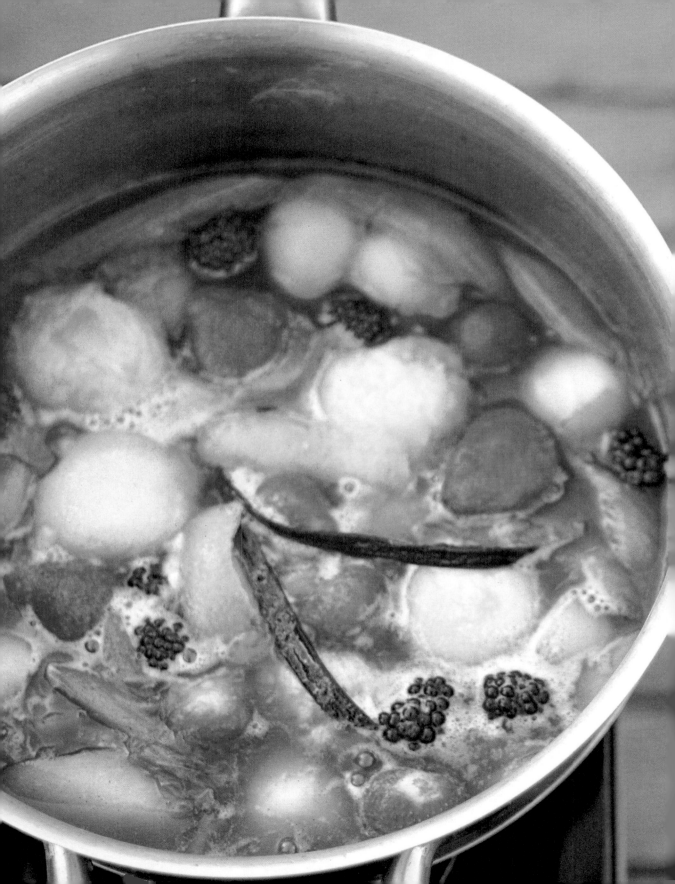

STEWED FRUIT

I know what you're thinking … stewed fruit = school dinners = not very exciting. But I'm here to change your mind – stewing, or gently poaching, fruit is a fantastic way of altering your perceived flavour of it. When stewed together with a little sugar and water (or maybe some alcohol like wine, port, brandy, rum or sherry) and other spices or flavourings, all types of fruit can take on a whole different vibe. Have you ever wondered where the inspiration and flavour combos came from for drinks like Dr Pepper and Vimto? Well, stewed fruit is the real McCoy because the juices can take on the most amazing flavours and it's completely good for you! Try a cinnamon stick or almonds with apricots and peaches, a couple of cloves with apples and pears, five-spice with plums, vanilla and orange zest with rhubarb (lemon zest and ginger are both good too!). But the one thing you have to remember is to try to keep as much of the fruit's shape and colour as you can, otherwise you'll end up with a jammy liquid.

I use all of the following fruits on a regular basis, depending on what's in season of course: rhubarb, peaches, pears, strawberries, plums, apples, cherries, figs, gooseberries, blackberries and blackcurrants. Now I would say stewed fruit is starting to sound a bit sexier! The other brilliant thing to bear in mind is that this is a dish that can be made very cheaply and it can also be easily transformed down the Family Tree, as you'll see. At the end of the day you can pick up boxes of slightly over-ripe or under-ripe fruit really cheaply, so this is a brilliant way of cooking on a budget.

SERVES 8
1 vanilla pod, halved
  and deseeded
255g/9oz caster sugar
optional: 1 clove
optional: ¼ of a stick of cinnamon
1 star anise
zest of ¼ of an orange

2 pears, each peeled and cut into eight
4 peaches, halved
4 plums, halved
500g/1lb 2oz rhubarb
a handful of strawberries, hulled
a handful of blackberries
optional: a small handful of fresh basil
  or mint, leaves picked

Score down the length of the vanilla pod and remove the seeds by scraping a knife down the inside of each half. Get yourself a high-sided pot and add the sugar and 255ml/9fl oz of water to it. Place on the heat, and when it starts to warm up add the vanilla pod and seeds, the clove, cinnamon stick, star anise and orange zest. Bring to the boil until the liquid becomes clear then remove the clove, cinnamon and star anise. Turn it down to a simmer and put your firmer fruit into the pot – in this case, the pears and peaches, followed by the plums and rhubarb a few minutes later. Simmer slowly for 5 or 6 minutes until tender. A couple of minutes before the end, add the strawberries and blackberries. Let the fruit sit in the syrup for all the flavours to develop. If I'm going to be serving it just as fruit with its flavoured syrup and ice cream I tend not to overcook it too much, as this way it stays fresh and light and colourful. However, if I want a pulp I will remove the lid and continue to cook it, stirring as often as I can. When done, remember to remove the skin and stones from the peaches and plums.

Divide the fruit into bowls, spoon over the hot syrup and, if you have some to hand, finish by sprinkling over some basil or mint leaves. Serve with a dollop of cream.

STEWED FRUIT

Crumble If you want to turn your stewed fruit into a crumble for 4, divide it between 4 ovenproof bowls. Top with a crumble mixture made by rubbing together 225g/8oz of plain flour, 115g/4oz of butter, 90g/3oz of sugar and a pinch of salt. Sprinkle the mixture over the fruit and bake in the oven at 180°C/350°F/gas 4 for 15 to 20 minutes until the top is crisp and the fruit is bubbling up at the sides. You can always make one large crumble if you would prefer.

Syllabub Syllabubs date back to the sixteenth century and are lovely cold desserts. They are made with cream and can be flavoured with sugar, wine or lemon juice. Stewed fruit is also a perfect flavouring. For 4 people, all you have to do is whip 565ml/1 pint of double cream to form soft peaks and, when it's nice and thick, pour your mushed stewed fruit on to it and mix together. Serve in individual glasses or bowls, with a little grated orange zest sprinkled over the top.

on Toast Stewed fruit is lovely with toast, although you may think it sounds a bit strange! All you have to do to make this simple dessert is butter some nice toasted bread, then smear over your stewed fruit, crumble over some ricotta or nice goat's cheese and spoon over some runny honey.

Filo Pastry Parcels Filo pastry is great to cook with. Buy a packet of fresh filo pastry sheets, then all you have to do is keep the pile of them underneath a damp cloth while you work with 2 sheets at a time. Take your 2 sheets and brush them with melted butter, then stick them together. Cut them into a square 20 x 20cm/8 x 8 inches and spoon 2 tablespoons of your stewed fruit into the middle of the square. Crumble over a little ricotta cheese and sprinkle over some muscovado sugar, then bring the sides of the filo pastry up and squeeze them together to make a little parcel. Brush the top with melted butter and place on to a baking tray. Repeat with the rest of your filo sheets and stewed fruit. Bake in the oven at 170°C/325°F/gas 3 for 15 to 20 minutes until golden and crisp.

with Yoghurt Stewed fruit is also really nice with a spoonful of natural yoghurt, some runny honey and a scattering of porridge oats. Great for breakfast.

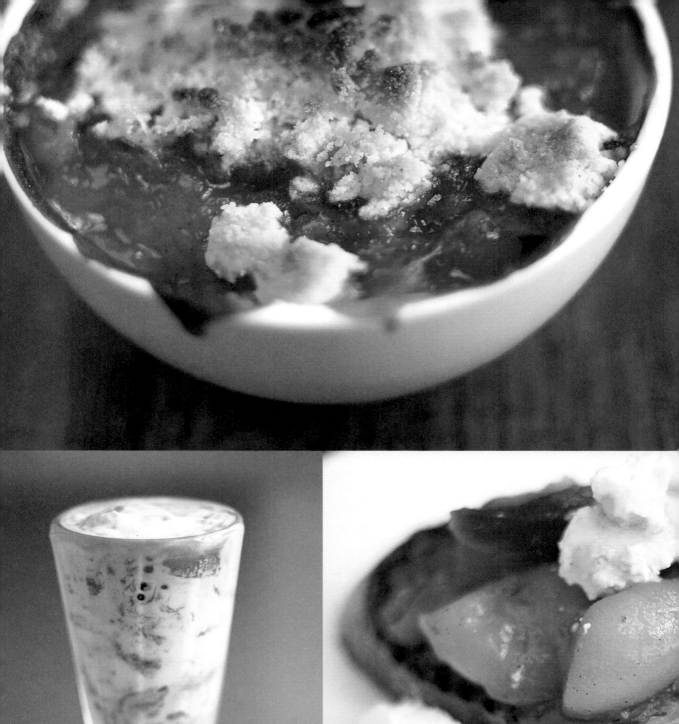

PUFF PASTRY

Frozen, pre-made puff pastry is available just about everywhere. Unlike shortcrust pastry, which is quite easy to make yourself, puff pastry is a real palaver at home unless you've got loads of time. So I would advise that you buy it, and the all-butter puff pastry is the one to look for. For those of you who aren't sure what puff pastry is, it's a type of pastry that has butter folded into it and is then rolled and folded with many layers, so that when it cooks it expands and you get the millefeuille effect, as the French call it (this means 'thousand-leaf', because this is what it looks like with all its layers). It looks great when it's all puffed up, and it has a fantastic crispy and chewy texture. Great for desserts, to go on pies and stews, stuff like that. Here are some Family Tree ideas for puff pastry . . .

Parmesan Twists One of the quickest and easiest things to do with puff pastry is to make these little 'twists' to have as munchies, to eat with salad or with drinks at a dinner party. These can be made and then frozen (uncooked) for when you have unexpected guests. Roll out your puff pastry to about 25cm/10 inches wide and about 0.5cm/¼ inch thick. Brush the surface with a little beaten egg. Sprinkle over a pinch of paprika (or try poppy seeds, sesame seeds or bashed fennel seeds), and cut across the width into 2cm/¾ inch wide strips. Then all you need to do is twist each strip about 4 or 5 times (see picture on page 57). They are now ready to freeze if you wish, or you can cook them straight away. Place them closely together on a roasting tray, grate over some Parmesan, and bake at 220°C/425°F/gas 7 for about 8 to 10 minutes, until golden and crisp.

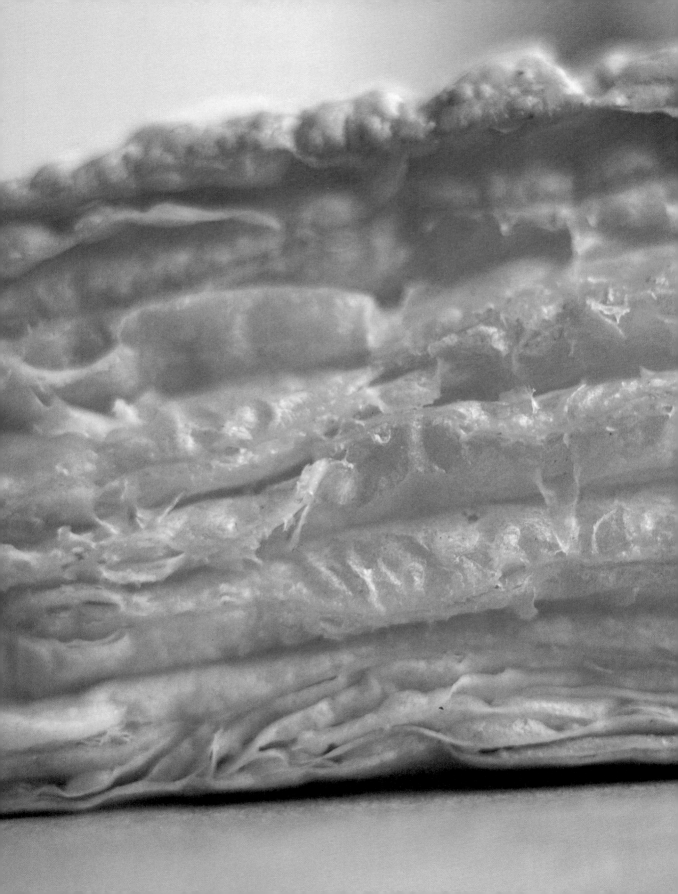

Quick Jammy Apple Tart

Roll out your puff pastry on a lightly flour-dusted surface until just under 0.5cm/¼ inch thick. Then get yourself an 18cm/7 inch plate. Using this as a template, place it on the pastry and cut out about 8 circles. Peel some apples or pears, quarter them, remove the cores and finely slice into slivers. Toss in a bowl straight away with just enough sugar to lightly coat the fruit, and a couple of tablespoons of freshly squeezed orange juice. This will make the sugar go syrupy so it will stick to the fruit. Then all you have to do is put a tablespoon of jam into the middle of each circle of puff pastry, and fan out your fruit slices on top. Fold in the sides to hold it all together, sprinkle over a little thyme, and bake in the oven at 220°C/425°F/gas 7 until the fruit has softened and the pastry is crisp and golden. Serve with crème fraîche or ice cream. Again, if you want to freeze these (uncooked) as last-minute lifesavers then feel free to. You can cook them straight from frozen at 220°C/425°F/gas 7, until the pastry is golden.

Mini Calzones with Prosciutto, Mozzarella and Tomato

Roll your puff pastry out into 8 x 18cm/7 inch circles, as above. On one half of each circle lay a slice of prosciutto, followed by a squash-ball-sized piece of mozzarella. Squash a cherry tomato on top, add a few basil leaves, and season with sea salt and freshly ground black pepper. Wrap the prosciutto around the filling to hold it together, then egg-wash the edges of the pastry and fold it in half, almost like a Cornish pasty. Pinch or crimp the sides together so the filling can't come out, and bake at 220°C/425°F/gas 7 until golden and crisp on the outside.

Sausage Rolls

It's a real shame that sausage rolls have become viewed as junk food over the years. You can make some really tasty ones using puff pastry. Buy some good sausages – Cumberland ones are great – rip them open and discard the skins. Put the meat into a bowl and add a handful of roughly chopped fresh herbs (try rosemary, sage, thyme). Then add one or two of the following: orange or lemon zest, some chestnuts, a little chopped apple or pear, and mix everything together to give you fantastically flavoured sausage meat. All you then need to do is roll out your puff pastry until it's 20cm/8 inches wide and just under 0.5cm/¼ inch thick, dusting with flour as needed. Cut the sheet of pastry in half, so you have two 10cm/4 inch wide strips. Now get your sausage stuffing and divide it in half. Roll each half into a sausage shape and lay these along the length of the two pastry strips. Egg-wash the pastry, roll it up, and then use the back of a fork to mark and seal the pastry so it is tightly wrapped up. Egg-wash the top of each, and cut the roll into shorter pieces if you want. Bake at 220°C/425°F/gas 7 until golden, crisp and puffed up. You can freeze the rolls uncooked – simply remove them from the freezer when you need them and cook them from frozen at 220°C/425°F/gas 7 until golden and crisp. Nice with some Branston pickle, a lump of Cheddar and a rocket salad.

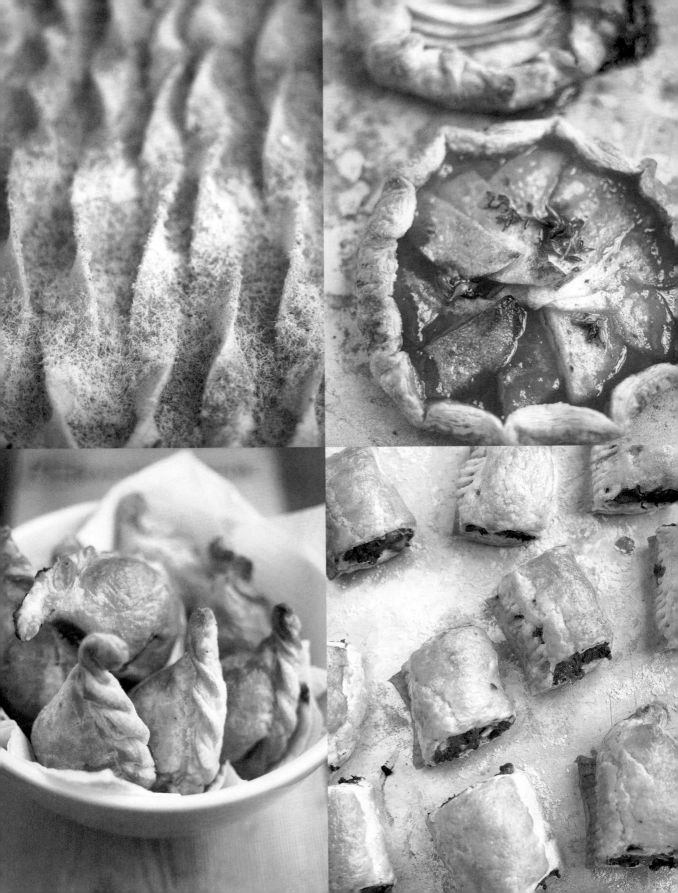

5 MINUTE WONDERS

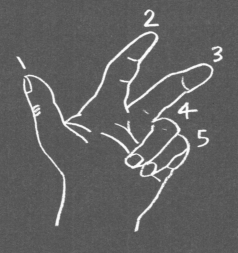

Just about everyone I know, including myself, comes home late and knackered quite a few times during the week. Did you know that fifteen years ago the average time spent making a meal for the family was an hour – nowadays it's a measly thirteen minutes! (And that's probably waiting for the microwave to go 'ding' while making a cup of tea.)

So I got to thinking that anyone making a quick dash round the supermarket on their way home from work could probably do with getting a little inspiration for dishes for one that can be made quickly when they get through the door. Bearing this in mind, the recipes here all use ingredients that you can pick up from any market or supermarket. I then decided to time myself making each of these dishes, which was fun! I tried to work reasonably slowly to give a realistic prep and cooking time. The results are pretty cool, especially considering that for some of the recipes, the time from the pan going on the heat to serving the food at the table was only 3 minutes! (My timing – you might need 5 to 10 minutes!) And nothing was compromised – all the dishes smelt great and tasted lovely. Each recipe has the time it took for me to make it – you never know, you might be able to beat me on some of them!

So if you're the kind of person who thinks they haven't got time to cook, or you run out of time (like we all do sometimes), then this chapter should be quite helpful to you. You know the thing: you're rushing around, you're busy, work seems to get later and later and on the way home you speed through the basket checkout, having picked up a chicken breast or some salmon and a selection of vegetables.

If you don't really find cooking all that relaxing, I hope these recipes will be fun to cook, and I hope they make you feel good and give you a nice dinner. It just goes to show that you don't need hours and hours to come up with some magic-tasting food.

A last note ... all the recipes in this chapter use pan-frying as the main method of cooking – I love this method, as it's totally immediate. But what you will need to get hold of is a large, non-stick pan – that will make your life even easier!

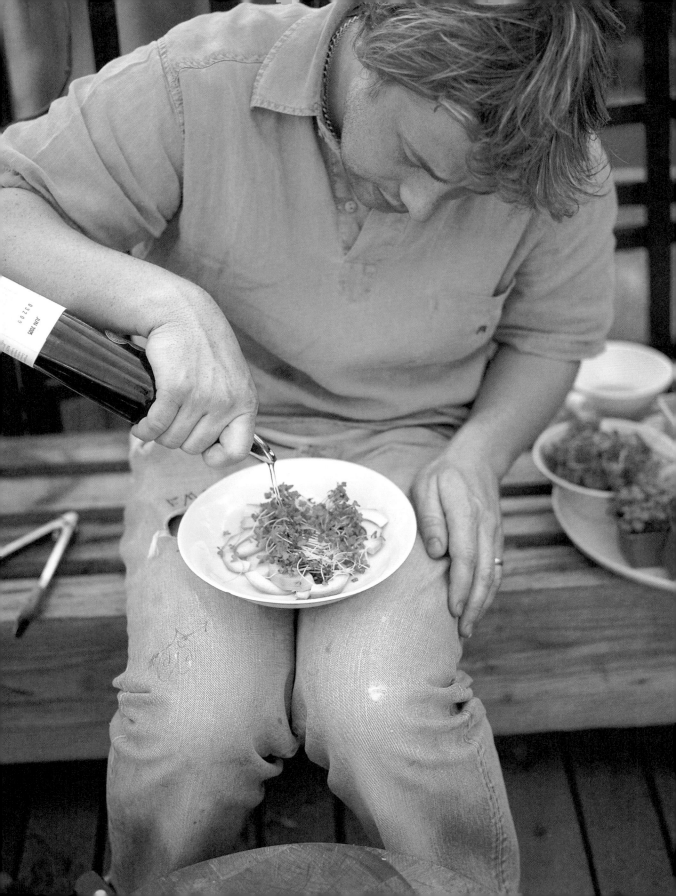

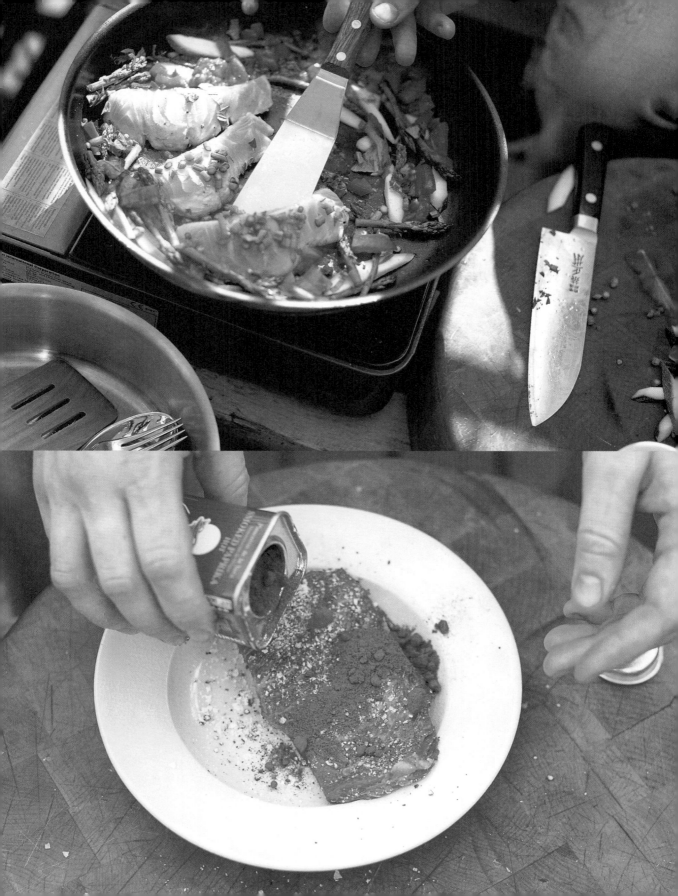

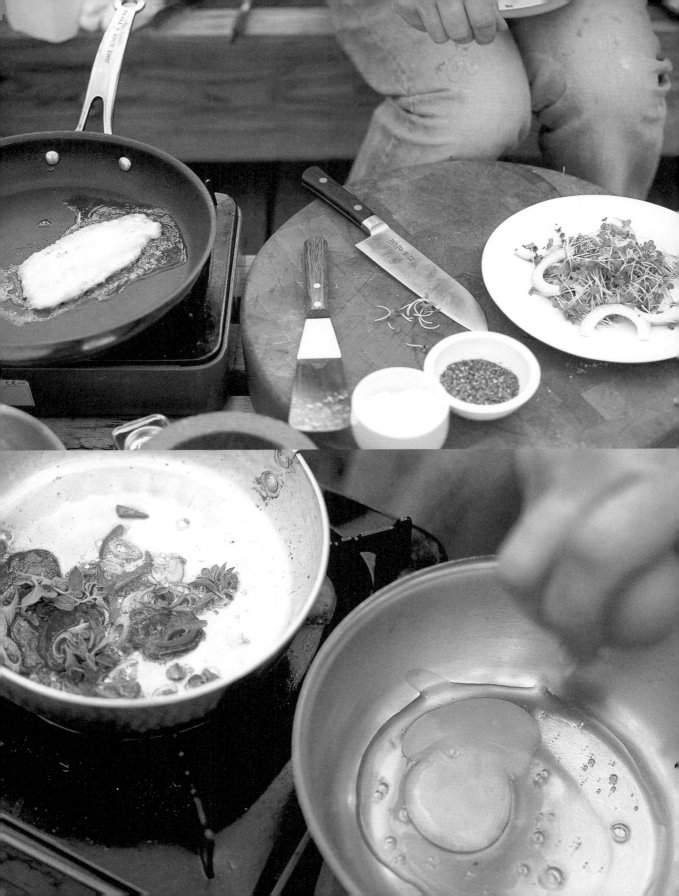

SALMON AND COUSCOUS (5m 48s)

SERVES 1 • 115g/4oz couscous • 1 x 200g/7oz salmon fillet, skin on, scaled and pinboned • extra virgin olive oil • sea salt and freshly ground black pepper • 1 small courgette, sliced into batons • 1 small handful of asparagus tips • 1 red chilli, deseeded and finely chopped • 2 ripe tomatoes, roughly chopped • juice of ½ a lemon • a small handful of fresh coriander, roughly chopped • 1 tablespoon crème fraîche

Put your couscous in a bowl, then pour over just enough boiling water to cover it. Set aside for 3 minutes to allow the couscous to soak up the water. Slice the salmon widthways into finger-size strips, drizzle with olive oil, and season with salt and pepper. Heat a small non-stick frying pan and add the salmon strips on their side. Scatter over the courgette, asparagus tips and chilli and cook for 2 minutes, turning the salmon over halfway. Mix the tomatoes, lemon juice, 4 tablespoons of olive oil and the coriander into the couscous and season to taste. Remove the salmon strips to a plate and add the couscous to the veggies left in the pan. Mix together and then put the salmon strips back into the pan on top of the couscous, place a lid on and put back on a high heat for a minute. To serve, slide everything on to your plate and spoon over some crème fraîche. Quick and tasty!

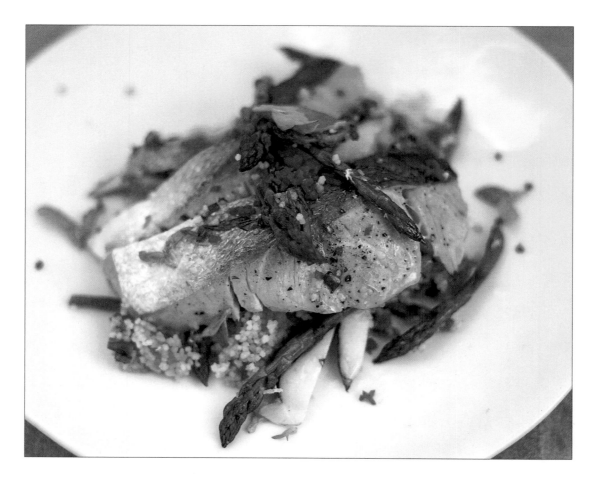

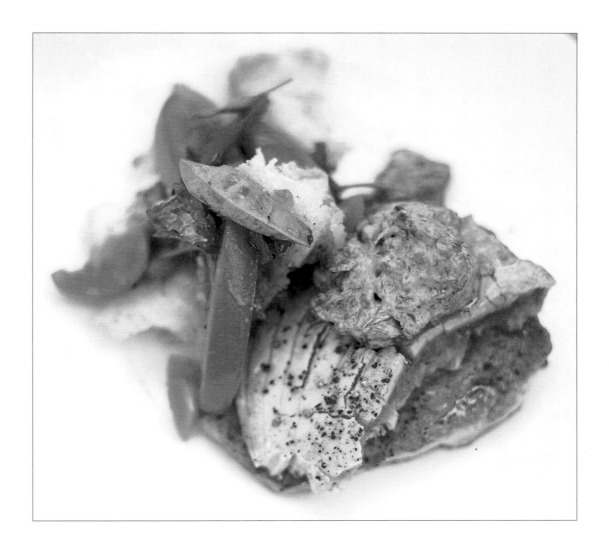

HOT TUNA SALAD (4m 5s)

SERVES 1 • 1 x 2cm thick tuna steak (200g/7oz) • extra virgin olive oil • sea salt and freshly ground black pepper • 3 ripe tomatoes, quartered • juice of ½ a lemon • a handful of chunky torn bread • a handful of fresh basil leaves • 2 tablespoons crème fraîche

Get a frying pan very hot. Rub the tuna with a little oil, season and sear for about 1 minute on each side (this will cook it rare). Crisp the bread until golden at the same time. Mix the tomatoes, crispy bread and 10 basil leaves in a bowl and stir in a little olive oil and half the lemon juice. Season and put on a plate. Pound the remaining basil in a pestle and mortar and mix with the crème fraîche. Season with salt, pepper and lemon juice. Place the tuna beside the salad and spoon over the sauce.

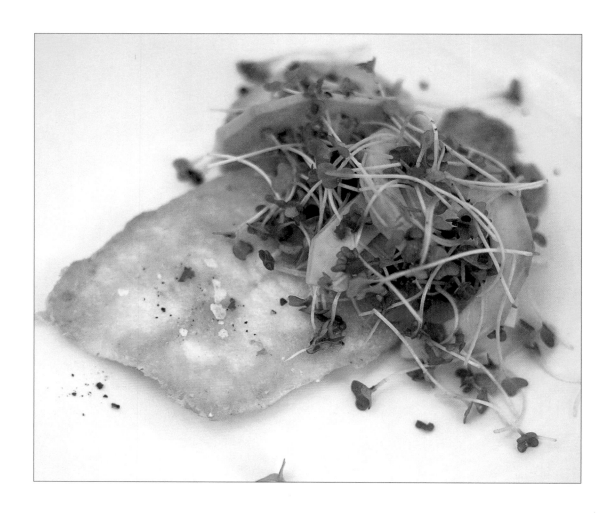

PARMESAN FISH FILLETS WITH AVOCADO AND CRESS SALAD (4m 58s)

SERVES 1 • 2 tablespoons flour • salt and freshly ground black pepper • 170g/6oz white fish fillets, skin removed • 1 egg, beaten • 55g/2oz freshly grated Parmesan cheese • olive oil • ½ a fresh red chilli, deseeded and finely chopped • 1 ripe avocado, peeled and sliced lengthways • 1 punnet of cress • 1 tablespoon extra virgin olive oil • juice of ½ a lemon

Get a frying pan really hot. Season the flour with salt and pepper. Dust the fish fillets with the seasoned flour, then dip into the egg and press into the grated Parmesan, making sure the fish is nicely covered. Add a little olive oil to the hot pan, and fry the fish fillets for a couple of minutes on each side until golden brown. Throw in the chilli. Mix together the avocado and cress with the extra virgin olive oil and lemon juice, and put on your plate with your fish fillets.

CHORIZO AND TOMATO OMELETTE (4m 58s)

SERVES 1 • extra virgin olive oil • 1 small whole Spanish chorizo sausage, sliced thickly • 1 ripe tomato, deseeded and sliced • 2 small sprigs of fresh marjoram or parsley, leaves picked and chopped • 3 free-range eggs • ½ a fresh red chilli, sliced • sea salt and freshly ground black pepper • 1 spring onion, finely sliced

Heat a little extra virgin olive oil in a small frying pan, then add the chorizo and fry for a minute before adding the tomato and the marjoram or parsley. Whisk the eggs in a small bowl, add the chilli, season with salt and pepper, and pour into the pan with the chorizo and tomato. Using a fork, mix the eggs around in the pan a little, and then throw in the spring onion. Continue to fry until the eggs set, giving you a lovely little omelette. Great served with some rocket dressed with a little olive oil.

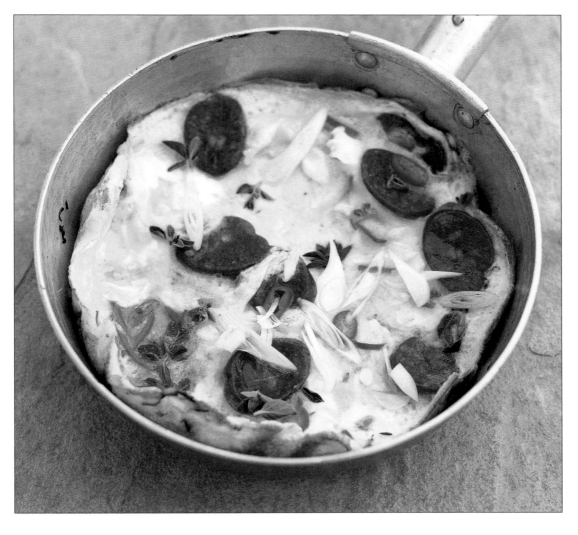

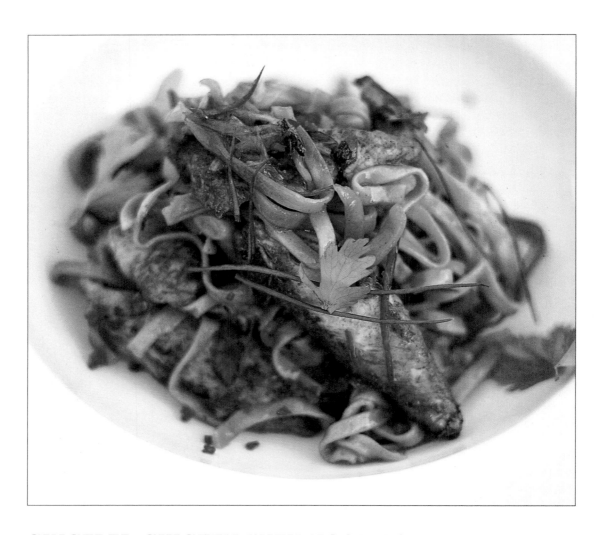

GINGERED CHICKEN WITH NOODLES (4m 41s)

SERVES 1 • 115g/4oz dried medium egg noodles • 2 tablespoons oil • 1 free-range organic chicken breast, cut into strips 2.5cm/1 inch wide • a thumb-sized piece of fresh ginger, peeled and thinly sliced • 1 fresh red chilli, deseeded and finely sliced • 1 teaspoon five-spice • 3 spring onions, finely sliced • a dash of soy sauce • 1 tablespoon runny honey • a small handful of fresh coriander, roughly chopped • sea salt and freshly ground black pepper • ½ a lemon

Drop the noodles into a pan of boiling water and cook according to the packet instructions – they should only need a couple of minutes. While the noodles are cooking, get a frying pan very hot, add the oil and let it heat through. Then add the chicken strips, ginger and chilli. Toss together, then add the five-spice. Once the chicken is browned, add the spring onions, soy sauce and honey. Drain the noodles using a colander, then add the noodles and coriander to the chicken. Season to taste and serve immediately with a squeeze of lemon.

BEEF WITH PAK CHOI, MUSHROOMS AND NOODLES
(5m 12s)

SERVES 1 • 115g/4oz thin rice noodles • 115g/4oz beef sirloin • olive oil • 1 teaspoon ground cumin • sea salt • ½ a red onion, finely sliced • a thumb-sized piece of fresh ginger, peeled and finely sliced • 1 fresh red chilli, deseeded and finely sliced • a small handful of shitake and oyster mushrooms, brushed clean and torn up • 200ml/7fl oz chicken stock • 1 pak choi, quartered

Boil the kettle and soak the noodles in the boiling water according to the packet instructions. Meanwhile rub the beef with olive oil, sprinkle with the cumin and a pinch of salt and rub all over. Place in a really hot frying pan and sear on all sides. Add the onion, ginger and chilli and cook for a couple of minutes, then add the mushrooms, stock and pak choi. Drain the noodles and add them to the pan. Stir around, and correct the seasoning. Slice up the beef and serve the noodles and pak choi in a big bowl, with the beef slices on top. Pour over the broth from the pan.

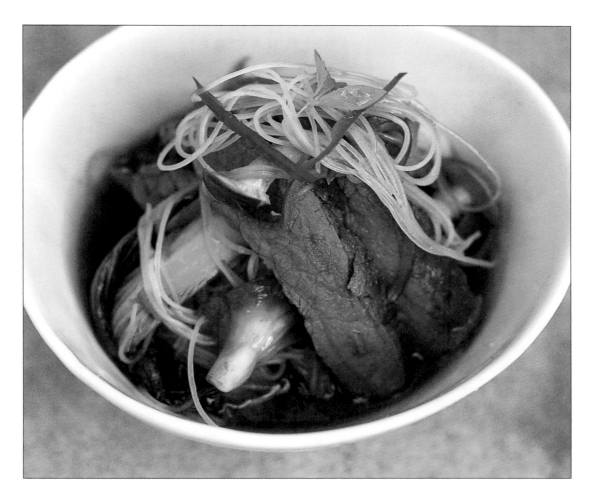

PAPRIKA SIRLOIN STEAK WRAP (5m 45s)

SERVES 1 • 1 sirloin steak, fat removed • extra virgin olive oil • 1 teaspoon smoked paprika • sea salt and freshly ground black pepper • a handful of rocket • 2 ripe tomatoes, roughly chopped • juice of 1 lemon • 2 tortilla wraps • 1 punnet of cress • 2 tablespoons hummus • 1 tablespoon soured cream

Heat a griddle pan or frying pan until very hot. Meanwhile, score each side of the steak and rub with olive oil. Sprinkle over the smoked paprika and season with salt and pepper. Place on the griddle and cook for about 2–3 minutes on each side, depending on how thick your steak is and how you like it cooked. Mix the rocket with the tomatoes, and dress with lemon juice and extra virgin olive oil. Wipe the pan clean with some kitchen paper, place the tortilla wraps in it and heat on both sides, but don't let them go crispy. Slice up the steak and serve it on the tortillas with the salad, cress, hummus and soured cream.

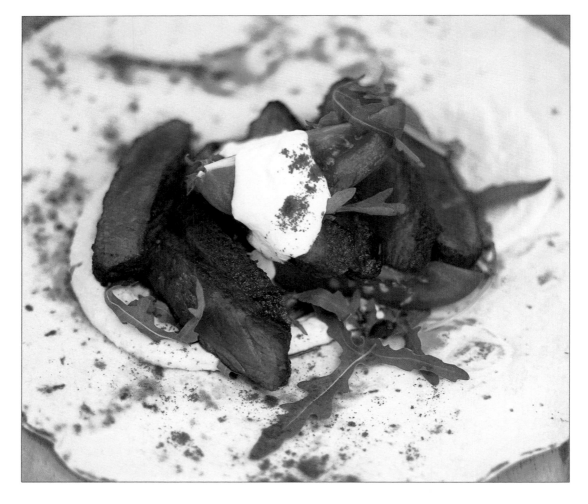

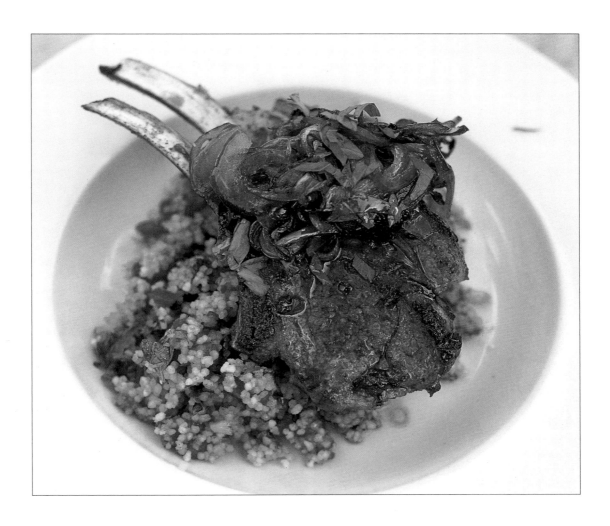

SUPER TASTY LAMB CUTLETS (4m 31s)

SERVES 1 • 115g/4oz couscous • 2 or 3 lamb cutlets, French-trimmed • sea salt and freshly ground black pepper • 1 teaspoon ground cumin• extra virgin olive oil • ½ a red onion, finely sliced • a sprig of fresh thyme, leaves picked and chopped • ¼ of a fresh red chilli, deseeded and finely chopped • 2 ripe tomatoes, chopped • 1 handful of fresh flat-leaf parsley • juice of 1 lemon

Get your frying pan hot. Place the couscous in a bowl and just cover with boiling water. With the palm of your hand bash the cutlets to flatten. Dust on both sides with salt, pepper and cumin and add with a little olive oil to the pan. When the cutlets have browned on one side, turn them, adding the onion, thyme and chilli and moving the ingredients around so they cook evenly for the next couple of minutes. Finely chop the tomatoes and most of the parsley and mix into the couscous with a good lug of olive oil and a squeeze of lemon. Season carefully to taste. Serve the couscous with the lamb and onions on top, and an extra sprinkling of parsley.

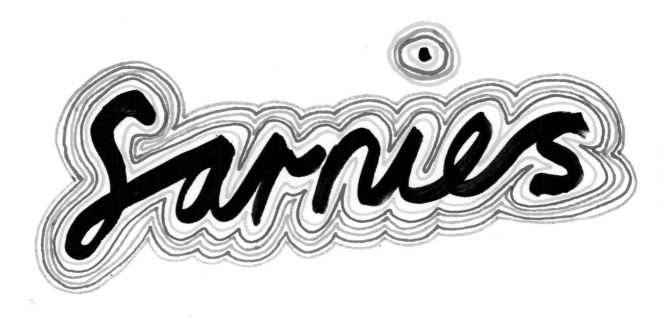

JAMIE'S LUNCHBOX

CIABATTA SANDWICH of GRILLED VEGETABLES WITH PESTO AND MOZZARELLA

SQUASHED FIG BASIL AND PARMA HAM SARNIE IN TOMATO BREAD

THE BEST PRAWN SANDWICH WITH BASIL MAYONNAISE AND CRESS

THE BEST BEEF SANDWICH WITH CRUNCHY LETTUCE ENGLISH MUSTARD AND GHERKINS

SMOKED SALMON LEMON AND CREME FRAICHE

CHEESY STEAK SANDWICH

DOUBLE-DECKER CHEDDAR CHEESE SANDWICH WITH PICKLED ONION AND CRISPS

BANANA AND BLUEBERRY FRENCH TOAST

QUESADILLAS WITH GUACAMOLE

CRISPY PEKING DUCK IN PANCAKES

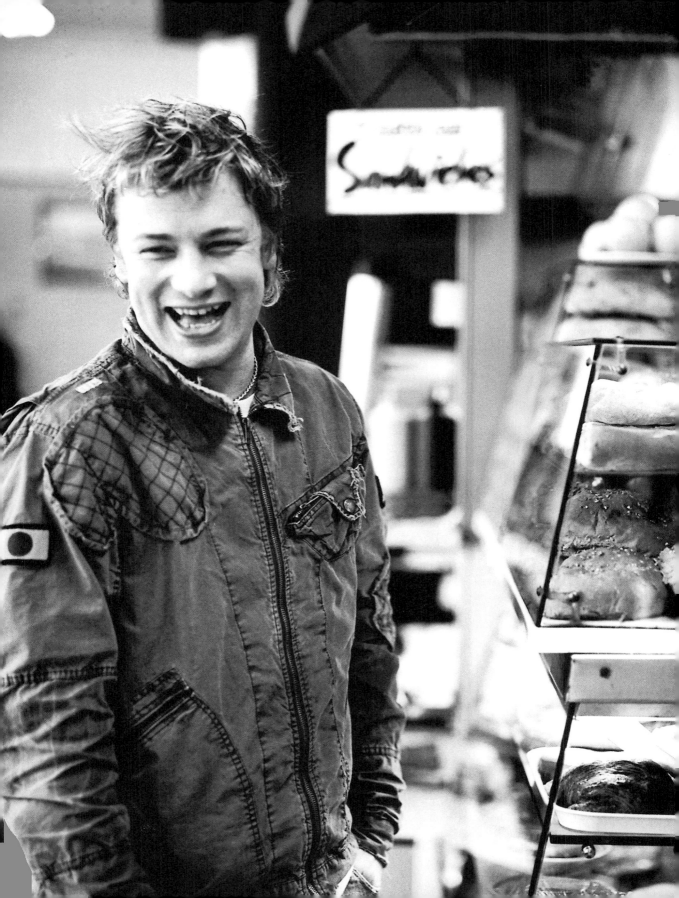

Sandwiches are the most widely eaten type of food in the UK, and probably in most western countries. Every country seems to have its own style of sandwich, from the croque monsieur in France, to the hamburger in America, to the quesadilla in South America, to Peking duck pancakes in China. And of course there is the good old doner kebab from Turkey!

I feel quite strongly about this chapter, because even though lots of people turn their noses up when it comes to sandwiches or think they are cheap and nasty and naff, or even a bit of a joke in the culinary world, the truth is they don't have to be.

You might think there's nothing remotely exciting about sandwiches, but the fact is that you can make them in seconds, they're really portable and there's no excuse for them not to be damned tasty.

If you talk to your friends about their favourite sandwiches you may agree on some, like a bacon sarnie for instance, but when you carry on talking you realize that actually you've all got your own way of making it. A discussion will no doubt follow, with remarks like, 'You want to toast the bread,' 'Gotta have brown sauce,' 'No, ketchup,' or that there's got to be melted cheese or a soft fried egg on top. In one particular conversation, with my friend John, things went downhill when he confessed that he has peanut butter, banana and bacon sandwiches and swears it's the best in the world – freak! But if he's happy with it that's fine. Another old chef mate, Chris, likes a triple-decker with bacon, beetroot and lettuce. And my thing is that I like to cut my loaf lengthways, using just thick smoked bacon. I cook the bacon first in the griddle pan and then toast the bread in the juices in the pan to give a kind of fried bread.

I think the reason some people aren't too keen on sandwiches is because they are often very similar and can get boring, but there's no need to make or buy the same ones all the time. Here's a collection of all the sandwiches that make me smile and make my tummy rumble when I think about them. Some of them make me want to be back on holiday, and others make me want to come home. In this chapter I'll also give you some hints and tips on how to turn your boring old lunchbox into a portable gourmet restaurant, so you can be a healthy and balanced VIP.

MY KINDA LUNCHBOX

- A really nice sarnie made with your favourite filling. Try using brown or wholemeal bread instead of white, and try not to stick to the same filling every day, if poss.

- Have a couple of cartons of pure unsweetened fruit juice or water – one for breaktime and one for lunch.

- Instead of the usual apple, which can become a bit boring, try a little bunch of grapes, half a melon, some sliced mango, half a papaya with a wedge of lime, or a kiwi, and include a spoon.

- Try and get your kids eating a little dried fruit – there is such a big choice now . . .

- I believe that a little healthyish chocolate treat is fine if you've got a balanced lunch.

- If you want to embarrass your kids, leave a little note for them in their lunch – like my mum used to do with me!

- While your kids are young, make a little salad an everyday thing, not a 'healthy' thing that is only eaten occasionally.

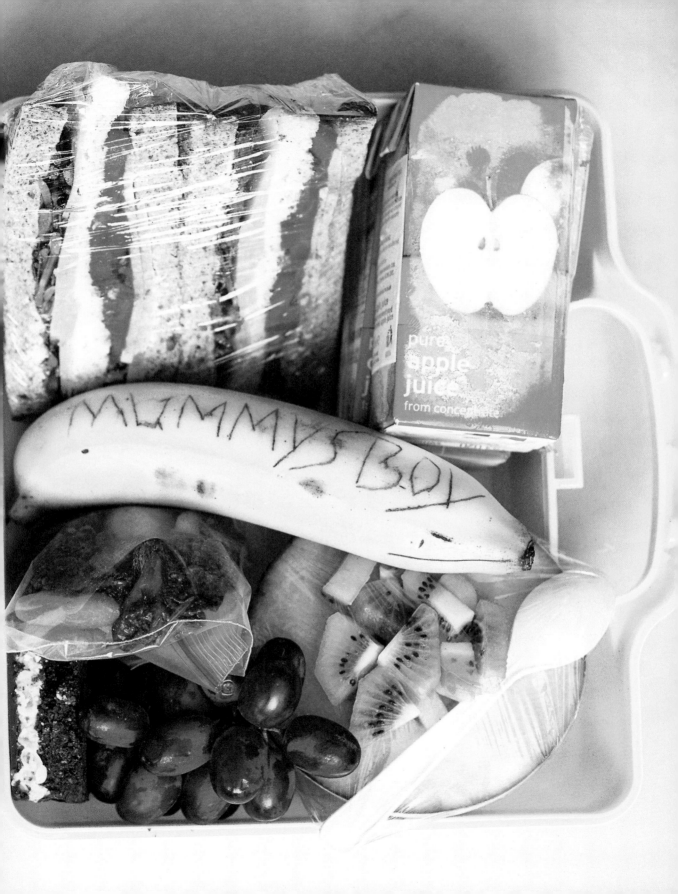

SOME LUNCHBOX TIPS

DID YOU KNOW ...

• If one of your two cartons of drink is frozen it will make your lunchbox into a mini coolbox – both hygienic and great, because by lunchtime it will have melted, giving you a lovely slushy cold drink.

• It's so important to spread your butter evenly from corner to corner, to act as a waterproof layer – this will help to prevent soggy sandwiches!

• There are so many different types of bread available these days, so ditch your plain white or wholemeal every now and again and give these a go with different fillings: rosemary and raisin with cheese, ciabatta with mozzarella and prosciutto, sun-dried tomato bread with ham, or poppy-seed rolls with chicken.

• A little fruit eaten every day will give your immune system a boost and make you feel more energetic. If you wrap your fruit in a napkin, you'll find that it won't get bruised.

• Kids can enjoy salads if they taste nice, if they're not soggy and if they're fun and a little interactive. So put a few slivers of Parmesan or some crumbled feta in a bag with a few cherry tomatoes and some nice mixed leaves. Make a separate wrap of dressing – 1 teaspoon of lemon juice with 3 of olive oil wrapped in a little clingfilm. Kids can squash the tomatoes up in the bag, add the dressing and shake it up – they'll love it!

• Thermos flasks are great to use – you can buy small ones which are perfect for taking hot food with you like soup or meatballs or sausages in tomato sauce. The possibilities are endless ...

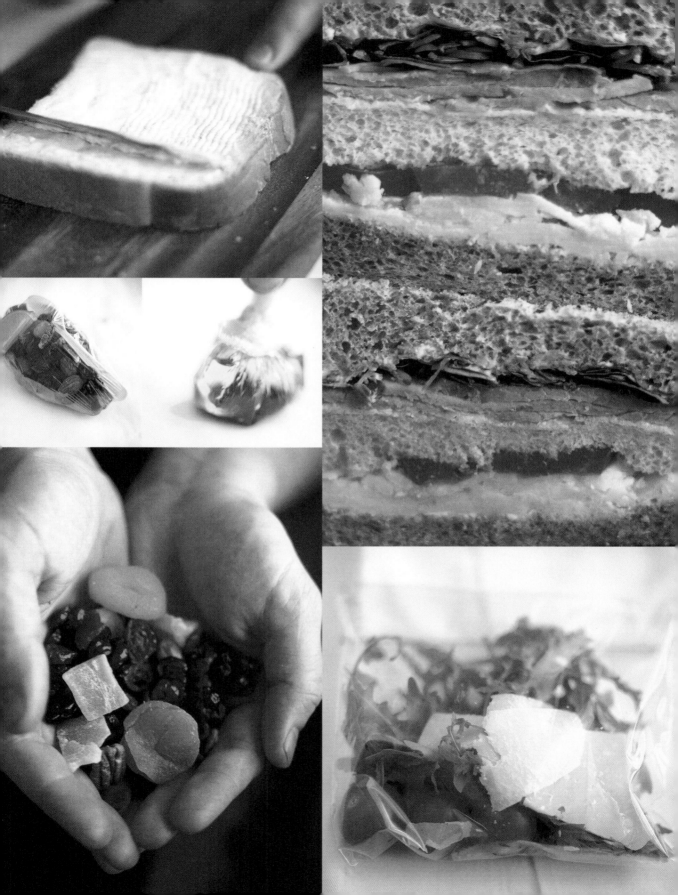

CIABATTA SANDWICH OF GRILLED VEGETABLES WITH PESTO AND MOZZARELLA

This sandwich is good for using up grilled veg like asparagus, courgettes, fennel and aubergine – wonderful just griddled on a griddle pan and dressed with some good olive oil, a squeeze of lemon, salt, freshly ground black pepper and fresh herbs. I keep any leftovers, stuff them into a chunk of ciabatta smeared with 1 tablespoon of pesto (see page 34) and add a little torn-up mozzarella. You could also add some grated Parmesan. Slices of prosciutto or grilled chicken pieces go really well too.

Wrap your sandwich up tightly in greaseproof paper and tinfoil before putting it in your lunchbox. Usually some juices come out of the mozzarella, so give the sarnie a good press down when you've finished making it to let the bread soak up the moisture and actually become more tasty because of it. When I eat this sandwich, I peel off the paper and foil from one side and then keep peeling back as I eat. This way I don't get juice all over myself!

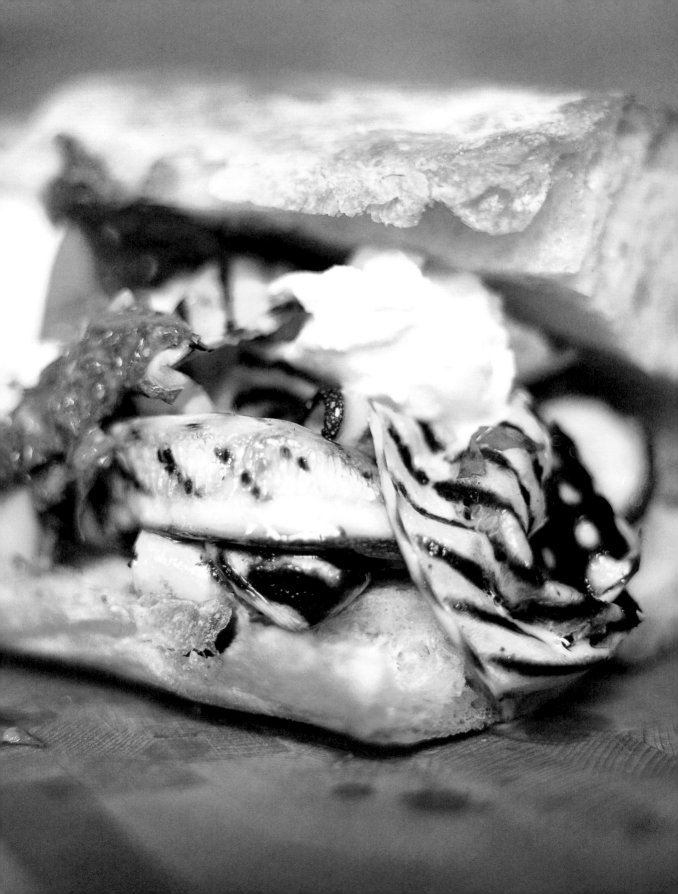

SQUASHED FIG, BASIL AND PARMA HAM SARNIE IN TOMATO BREAD

This filling is great with all kinds of bread. Here I've used it in some lovely tomato bread. Lightly butter the bread, tear open a beautifully ripe, sticky fig – generally when you think they are a little over-ripe and their skins have started to crack they are perfect – and squash it into one side of the bread. Rip over some fresh basil, then lay over some Parma ham, and even some mozzarella or shaved Parmesan if you like. This also works well if toasted or Brevilled and it's best served fresh, with an Italian beer.

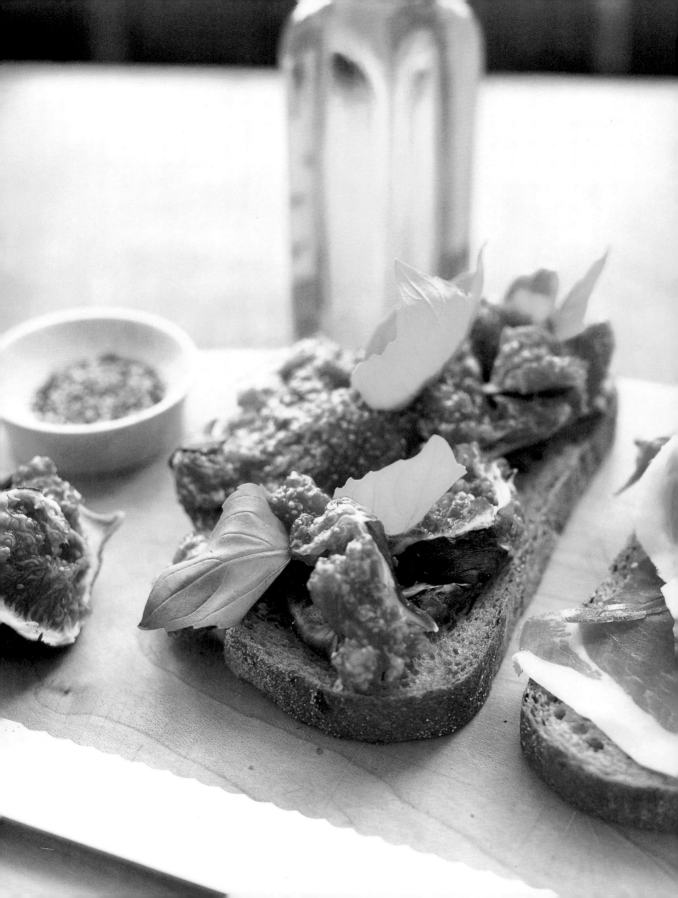

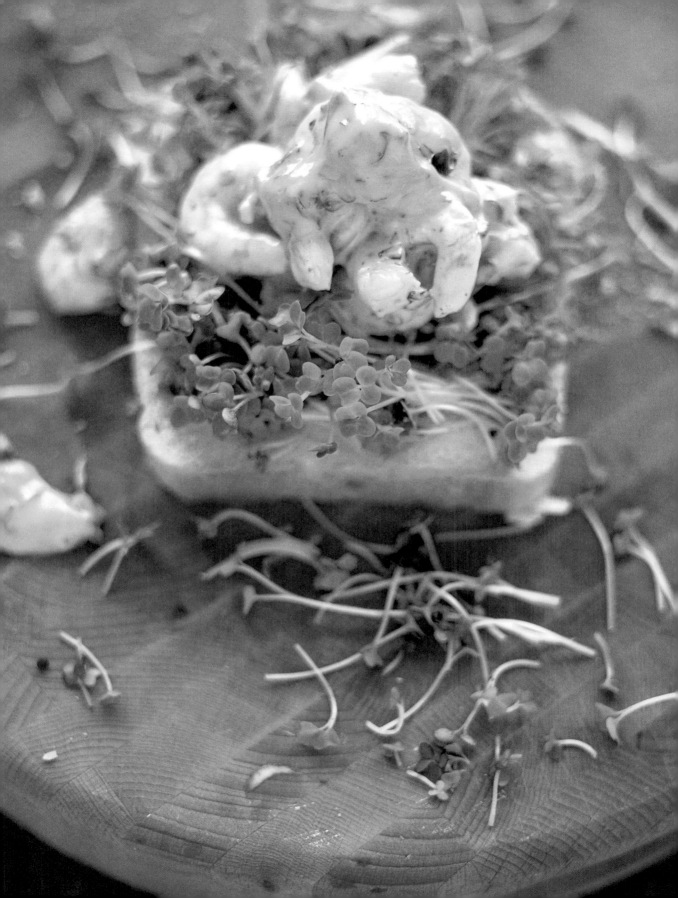

THE BEST PRAWN SANDWICH WITH BASIL MAYONNAISE AND CRESS

Obviously this is best made with great cooked prawns and a tablespoon of homemade mayonnaise or aïoli. But I know that you may think, 'I can't be bothered to make my own.' Is it worth it? Yes, definitely. However, you will still get good results using jarred mayo (although homemade is much more of a treat) if you smash up a small handful of fresh basil and mix it in. Add a squeeze of lemon juice, and salt, freshly ground black pepper and cayenne to taste. Toss the prawns in the basil mayo till they're well coated (you can chop some of them up if you like).

Get yourself two slices of decent white or brown bread and butter them well. Then take a punnet of sandwich cress, which is nice and crunchy and peppery. Put half the cress on the bread, with the prawns on top, followed by the rest of the cress. Put the other slice of bread on top of that, squeeze down, and cut diagonally into four. Great served with a few plain Kettle chips. And you know what? This sandwich is so good that it would even go down well with a glass of wine.

PS If you're going to have this sarnie in your packed lunch, wrap the prawns and mayo in some clingfilm and make the sarnie up just before eating so it doesn't go soggy. To do this, lay some clingfilm out and dollop your prawn mixture in the middle, then gather the clingfilm up and tie it in a knot. When you're ready to make up your sandwich, pop the clingfilm open and squeeze your prawns and mayo out. What will the office say about that?!

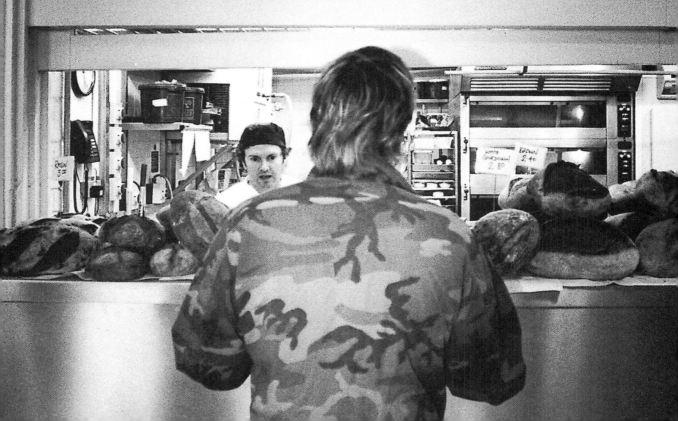

BAKERY

st john bread and wine, commercial street, london
amazing eccles cakes and bread

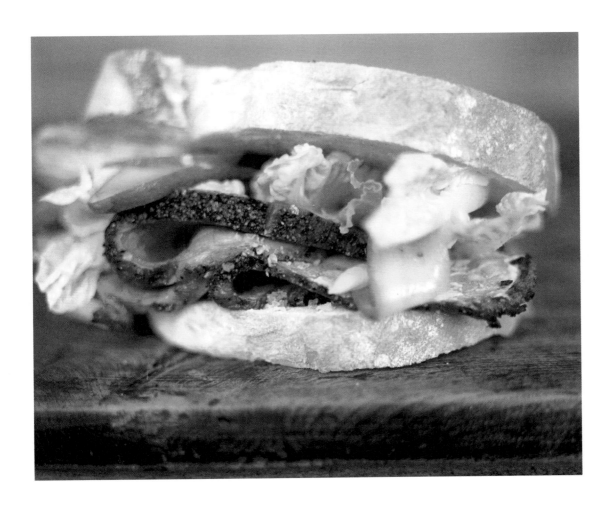

THE BEST ROAST BEEF SANDWICH WITH CRUNCHY LETTUCE, ENGLISH MUSTARD AND GHERKINS

This sarnie is best made using a really fluffy loaf with a crispy crust. I like to butter two slices well, then lay ragged slices of cold, rare roast beef – or you could use pastrami if you like – over one slice. Place a small handful of crunchy lettuce, such as Romaine or cos, over the top, then some thin slices of large sweet and sour gherkins. I like to spread the other slice really generously with strong English mustard, add plenty of sea salt and freshly ground black pepper, then place it on top of the first slice and serve with chips. (And if your eyes don't water you need more mustard!)

DOUBLE-DECKER CHEDDAR CHEESE SANDWICH WITH PICKLED ONIONS AND CRISPS

By no means am I condoning this as a 'healthy' meal, but once in a blue moon I make this sandwich for myself. The texture and crunch of the crisps takes me straight back to being seven years old when I used to make picnics for my mates Jimmy, Andy the gasman and Guy Allum. I have the good fortune of being able to visit two of the best cheese shops in England – Neal's Yard and La Fromagerie – both of which are a constant source of information and inspiration to me when it comes to new cheesemakers. Even though their advice, suggestions and knowledge are genius, I find it hard to resist my own addiction to something which would make their hair stand on end . . . a sandwich lightly buttered and layered with finely sliced pickled onions and the best Cheddar I can get my hands on, cut into 3mm slices. As I construct the layers, I put six or seven plain or salt and vinegar crisps in between the bread and, like popping those plastic air bubble things, I have rather too much pleasure in pushing down on the bread and hearing them crush. Give me a pint of Hoegaarden and two minutes and it's all over! I know for a fact that Patricia from La Fromagerie would say that the vinegar from the onions would kill the cheese and give you indigestion, but somehow I don't care! Sorry Pat! xxx

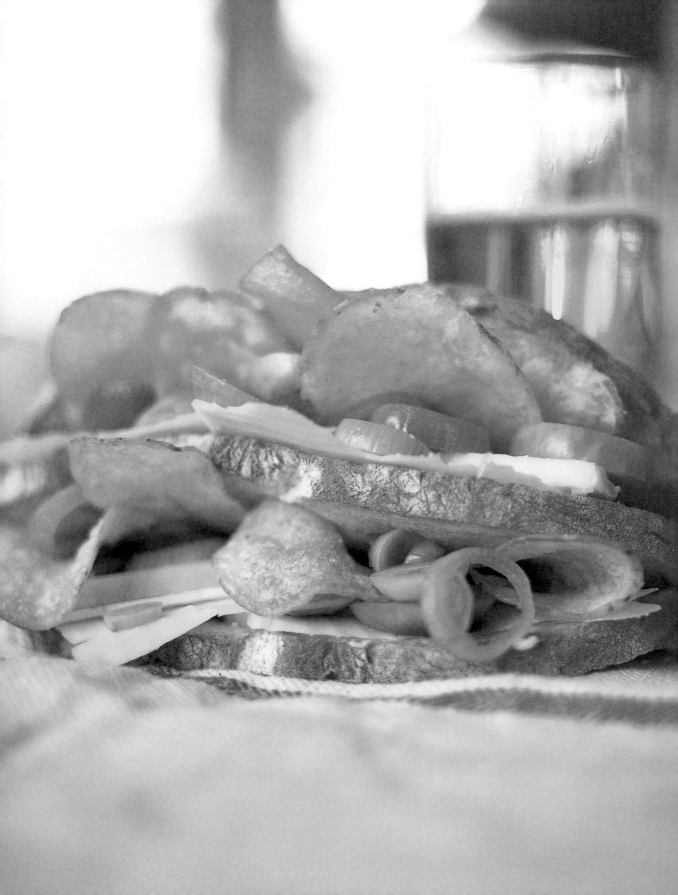

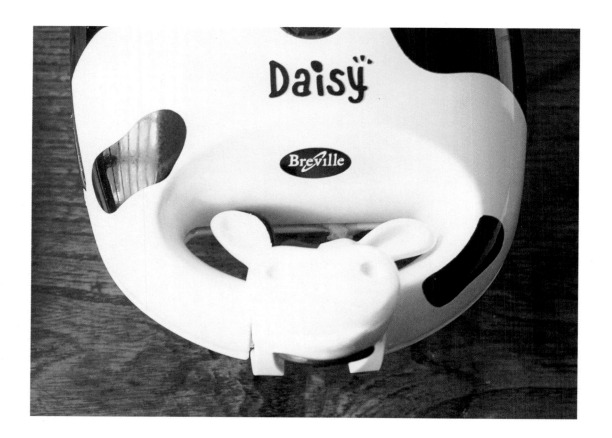

RETURN OF THE BREVILLE

The other day I was in Argos getting some bits and pieces when I saw this sandwich Breville in the shape of a cow, called Daisy. With my youngest daughter being called Daisy, and with writing this chapter, I thought I'd buy one. And it actually moos when I open it – I'm not kidding! Even though I'm not really a fan of kitchen gizmos, the actual end result from toasting a sandwich in a Breville is fantastic, as you have wonderfully crisp outsides but with a lovely oozy filling. They are also incredibly quick to use. I always get caught out, though, as toasted sandwiches can be dangerously hot inside. I always end up burning my tongue if I'm too hungry. Like pizzas, all Breville sandwiches are pretty damn good when eaten cold too.

Things to bear in mind when making a good old Breville sarnie:

- Don't go too thick on the bread.
- Square bread fits the best.
- Lightly butter the bread on both sides, or use some olive oil, so it goes really golden and chewy.
- Whatever combination you go for, a nice stringy cheese is essential and it's best to have it on the top and bottom pieces of bread with your other fillings in the middle.

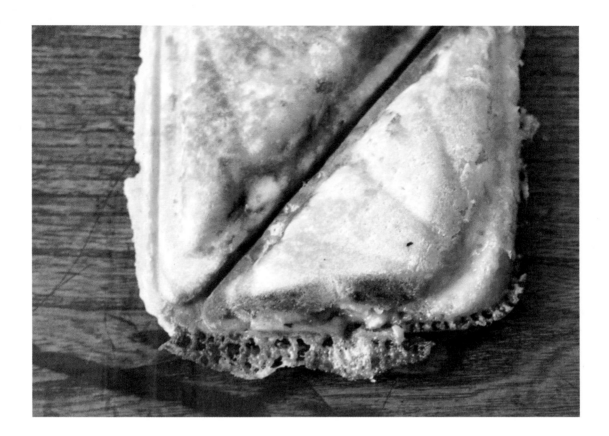

Just to get you thinking, here are some great combos:

- Leftover roast pork, taleggio cheese. Dress a few leaves of fresh sage with some olive oil and place on the outside of the bread before toasting. They will go crispy and taste fantastic.
- Tacky but nice – ham with mustard or pineapple and red Leicester cheese.
- Cooked cold sausage sliced up with Cheddar cheese and Worcestershire sauce.
- Tomato, mozzarella and pesto – a good tip is to squeeze the tomato seeds out before slicing it up as this makes the sandwich less soggy.
- One of the best indulgences is leftover meatballs with fresh basil and mozzarella really squashed down. Heat the meatballs up first before using them.
- Cheddar and Stilton with red onion chutney.
- Leftover mashed potato with sliced spring onions, Cheddar cheese and mustard.

PS Even though my Breville is very cute and funny and it draws a lot of interest from my little kiddies, I don't think it's very wise to keep it out on the worktop as it gets so hot. Always remember to unplug it, make sure your kids can't reach it while it's cooling down, then pack it away. (Maybe I've turned into the worrying parent I thought I'd never be!)

SMOKED SALMON, LEMON AND CRÈME FRAÎCHE SANDWICH

This is my favourite sarnie ever! Even from a very early age I knew it was something special. My family ran a pub restaurant in the countryside, so we always had lovely smoked salmon. When I was about ten I used to play with the gypsies who came to our village every summer to dig potatoes. One of them, Guy, used to have jam sandwiches every day, and one day I gave him one of my smoked salmon ones. I told him to squeeze on some lemon juice before he took a bite, and his face was just a picture! It was one of those defining moments that really inspired me to cook for ever. His tastebuds were obviously saying 'wake up, this is Heaven!', and he loved it.

I am a firm believer in the simple smoked salmon sarnie: all you need is thinly sliced wholemeal or rye bread and cured wild salmon – an absolute joy. To make this perfect sarnie, butter your bread, then get a tablespoon of crème fraîche and squeeze in the juice of half a lemon, with salt and plenty of freshly ground black pepper to taste. I like to place a layer of salmon on a piece of the bread, smearing over the lemony crème fraîche, then place the final layer of smoked salmon over the top with the other piece of brown bread. For an extra twang, you can sprinkle the salmon with very finely grated lemon zest. If you want to, you can cut the crusts off and quarter the sandwich, but I just like to tuck into the whole thing. The crème fraîche really finishes it off and it explodes in your mouth. Lovely.

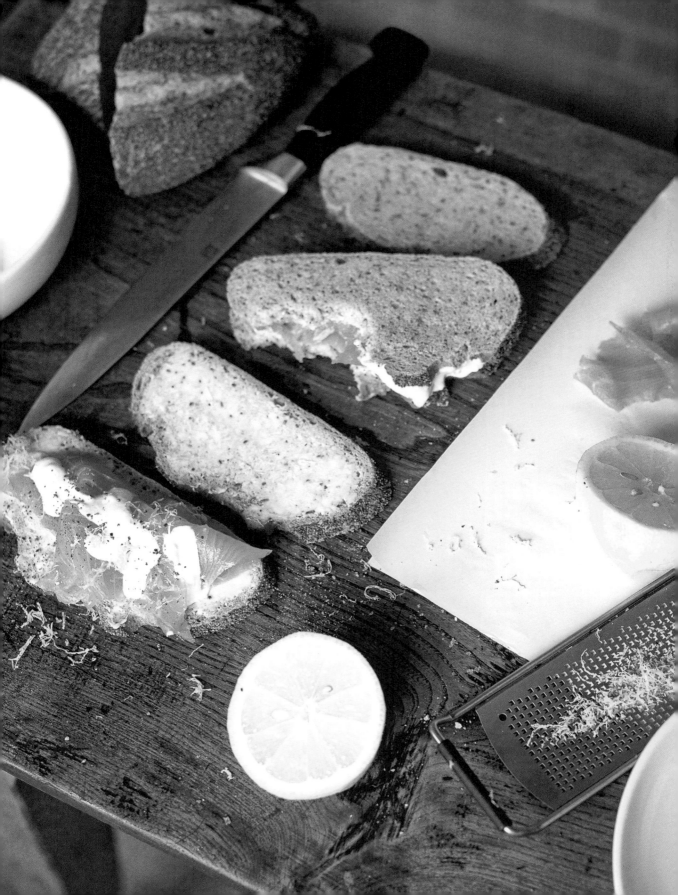

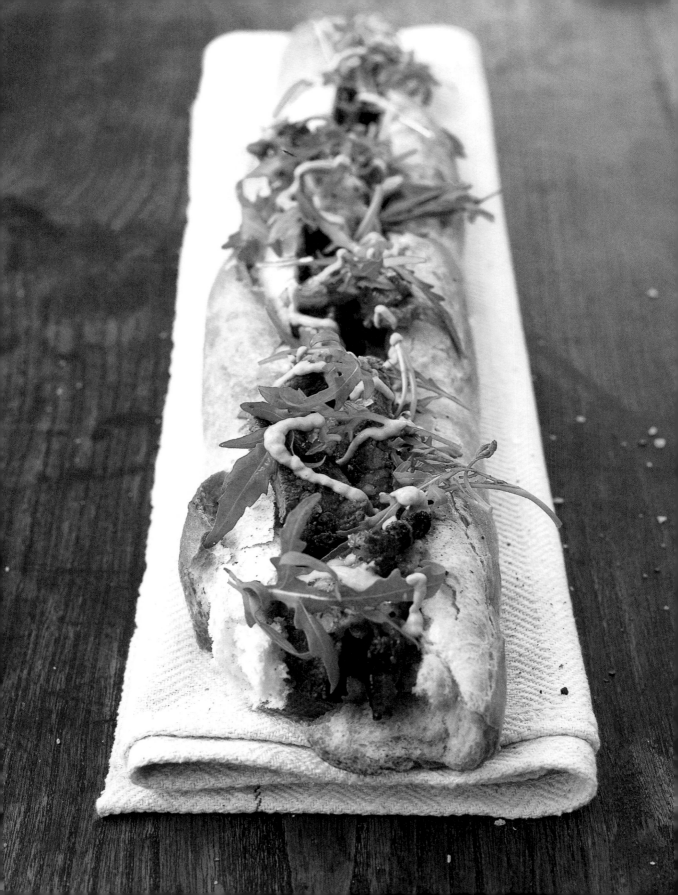

SCOTTISH PETE'S CHEESY STEAK SANDWICH

My mate Peter Begg is one of my best friends and a fantastic cook. He used to work in the circus when he was younger, where he ran a kind of roulette stall, and this kept him busy for a few months travelling round America. Apart from some of his colourful stories about the bearded lady and the tattooed man, I remember the passionate way he talked about the cheesy steak sandwiches. Apparently thousands of these sandwiches would be sold from stalls in this travelling circus.

It basically involves getting a long submarine or baguette type roll and heating it in the oven at 150°C/300°F/gas 2 for 5 minutes or so until it's just warmed through and not too crispy. Then get yourself a nice piece of rib eye, sirloin or rump steak – not too thick – and bash it out with your fist or a rolling pin to make it a little thinner and tenderize it. Season it with sea salt and freshly ground black pepper and lay it on a very hot griddle pan. Obviously you can cook it to your liking, but I do mine medium rare.

Once the steak is nicely seared on one side, turn it over and immediately grate Provolone cheese over the top so it melts from the heat of the steak and mixes with the juices. Once the other side is done, place it on a board, slice it up, and stuff it into your baguette or submarine roll with some wild rocket. Pour some of the steak juice over the bread, squeeze over some yellow American mustard and tuck in. Sliced onions also go really well with it, so if you have some they can be cooked next to the steak in the pan.

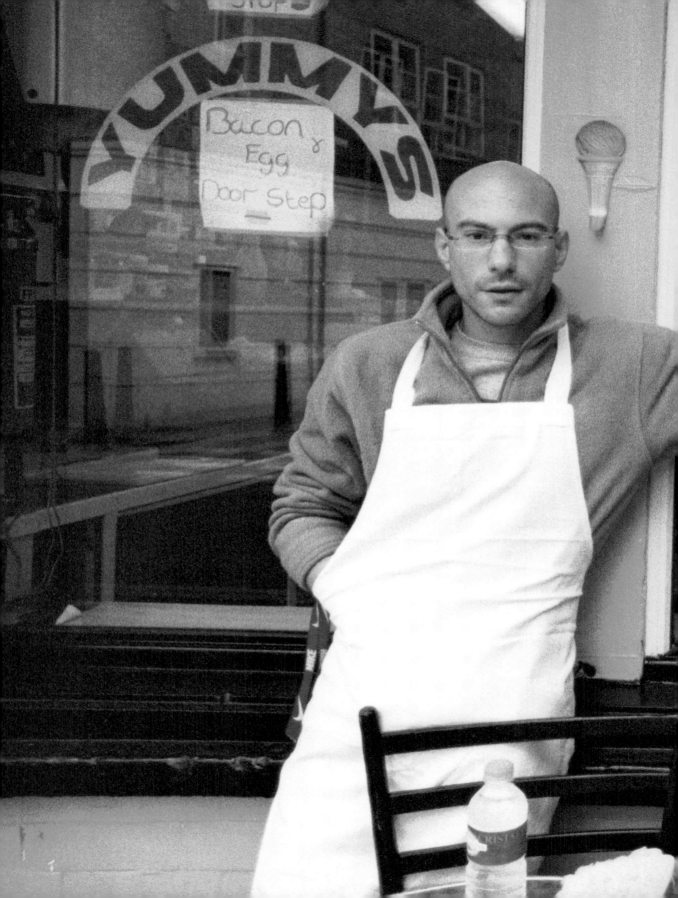

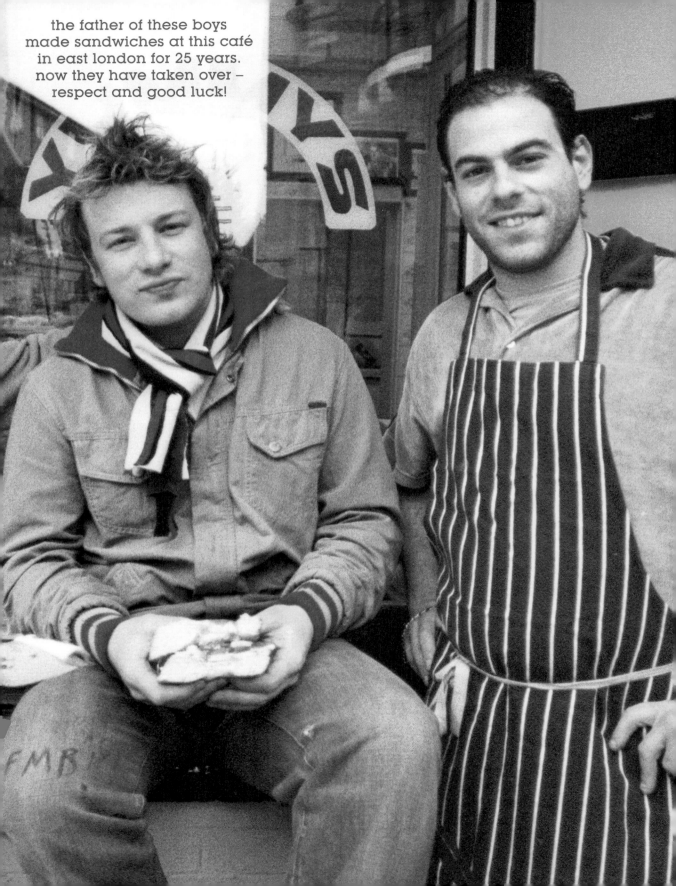

the father of these boys
made sandwiches at this café
in east london for 25 years.
now they have taken over –
respect and good luck!

BANANA AND BLUEBERRY FRENCH TOAST

This is the kind of sandwich that can be eaten for breakfast or even for dessert. Feel free to vary the fruit that you use – my missus likes strawberries and bananas, while my daughter Poppy likes banana with blackberries and blueberries.

All you do is get two slices of nice medium-cut white bread and butter them thinly on both sides. Toss your fruit combination in a little honey or sugar just to sweeten it a bit. A little mashed banana holds it all together quite nicely.

Beat a couple of eggs up in a bowl with a couple of tablespoons of caster sugar, then dip both slices of bread in the sweet egg mixture so it's egged on both sides. Let the excess drip off then smear the fruit mixture on one slice, leaving a slight space around the edges of the bread. Put the other slice on top and press down. The egg will help the fruit to stick. Fry in a little butter in a medium hot pan on both sides, pushing down so that the fruit is pressed into the bread. Once the bread is golden and slightly crisp, dust with icing sugar and serve with a dollop of crème fraîche, cream or ice cream and any remaining fruit mixture spooned over.

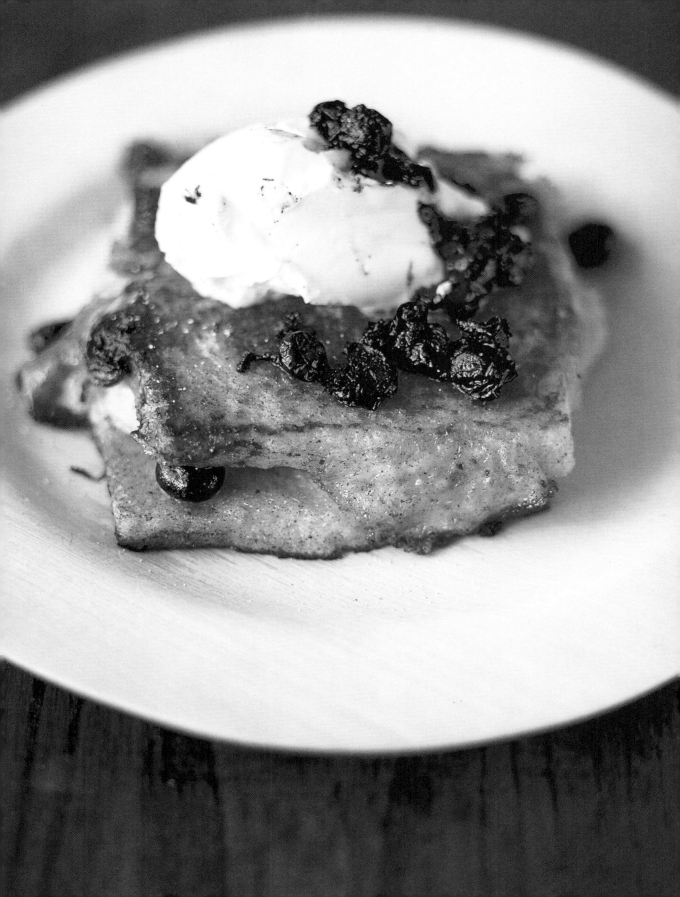

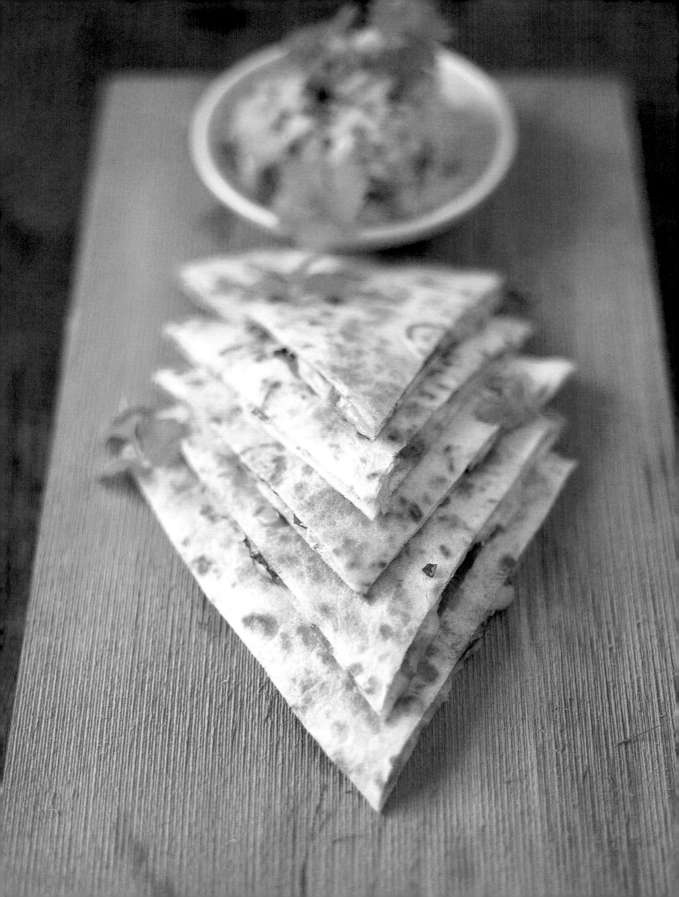

QUESADILLAS WITH GUACAMOLE

A quesadilla is basically a Mexican-style stuffed pancake, like a toasted sandwich, made with two tortillas sandwiched together with a cheese-based filling. They are warmed through and served with guacamole and sour cream. They are one of my favourite things to eat – Jools and I tend to have them every Saturday because we love them!

To make the guacamole I use 2 or 3 ripe avocados, 2 or 3 ripe deseeded tomatoes and a couple of deseeded red chillies, and I throw all this into a food processor with a handful of peeled and chopped spring onions and a good handful of fresh coriander. Once this has been chopped up nice and fine, I add a couple more chopped tomatoes, a good pinch of salt and half of another avocado, chopped, to give it a nice chunky texture. Transfer everything into a bowl and season carefully with sea salt, freshly ground black pepper and a good squeeze of lemon or lime juice. If you decide to buy ready-made guacamole, which is a bit lazy but probably very realistic, you can put it into a bowl and chirp it up a bit with a squeeze of lemon juice, a little extra salt and a bit of chilli to give it a kick.

To fill the quesadillas you will need a couple of big handfuls of grated Cheddar and/or red Leicester cheese, some finely sliced spring onions, a couple of handfuls of chopped fresh coriander, and a red pepper and some red or green chillies all deseeded and finely chopped. Mix all this up in a bowl and then sprinkle a handful between two layers of tortilla and press down. You can make up 4, 10 or even 20 quesadillas and keep them in the fridge until you need them if you want.

Some people like to fry them in oil, but this makes them greasy and is not all that healthy. You can grill them, but I like to put them in a dry non-stick frying pan on a medium heat, so that after about a minute and a half on each side you are left with a really crispy outside and an oozy, stringy filling. Serve the quesadillas cut into quarters, with the guacamole, sour cream and a beer.

PS You can also posh them up a bit using grilled chicken or seafood, leftover pork, shellfish, or a selection of grilled vegetables.

CRISPY PEKING DUCK IN PANCAKES

Peking duck is something that has always been very close to the Oliver family. Bizarrely enough, the fact that my parents ran a pub restaurant meant that we very rarely went out for dinner as a family, but when we did, my old man used to take us out to this Chinese restaurant in Sawbridgeworth where we all fell in love with Peking duck.

You probably don't think that a Peking duck pancake is a sandwich, but it is really. Everyone has their own little thing about it – Jools loves the plum sauce and can just eat it on its own; I love the crispy skin on the duck; and my Grandad, bless his cotton socks, could not use chopsticks and thought he'd never get fed, because I would spin the round table in the middle to make sure I got the prime piece of duck before anyone else. There are hundreds of ways of cooking duck in Asian cultures – steamed, roasted, pumped up with bicycle pumps to remove the meat from the skin – but we're at home and so we can't do with all this mucking about. My way is simple and it works . . .

Preheat the oven to 170°C/325°F/gas 3. Rub a nice duck with loads of salt, inside and out. Dust the bird all over with five-spice and, if you've got any, grate some fresh ginger and rub it round the cavity, leaving the ginger inside to flavour. Place the duck in a roasting tray and put it in the oven. All you need to do is check on it every so often and spoon away the excess fat that has rendered out of the duck. This will make the skin go wonderfully crispy. Generally, after a couple of hours it will be perfect – the leg meat will pull off the bone and the skin will be wonderfully crisp. You don't always need to, but I sometimes turn the heat up to 200°C/400°F/gas 6 for a short while until it's really crispy.

While this beautiful bird is cooking, you can make your plum sauce. Chuck 10 or 12 destoned plums into a pan with 5 tablespoons of sugar, a couple of pinches of five-spice, a couple of table-spoons of soy sauce, half a teaspoon of chilli powder and a splash of water. Bring to the boil, then simmer until you get a nice shiny pulp. You can remove the plum skins if you want to, but I usually leave them in. Sometimes I add a little grated orange zest, as this goes well with duck. Put the sauce to one side to cool before serving it, and taste to check the seasoning.

As for the spring onions and cucumber, that's straightforward. Finely slice them. I strongly advise buying pre-made pancakes which you can place in a steamer or microwave and slowly steam until nice and hot. The bamboo steamers are only a few quid from Chinese supermarkets, so it's worth getting hold of some and they're great to serve at the table.

Once the duck has cooled a little bit, use two forks to shred all the meat off the carcass. I remember the Chinese lady at the restaurant in Sawbridgeworth doing this. You can do the same, putting all the meat with its crispy skin on to a serving plate. Take a pancake, place some duck, a bit of spring onion, a little cucumber and a dollop of plum sauce on to it, then roll it up – lovely.

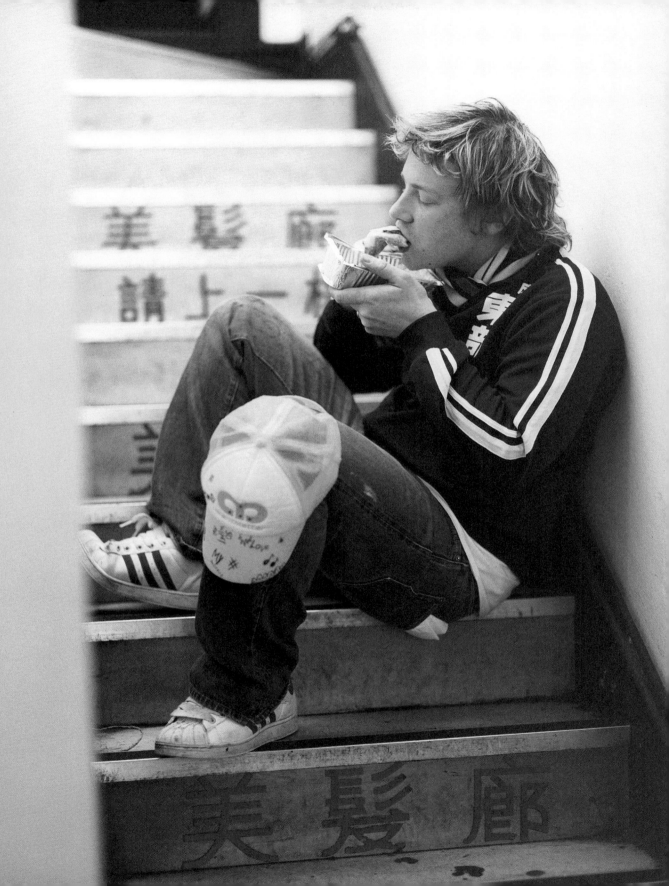

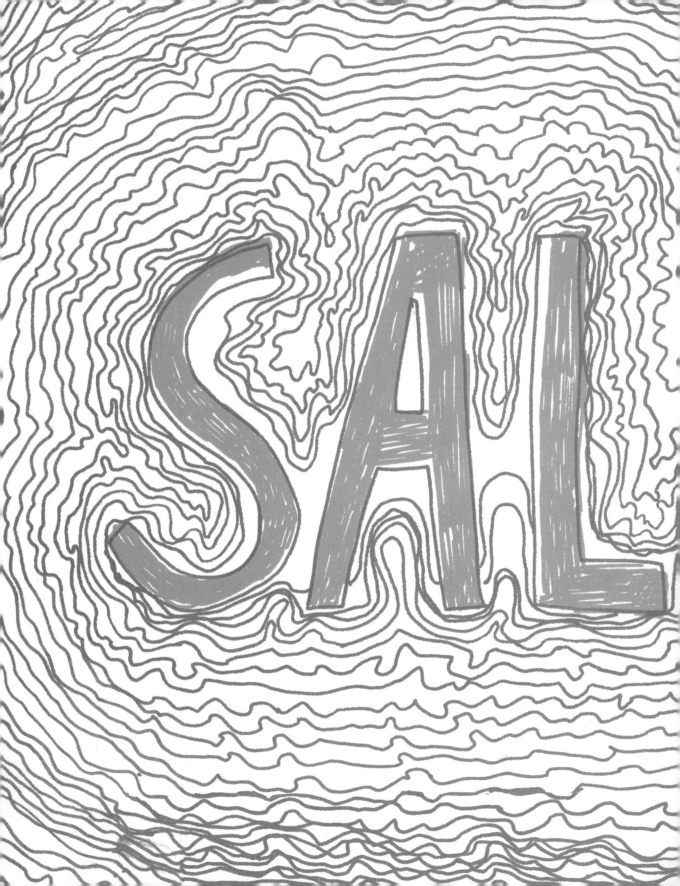

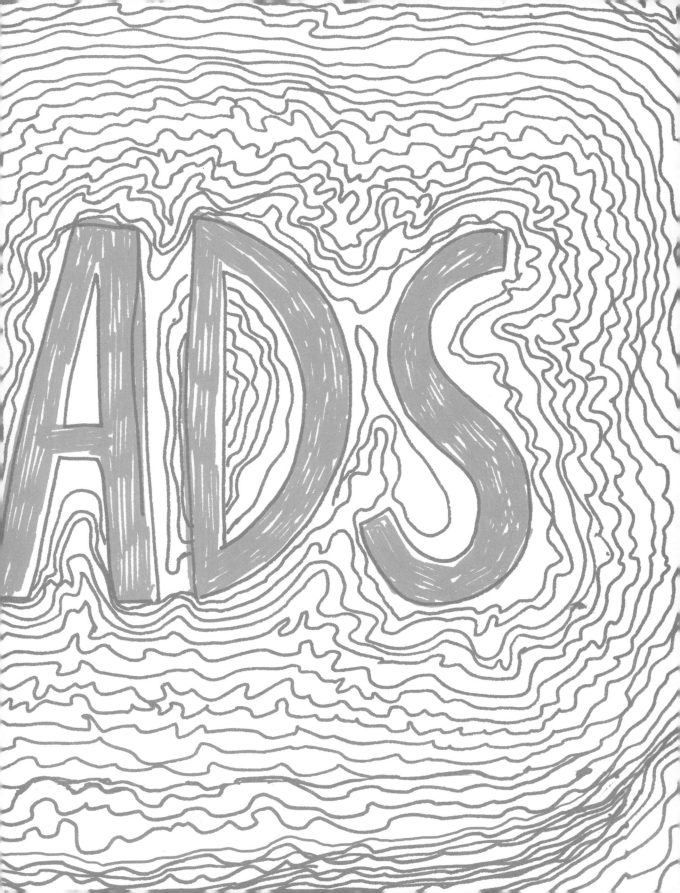

I'm really pleased with this chapter because I was thinking that I'd covered just about every great salad in my previous books, yet this year I've been completely inspired by salads from all over the world – India, Morocco, France, Japan, America – so I've included them here. Most of them are really simple and cheap to make, but they're some of the best salads I've ever had, whether served as a starter, or as a side dish with something else. From the chop salad on page 111, which is really fun and quick to make, to really unusual things like the veggies with the mint and pea yoghurt on page 129, which involves everyone getting stuck in and looks totally different to any other salad you've ever seen.

I've used fresh horseradish in a few of the recipes as I have a real thing about it. It's a fantastic root that grows absolutely everywhere. I keep a spade in the back of my car at all times, just in case I come across a nice clump of wild horseradish! If you get a chance go and dig some up. A horseradish root looks like a parsnip and once you cut into it you'll get the smell straight away – like English mustard.

To prepare horseradish, all you have to do is wash the root, peel it, and grate it finely. Add as much or as little as you like, to any recipe, but its best friends are tomatoes, fish, beef and beetroot. Mixed with crème fraîche or double cream with some lemon juice and seasoning it's great with beef, used in a Bloody Mary it's genius, and grated over preserved meats like bresaola or prosciutto it's fantastic.

PS My salads have taken a turn of genius lately because I planted some herbs that I got from www.jekkasherbfarm.com . . . I suggest that you do the same as they are superb!

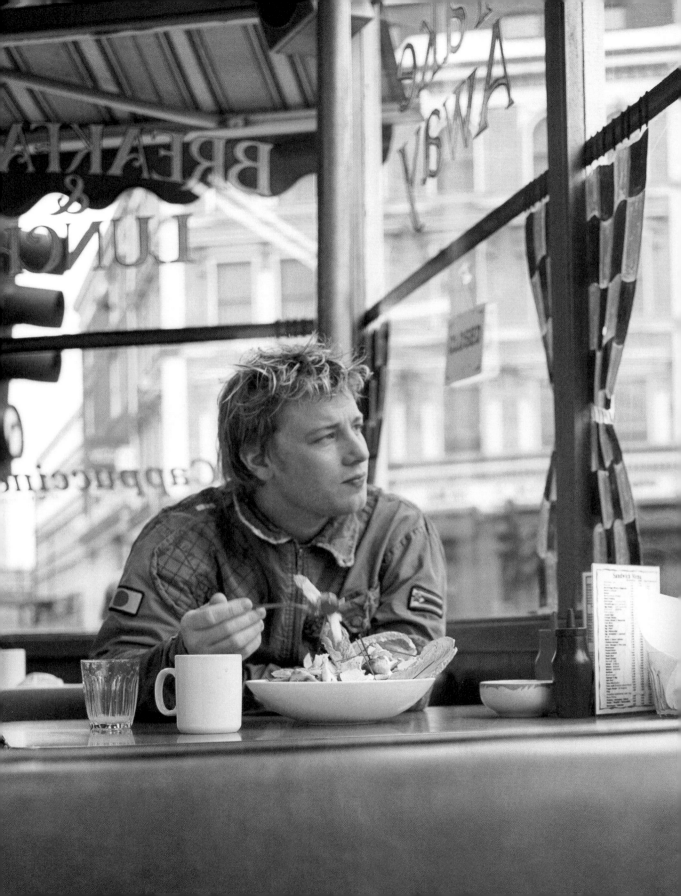

MOROCCAN STYLE BROAD BEAN SALAD WITH YOGHURT AND CRUNCHY BITS

This is a really great combination of flavours, colours and textures and, of course, is best made with fresh broad beans in season. The smaller beans can be used as they are, but the mid to large ones, with tougher skin, will have to be peeled after cooking. Just pinch the skin between your nails and the bean will pop out – simple. I think my broad bean combo is pretty much perfect, but you can try it with fresh cannellini beans as well if you fancy a change.

SERVES 4

4 large handfuls of podded
  broad beans
2 lemons
extra virgin olive oil
sea salt and freshly ground
  black pepper
a handful of fresh mint,
  leaves picked

1 small red onion, peeled and
  finely chopped
1 teaspoon cumin seeds, bashed
a pinch of dried chilli
2 handfuls of stale breadcrumbs
285ml/½ pint creamy live yoghurt or
  soured cream

First of all pod your beans. When I'm doing mine I round up friends and family to get the job done quicker. I also put the larger ones in one bowl and the smaller ones in another – they'll need different cooking times. Blanch the beans in unsalted boiling water for a couple of minutes, giving the large ones a bit longer (don't add salt, as this will toughen the skins). Drain them and lay them flat on a tray to cool down slightly. This salad always works best when the beans are eaten slightly warm. If you're making it in advance, though, you could always give them a quick flash in the microwave just before serving. Remove the skins from the larger beans if necessary. Place in a bowl and dress with the juice of 1 lemon and three times as much extra virgin olive oil. Season with salt and freshly ground black pepper to taste. Add a little more lemon juice if needed – feel free to adjust to your taste. At this stage I like to finely slice half the mint and add it to the beans while they sit and marinate for a little while.

In a shallow pan, on a medium heat, fry the chopped onion, cumin seeds and chilli in a little olive oil. Stir and cook until softened. As the onions start to colour, add your breadcrumbs and mix these really well into the onions. Continue to cook until the crumbs are crispy and golden, then season them to taste and put to one side. To serve, divide the yoghurt or sour cream between four plates or bowls. Give the broad beans a final toss, add the rest of the mint leaves, and divide between the plates on top of the yoghurt. Finally, sprinkle over the warm spiced crunchy bits.

Sometimes I like to zest a bit of lemon over the top to give a little edge. Fantastic served with grilled chicken or as a tapas or antipasti style thing. Also great with flatbreads like pitta.

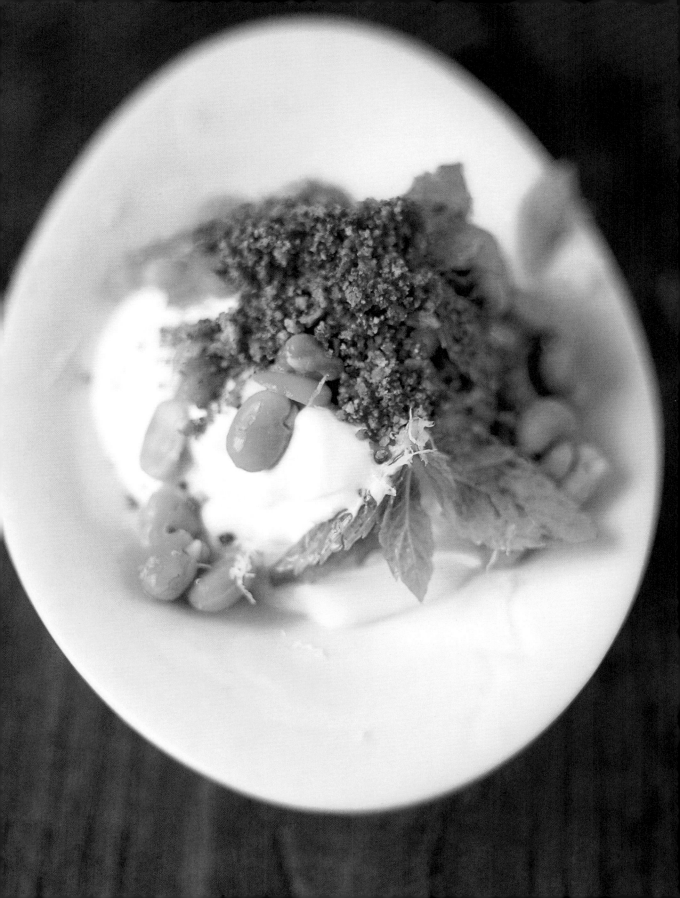

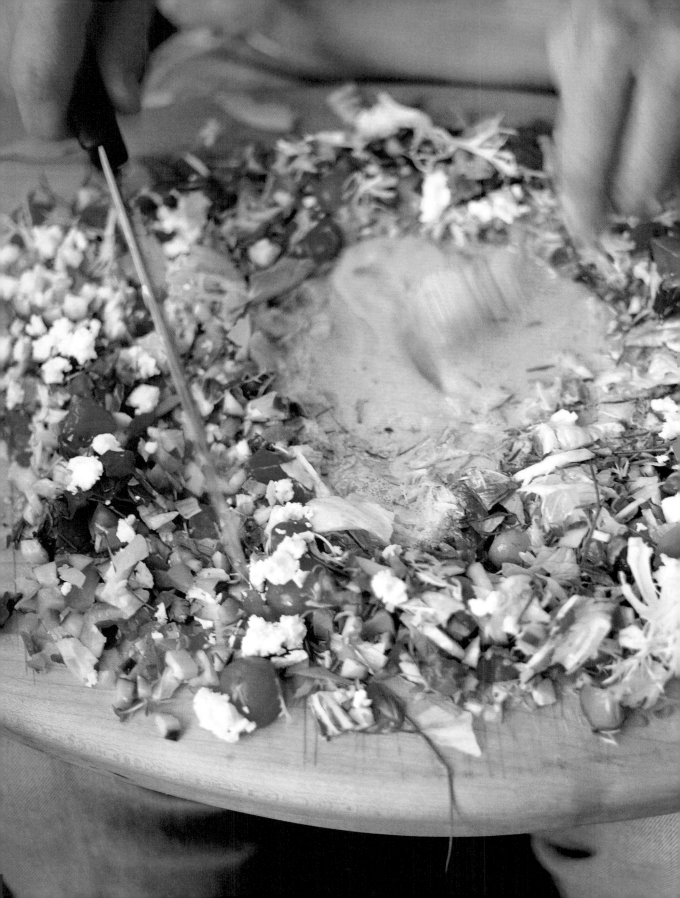

MY FAVOURITE AMERICAN CHOP SALAD

I've had this salad loads of times in the States – the best place to try it. Especially in really cool, quaint 1930s style diners, or what are called 'chop houses'. You can order not only a salad, but a 'chop steak' as well. This is kind of like a burger but the meat is cut a lot coarser and is then pressed back into a steak shape, as opposed to a burger. It's served with fries and salad.

Moving on to the chop salad, I've asked many people in diners why it's called this and the only conclusion we could come to is that they chop all the ingredients up, which is fair enough! I've had fantastic ones and I've had really bad ones. The only defining point between the two is the combination of ingredients and the fact that the good ones are not wilted and horrible, but nice and fresh. The salad should be eaten immediately after it has been chopped and dressed. It shows that you can make everyday ingredients seem a bit special, and the picture even makes it look a bit posh! You'll notice that I dress it at the same time as making it, which I think is the best way of doing it.

Just think about it: instead of having a dinner party where you bring out six plates of salad, one for each place mat – a bit boring – you can add a bit of theatre by bringing out a chopping board with a mezzaluna (rounded chopping knife), along with eight or nine individual whole ingredients. Start chopping these up and everyone will be wondering what's going on. And then you serve it and it will be fantastic. As well as being cool, it takes away the stress of trying to plate it up all prettily.

SERVES 6

1 red pepper, halved
1 fresh red chilli, halved
1 red onion, peeled
5 or 6 ripe tomatoes
½ a cucumber
200g/7oz feta cheese
2 Romaine or cos lettuces, or
   4 little gem lettuces

1 radicchio
2 or 3 handfuls of mixed fresh herbs
   (parsley, basil, chives, mint)
2 teaspoons English mustard
3 tablespoons white wine vinegar
8 tablespoons extra virgin olive oil
sea salt and freshly ground
   black pepper

Remove the seeds from the pepper and chilli. Wash all your other salad ingredients and drain, then get a large chopping board and either a mezzaluna (a double-handed rounded knife) or a chef's knife, and get ready to chop! It is important to chop the onion and chilli finely and to dice the tomatoes, pepper, cucumber and feta into 1cm/½ inch pieces, as this will help to bind with the dressing when you come to mix it in. With the lettuce, radicchio and herbs, just make sure you chop them all into 1cm/½ inch strips.

Make a well in the centre of the ingredients on your board. Add the mustard and stir it in with a teaspoon while you add the vinegar and oil. Keep tasting to balance the flavours, and remember some vinegars can be harsher than others – just add a little more or less to your taste. Season well, taste, then add a tiny bit more seasoning before bringing all the salad into the centre of the board. Mix it up and serve. Great with steak, fish or burgers.

CRUNCHY KERALAN SALAD

This is a fantastic and really unusual salad that was inspired by a friend of mine called Das who runs the most terrific Indian restaurants in London, called Rasa. Although I have called it 'Keralan', it isn't really a true salad from there as you'd never find cress in Kerala! In Rasa, Das uses a lot of fresh coconut – which really is one of the most incredible flavours for making dishes like curries, or mixed into rice, breads, desserts and salads. You can now buy coconuts from most supermarkets, but if you can't find one, feel free to make this salad without it – it will still be pretty good but it won't have that special edge to it. Only make this when the mangoes are silky smooth and not at all stringy. You should be able to cut through them like butter.

SERVES 4

1 coconut
2 red peppers
4 punnets of cress
1 bunch of spring onions
2 ripe mangoes, peeled

FOR THE DRESSING
a thumb-sized piece of fresh ginger, peeled
zest and juice of 3–4 limes
7–8 tablespoons extra virgin olive oil
sea salt and freshly ground black pepper

First of all you need to crack open the shell of the coconut. I normally do this by placing it on a tea towel on a hard surface and then giving it a wallop with a rolling-pin or a hammer. Once you've cracked it open you can pull it apart (being careful not to spill the milk everywhere!), discarding the hard outer shell. The dark skin on the outside of the coconut's flesh doesn't bother me, especially if I'm grating it. But if you want to remove it, a speed peeler works quite well.

Once you've got into your coconut, cut the peppers into quarters, remove the stalks and seeds, then finely slice. Trim your cress directly from its punnet (the easiest way to do this is to take the cress out of the punnet, wash the leafy end and stalks under a tap, then slice the stalk end off and discard it). Trim your spring onions and finely slice them. Cut the mango flesh off the stones and finely slice it (there is a knack to doing this properly – if you look at the shape of the mango, the flat stone always lies the same way, parallel with the flattest sides, so you should be able to slice the flesh off with not too much wastage). Get your pieces of coconut and grate them finely. Put all these ingredients into a large salad bowl.

Lime and ginger work together really well in the dressing. Finely grate the ginger and lime zest into a small bowl, then add the lime juice and olive oil. Season to taste, and add more oil as necessary to balance the flavours of your dressing. Limes can be different strengths depending on their juiciness and size.

Dress the salad just before serving, saving any extra dressing for another day, and eat straight away. Great just as it is, or with some grilled prawns or satay chicken. Also lovely as a snack inside a wrap or flatbread. So even though the coconut may be a pain to prepare it's well worth it . . .

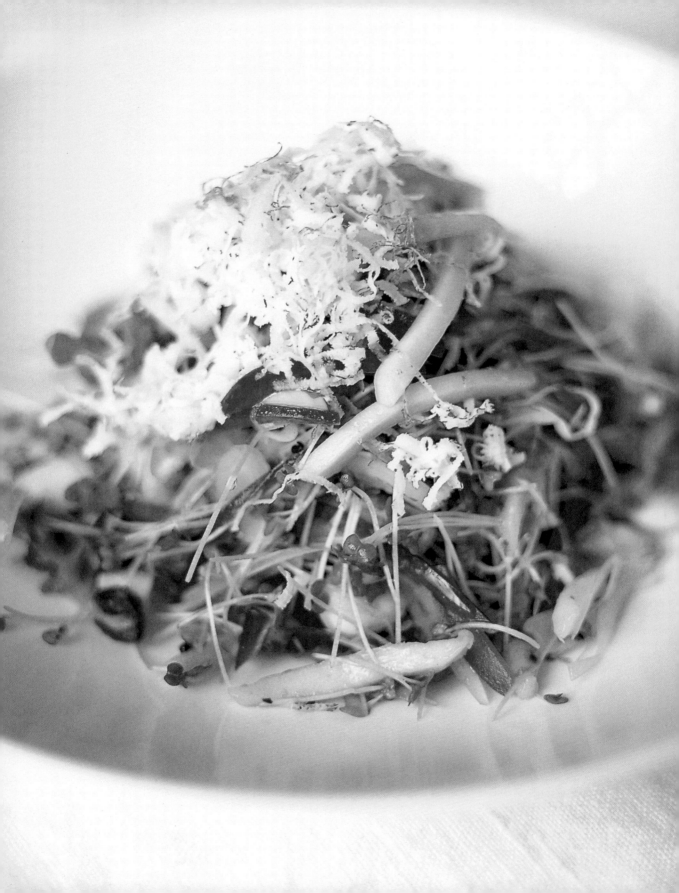

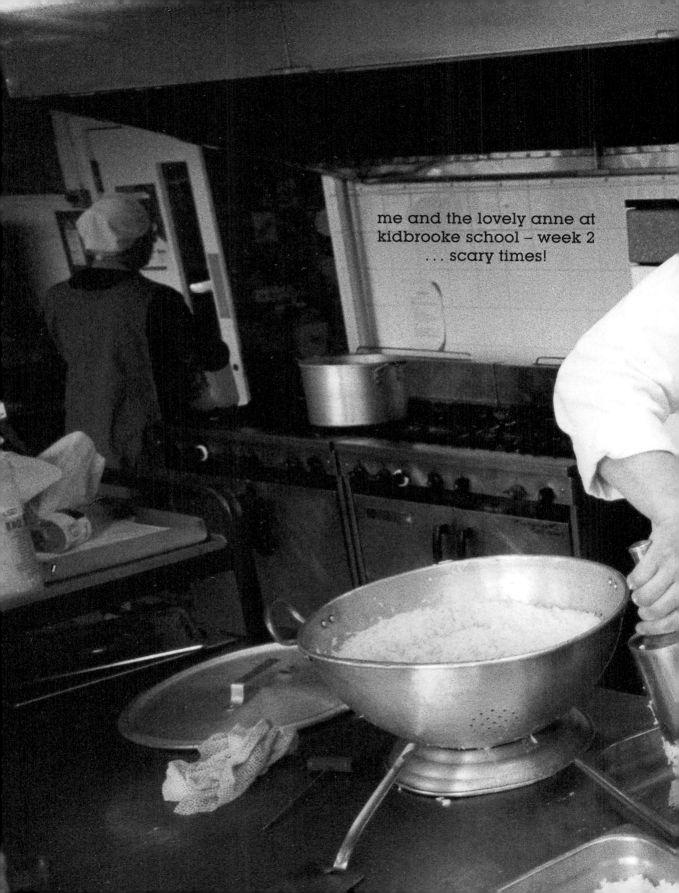

me and the lovely anne at
kidbrooke school – week 2
. . . scary times!

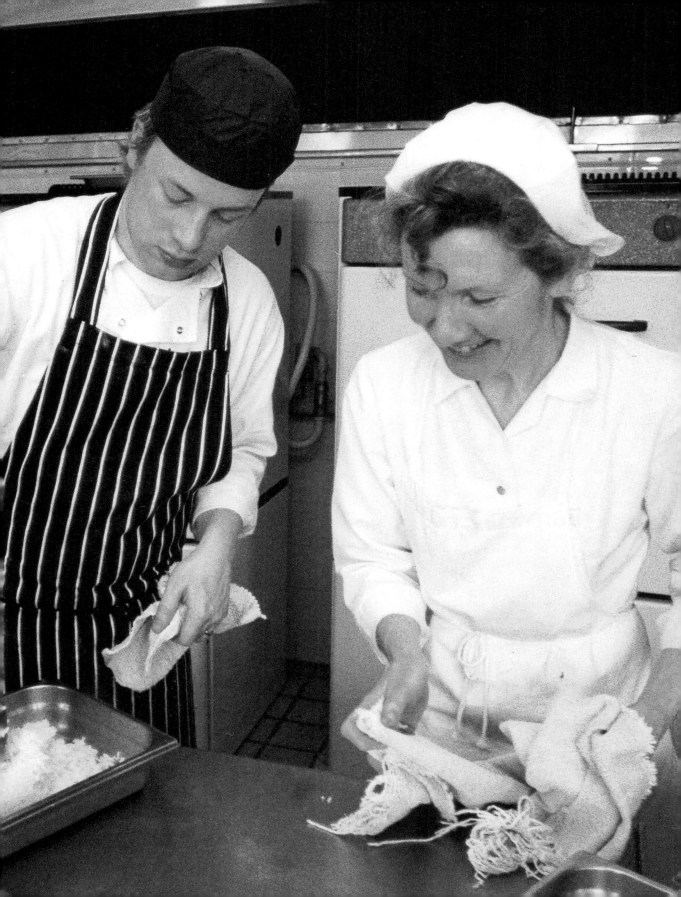

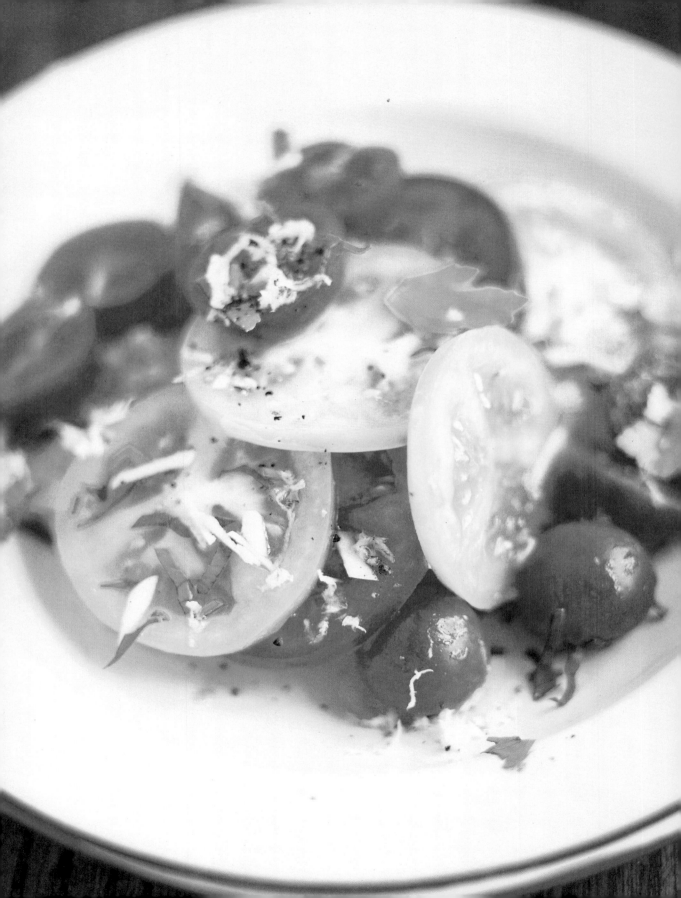

SUMMER TOMATO AND HORSERADISH SALAD

For this salad it's great to try and get a whole mixture of different tomatoes, at room temperature, nice and ripe. Let them sunbathe on the window ledge if need be! Try and get hold of fresh horse-radish – give your greengrocer a challenge to get some in.

SERVES 6
4 large handfuls of mixed tomatoes
sea salt and freshly ground black pepper
extra virgin olive oil
good red wine vinegar
½ a clove of garlic, grated
2 teaspoons fresh horseradish, grated, or jarred hot horseradish
a small handful of fresh flat-leaf parsley, finely sliced

Cut the bigger tomatoes into slices about 1cm/½ inch thick. You can halve the cherry tomatoes or leave them whole. Then sprinkle them all with a good dusting of sea salt. Put them in a colander and leave them for 30 minutes. What's going to happen here is that the salt will draw the excess moisture out of the tomatoes, intensifying their flavour. Don't worry about the salad being too salty, as a lot of the salt drips away.

Place the tomatoes in a large bowl and dress with enough extra virgin olive oil to loosen (approximately 6 tablespoons), and 1–2 tablespoons of vinegar, but do add these to your own taste. Toss around and check for seasoning – you may or may not need salt but will certainly need pepper. Add the garlic. Now start to add the horseradish. Stir in a couple of teaspoons to begin with, toss around and taste. If you like it a bit hotter, add a bit more horseradish. All I do now is get some finely sliced flat-leaf parsley (stalks and leaves) and mix this into the tomatoes. Toss everything together and serve as a wonderful salad, making sure you mop up all the juices with some nice squashy bread.

This salad is fantastic with roast beef, goat's cheese or jacket potatoes. And to be honest, even if you put these tomatoes in a roasting tray and roasted them with some sausages scattered around them it would be nice.

SMOKED TROUT, HORSERADISH AND NEW POTATO SALAD

I'm pretty sure that smoked fish and new potatoes are a match made in heaven, but there are a few extras that can turn it into something even more memorable and comforting. A squeeze of lemon is one example, but horseradish is even better! Of course you can use the jarred stuff, which you can get creamed or preserved. But remember that you'll have probably driven past a hundred jars of the stuff growing wild, on the way to the market!

SERVES 4
700g/1½lb new potatoes, scrubbed
4 heaped tablespoons crème fraîche or soured cream
zest of 2 lemons and juice of 1
4 tablespoons good extra virgin olive oil
sea salt and freshly ground black pepper
4 heaped teaspoons horseradish, preferably fresh
a handful of fresh parsley
a small handful of fresh chives
a small bunch of spring onions, washed and finely sliced
400g/14oz hot-smoked trout or eel

First of all cook the potatoes in salted boiling water until they are tender, then drain them. While they are still warm, and when they're cool enough to handle, either cut them in half or squash them into a large salad bowl. Add your crème fraîche, the zest and juice of 1 lemon and your olive oil. Toss around, then season to taste. Add or grate in your horseradish, tasting as you go, then chop up the parsley and chives and throw these into the bowl. Add the spring onions, tear in your smoked trout or eel, and mix everything together. Now it's very important to balance your salad with more seasoning and maybe an extra squeeze of lemon. You may even want to give it more of a kick by adding some more horseradish. Personally, I love to add a lot of horseradish and make it really hot. Great served as a starter, salad or even dinner if you love it as much as I do.

PS It's nice to try lightly grilling your fish if you prefer to eat it warm.

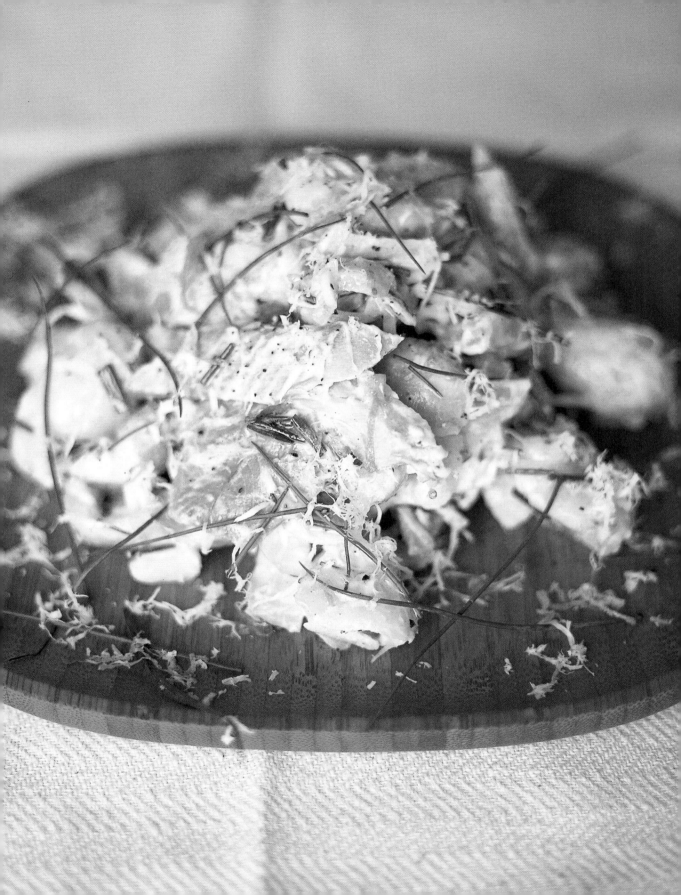

RAW BEETROOT SALAD

The other day I had a nice little roast in the oven – comfort food for a great Sunday afternoon. I had a bunch of raw beetroot to use up, so I thought it would be good to have something nice and zingy to munch on while I was waiting for the chicken to cook – like some tapas or antipasti to get my tastebuds going. You can get some great beetroots these days – fantastic colours.

I took the leaves off the beetroots and threw them away, as I didn't need them for this salad (although it's worth remembering that they're edible and that they taste nicer than Swiss chard or spinach!). I washed the beetroots and then, using a speed peeler, I peeled them all down into really thin slices and flavoured them with salt, pepper, chopped flat-leaf parsley and a little grated fresh horseradish to give a nice bit of heat. Then I left them for 5–10 minutes so that the acid from the horseradish would soften the beetroot. The horseradish is optional, but it gives a good twang.

This salad is lovely on a bit of toast, with maybe a splash of vodka or a little block of crumbled feta cheese. Really nice to pick at before you have dinner.

beautiful beetroots
picked fresh from
prince charles'
back garden
at highgrove.
can't be bad!

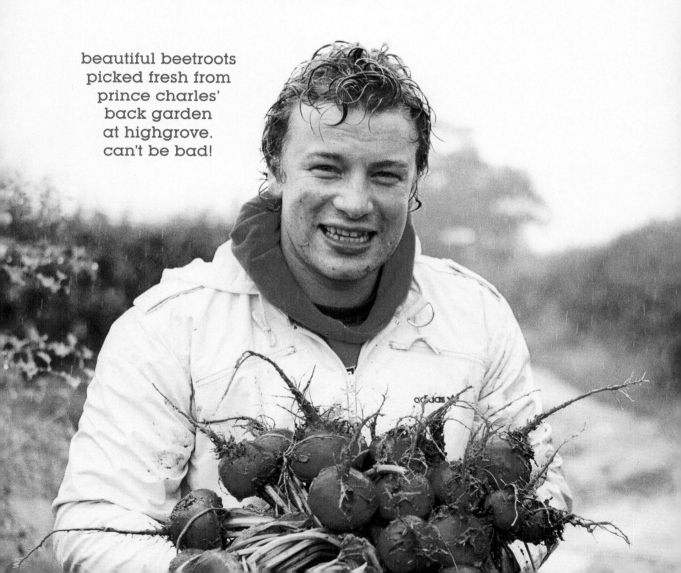

SUMMER CHICKPEA SALAD

Chickpeas are pretty under-used in this country, to be honest. In places like Morocco, Italy and Spain they are prized like our Jersey new potato. Still, we have a lot more choice now than we used to have. If you go to a Spanish deli or specialist counter, you will generally be able to find jars of cooked chickpeas in water and these are the ones you want to make this salad really good. They should look a little plumper than tinned chickpeas but, of course, both tinned ones or dried ones can be used successfully.

This salad is a great one for making up as you go along; you can use different spices, sun-dried tomatoes and spicy chorizo sausages, for instance.

SERVES 4
1 small red onion, peeled
1–2 fresh red chillies, deseeded
2 handfuls of ripe red or yellow tomatoes
2 lemons
extra virgin olive oil
sea salt and freshly ground black pepper
1 x 410g jar or tin of chickpeas, drained, or around 4 large
    handfuls of soaked and cooked chickpeas
a handful of fresh mint, chopped
a handful of fresh green or purple basil, finely ripped
200g/7oz feta cheese

First of all, finely slice your red onion. Once that's done, finely slice your chillies then roughly chop your tomatoes, mixing them in with the onion and chillies. Scrape all of this, and the juice, into a bowl and dress with the juice of 1½ lemons and about 3 times as much good extra virgin olive oil. Season to taste. Heat the chickpeas in a pan, then add 90 per cent of them to the bowl. Mush up the remaining chickpeas and add these as well – they will give a nice creamy consistency. Allow to marinate for a little while and serve at room temperature.

Just as you're ready to serve, give the salad a final dress with the fresh mint and basil. Taste one last time for seasoning – you may want to add the juice from your remaining lemon half at this point. Place on a nice serving dish and crumble over the feta cheese.

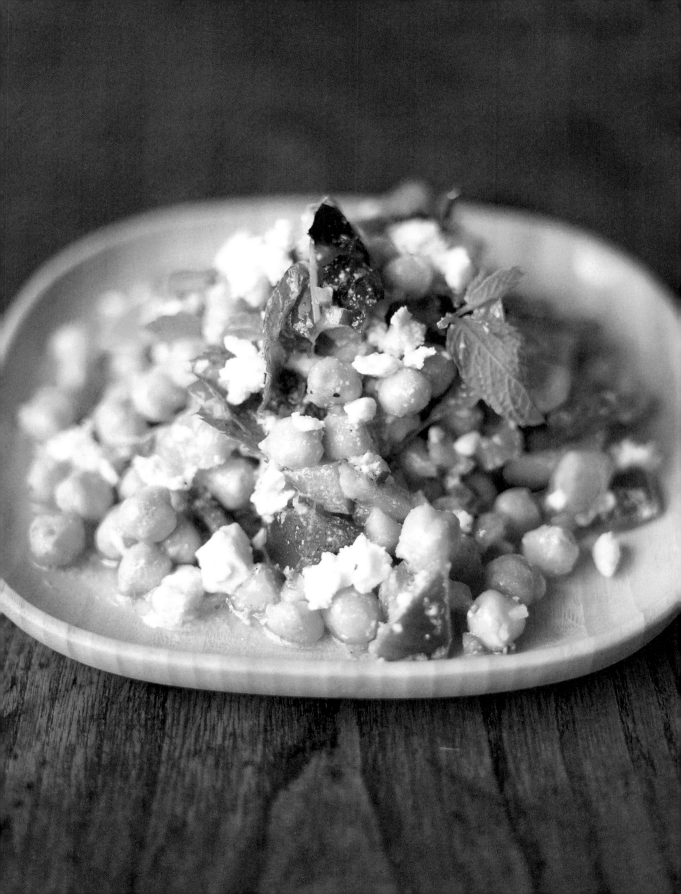

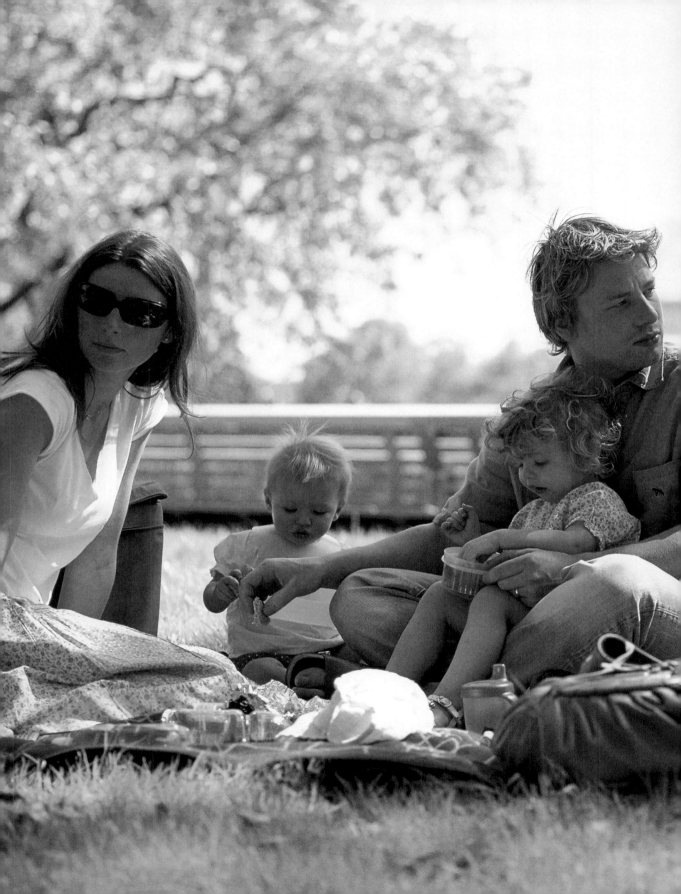

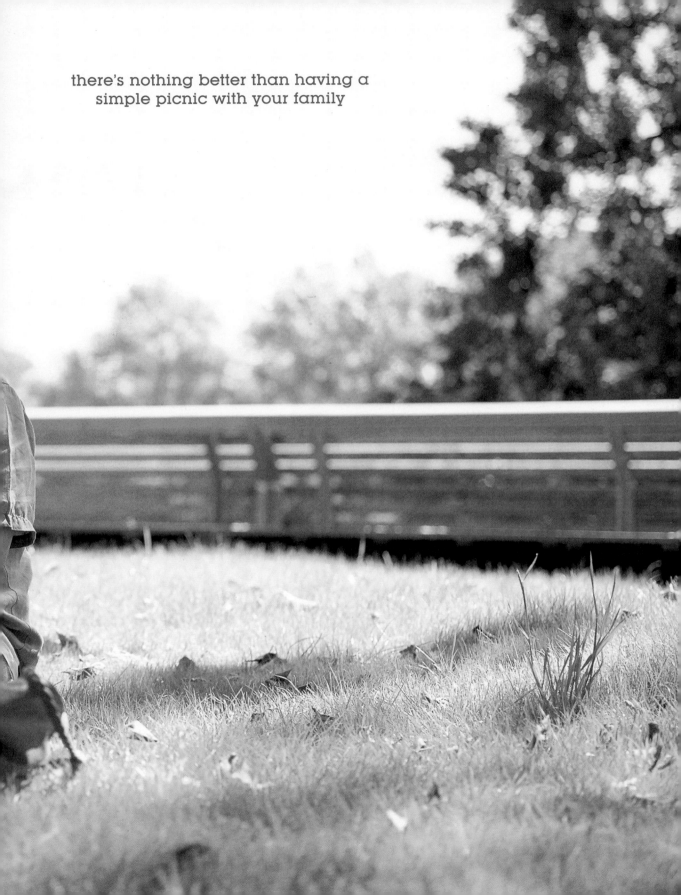

there's nothing better than having a
simple picnic with your family

THAI WATERMELON SALAD

Watermelons are a lovely summery fruit, but not all that useful as ingredients. However, you can sorbet them or fill them up with vodka, as I showed in my first book, *The Naked Chef*. And, bearing in mind that they are crunchy, watery and slightly sweet, they are fantastic in a salad with fish or even deep-fried squid. Or you could turn them into a snack, with some salt and crumbled feta cheese on top, as I have done here.

SERVES 4

¼ of a watermelon
2 handfuls of fresh coriander, leaves picked
2 handfuls of rocket
2 handfuls of fresh mint, leaves picked
1 small bunch of radishes, finely sliced
a handful of sunflower seeds or peanuts
115g/4oz feta cheese

FOR THE DRESSING

a thumb-sized piece of fresh ginger, peeled and grated
1 red, 1 yellow and 1 green chilli, deseeded and finely sliced
2 tablespoons soy sauce
6 tablespoons olive oil
1 teaspoon sesame oil
juice of 3–4 limes
sea salt and freshly ground black pepper

Remove the skin from the watermelon and cut the flesh into small cubes, removing as many seeds as you can be bothered to (but don't worry too much, as you can eat them and you'll hardly notice them in the salad).

When you pick the coriander leaves remove the stringier part of the stalks but keep the finer ones, as they are nice to eat. Place in a bowl with the rocket, mint, watermelon and radishes. Put the ginger, chilli, soy sauce, olive oil and sesame oil into a smaller bowl and add just enough lime juice to cut through the oil – the number of limes you use will depend on how juicy they are. Season to taste and make sure the dressing is well-balanced.

Place your sunflower seeds or peanuts in the oven or in a pan and warm through, then roughly pound them up in a pestle and mortar or in a metal bowl using the end of a rolling-pin. Dress the salad really quickly. (You can use more dressing if you wish, but any left over is great to keep in the fridge to use the next day.) Divide between the plates, sprinkle over the hot peanuts or sunflower seeds and crumble the feta cheese over the top.

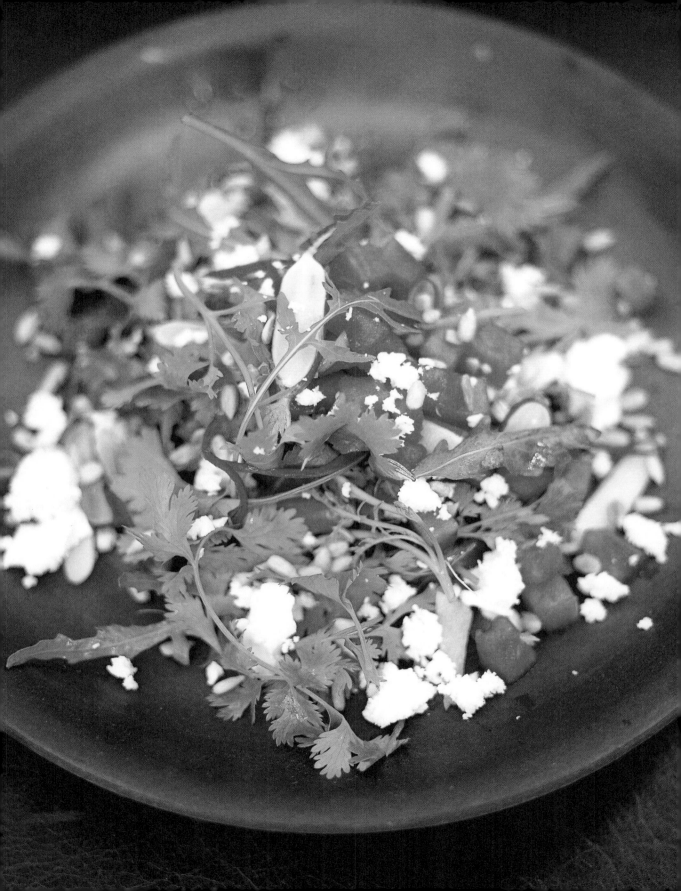

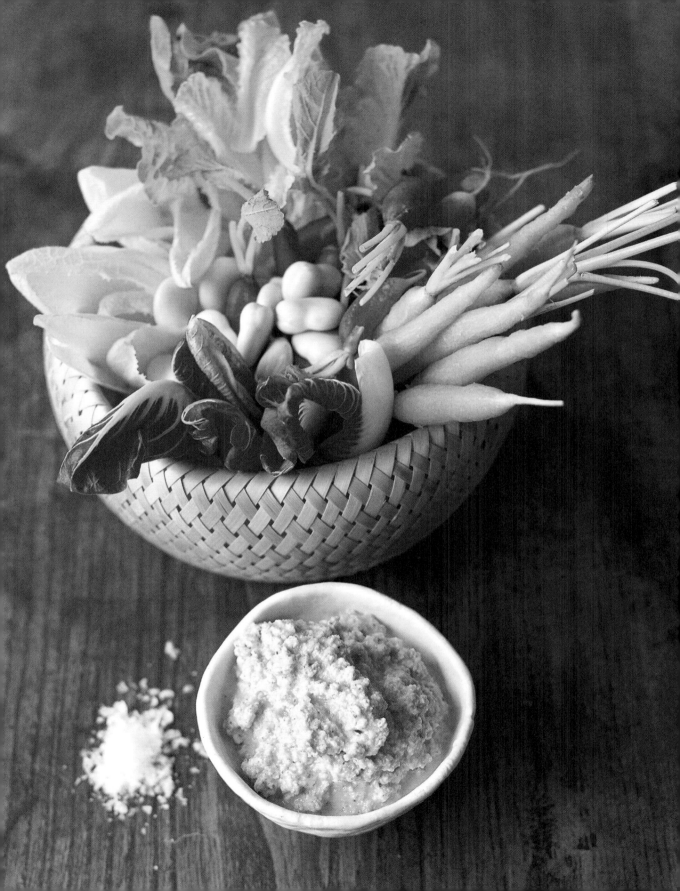

COOL CRUDITÉ VEGGIES WITH A MINTED PEA AND YOGHURT DIP

This dish is only as good as the vegetables you buy, so use that as your starting point and you'll be on to an absolute winner! Here are some tips on buying and preparing a selection of veg . . .

- In most supermarkets these days you can get fresh baby carrots with their green tops. Leave about an inch of the tops on and just give the carrots a scrub.

- Do the same with some lovely radishes. You can get some marbled pink and white oval ones now, which are crunchy and peppery. Again, leave the tops on as these make good handles when it comes to dipping.

- Use nice crunchy lettuces. Sweeter lettuces like cos and Romaine are good for dipping – I try to use the inner part, keeping the outer leaves for another salad. I leave the stalk on and then cut the lettuce into quarters, and that way they stay in one piece, but you don't have to do this. The important thing is to get good chunks of vegetables. I like to contrast the sweet lettuces with slightly more bitter ones like radicchio or endive.

- If you've got some young asparagus that's just come into season, it's really nice eaten raw. Feel free to use your imagination on the veggie side. Little fingers of celery or celeriac are also good. However, you often come across people who use raw cauliflower with dips – I personally would prefer colonic irrigation! I think cauliflower and broccoli are just awful eaten raw, so I wouldn't suggest using them here.

> FOR THE DIP
> 1 x 200ml tub of yoghurt
> 1–2 handfuls of fresh mint, leaves picked
> 2 handfuls of fresh podded peas
> a handful of freshly grated Parmesan cheese
> sea salt and freshly ground black pepper
> juice of ½ a lemon

Whizz the yoghurt and mint up in a food processor for half a minute or so. Add the peas and the Parmesan and whizz again – the peas will break down and the yoghurt will become green. Put into a bowl, correcting the seasoning with extra salt and pepper and a good squeeze of lemon juice. When you add the lemon juice and peas to the yoghurt, quite often it splits and turns into a kind of cheese, but this is absolutely fine. It depends on the type of yoghurt you use and how acidic your lemon is. Just pour away any excess water. Usually, though, it doesn't split and is more like a purée, but both ways are good.

The best way to serve this is to put the dip into a bowl and have a big board next to it with your veggies on. And have some salt and pepper to hand in case you need it. It's a good sociable way to start a meal.

JAPANESE STYLE SATURDAY NIGHT STEAK

This idea comes from a fantastic restaurant called Ima-Ha-N in the Asakusa district of Tokyo where they poach thin slices of very tender beef in seaweed stock for just a few seconds before dipping them in a special sauce made from sesame seed paste, lime and soy – so delicious! The meat really melts in your mouth. British beef is great to use for this dish, although it's not quite as tender as Japanese beef. However, it does have loads more flavour, so I decided to invent a dish along the same lines that works best using our meat.

> SERVES 2
> 2 sirloin steaks, about 2.5cm/1 inch thick
> ½ a mooli (also known as daikon)
> a bunch of fresh crisp radishes
> 1 fresh red chilli
> a small bunch of fresh coriander
> 2 tablespoons water
> 2 tablespoons tahini
> 1 teaspoon soy sauce
> juice of 1 lime
> sea salt and freshly ground black pepper
> olive oil

Take your steaks out of the fridge 15 minutes before you want to cook them. Put them on a plate and just put them to one side while you prepare the rest of the ingredients.

Peel the skin off the mooli, then continue to peel long strips off it and put these in a bowl. Slice the radishes into fine rounds, deseed the chilli and slice it thinly, and add both to the mooli strips. Tear the coriander leaves into pieces and throw them in too. Add the water gradually to the tahini and mix until you have a smooth paste. Stir in the soy and most of the lime juice, then taste and add a little more lime if necessary. Mix until smooth.

Heat a frying pan big enough to hold both the steaks at the same time without them touching. Season the steaks well with sea salt and freshly ground black pepper, rub them with a little olive oil, and place them gently in the pan. Fry for about 8 minutes, turning the steaks over every minute and lowering the heat to medium after the first minute. Rest the steaks for a couple of minutes before slicing them up thinly. Tip any juices from the steaks into the tahini sauce mix.

To serve, dress the salad with the sauce, mix in the slices of beef, and tuck in!

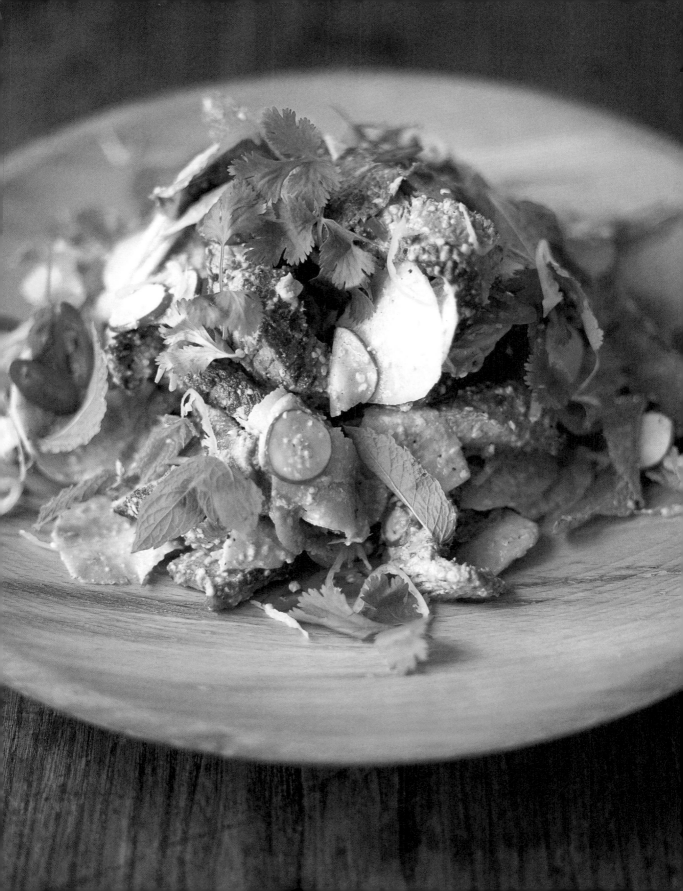

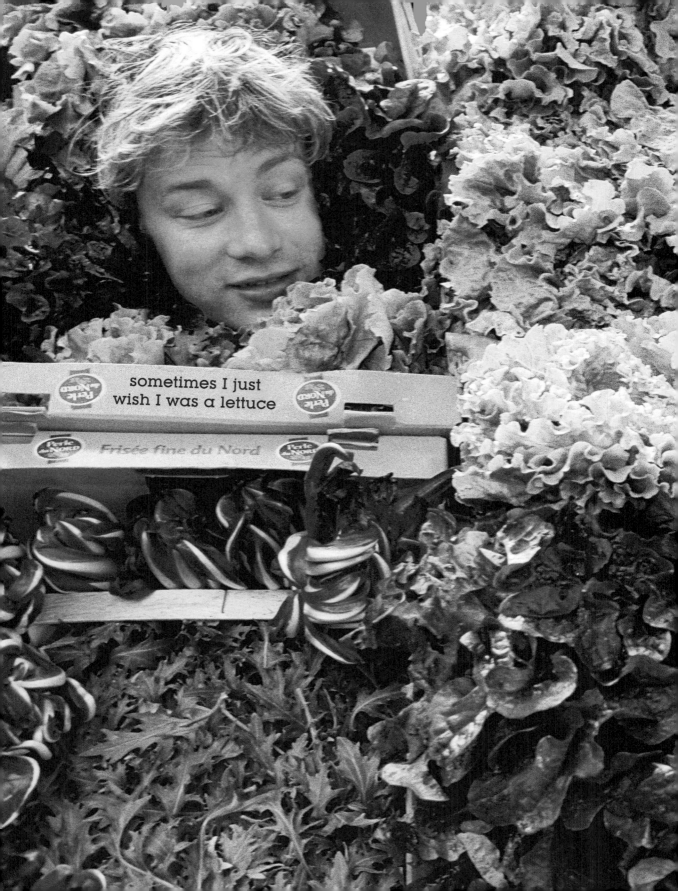

sometimes I just
wish I was a lettuce

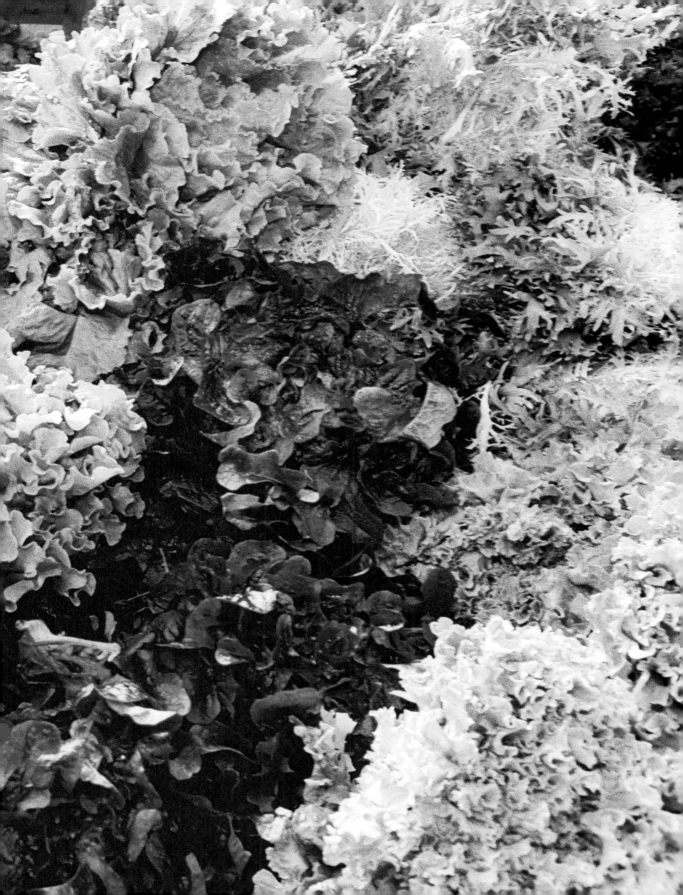

CARROT AND CORIANDER CRUNCH SALAD

I always think it's brilliant if you can turn the humble carrot into anything remotely cool or credible, especially in the salad world. You deserve to have a medal if you can come up with something amazing. If you're lucky enough to have vegetables in your garden you'll know what I mean when I say freshness is everything. But those of you who haven't got a garden should buy the freshest-looking organic ones that you can find.

I use a mandolin to slice the carrots for this salad – it will give you long ribbony slices – but you can use a speed peeler, a coarse grater or do it by hand with a knife instead. As long as your results are nice and crunchy, that's all that matters.

This is really good as a starter, or try eating it with some little kebabs if you're having a barbecue, or stuffed into some pitta bread with sliced grilled chicken.

SERVES 4–6
6 medium carrots, washed and peeled
a large handful of fresh coriander, leaves picked
4 teaspoons sesame seeds, toasted, or poppy seeds

FOR THE DRESSING
zest and juice of 1 orange
2 lemons
extra virgin olive oil
2 heaped tablespoons sesame seeds, toasted
sea salt and freshly ground black pepper

First of all, slice the carrots or cut them up into fine ribbons, matchsticks or batons. Put them into a salad bowl with the coriander leaves and the sesame or poppy seeds. To make the dressing, finely grate the zest of the orange into a bowl. Add the orange juice, the juice of 1½ lemons and about 4 times that amount of extra virgin olive oil. Lightly pound your toasted sesame seeds to a pulp in a pestle and mortar, then add to the dressing. Mix well, then season to taste with salt, pepper and possibly more lemon juice to make it nice and zingy so that you can taste it once you've dressed the salad. Once the salad is dressed, the flavour of the lemon will lessen, so get eating straight away.

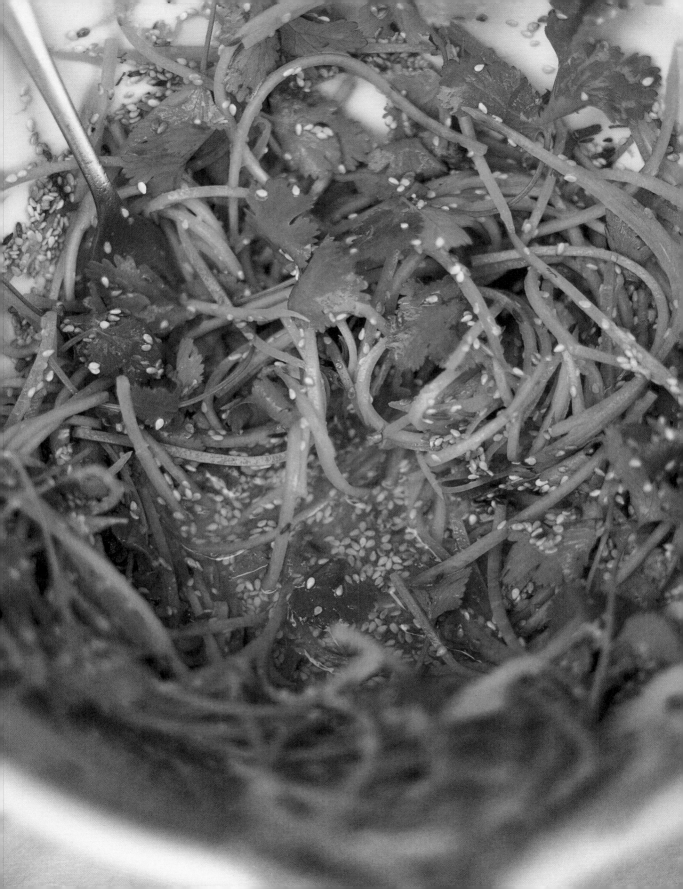

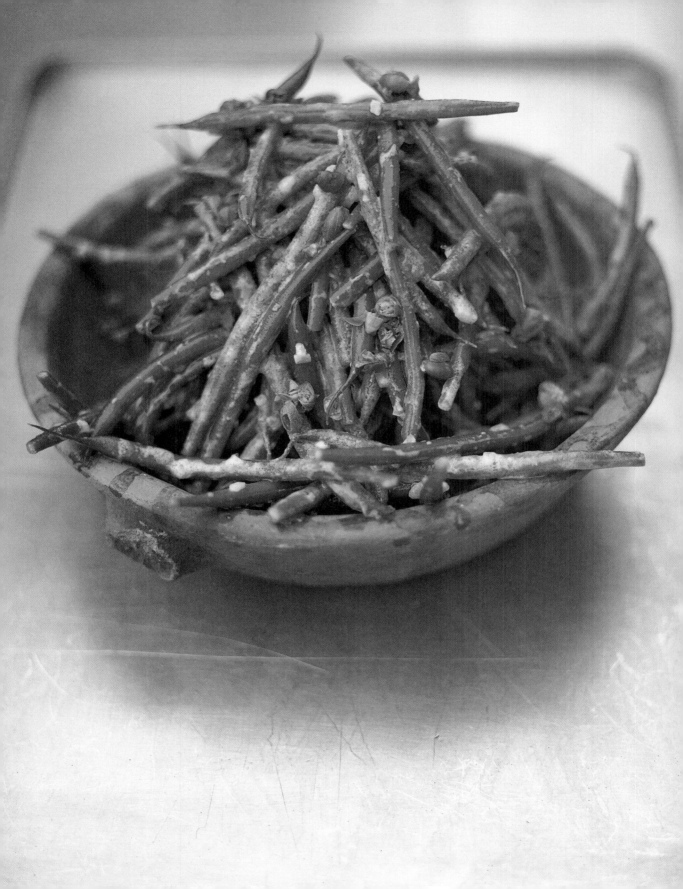

GOOD OLD FRENCH BEAN SALAD

I had this salad a while ago in a bistro in France and it was fantastic. You know, twangy and mustardy and so nice to eat as a starter before the main course arrived. It reminded me that sometimes cooking rules should be broken. We're told that beans should only be cooked until they're al dente, but I think we should cook them for a bit longer. I'd rather run my nails down a blackboard than eat a squeaky al dente green bean! So here's a recipe for properly cooked beans! Keep your eyes open for different coloured beans – green, yellow or black – as a mixture will make it even more interesting. And when preparing them, leave the wispy ends on as they look so nice.

SERVES 4
4 handfuls of French beans, stalk ends removed
2-3 heaped teaspoons good French mustard, to taste
2 tablespoons good-quality white wine vinegar
7 tablespoons extra virgin olive oil
sea salt and freshly ground black pepper
1 medium shallot, peeled and finely chopped
optional: 1 tablespoon capers
½ a clove of garlic, finely grated
optional: a small handful of fresh chervil

Bring a pan of water to a fast boil, add your beans, put a lid on the pan, and cook for at least 4 to 5 minutes. Boiling the beans fast like this helps them to retain all their nutrients. Meanwhile, put the mustard and vinegar into a jam jar or bowl and, while stirring, add the olive oil to make a good hot French dressing. Season carefully with sea salt and freshly ground black pepper, then add the finely chopped shallot, the capers if you're using them and the garlic.

Remove one of the beans from the pan to check if it's cooked. If it holds its shape but is also soft to the bite, it's perfect. Drain in a colander. Now, while the beans are steaming hot, this is the perfect moment to dress them – a hot bean will take on more of the wonderful dressing than a cold one. It is best to serve the beans warm, not cold, and certainly not at fridge temperature because the flavours will be muted and boring. Serve the beans in a bowl, sprinkled with chervil if you like – it's a delicate, crunchy herb that goes well with beans. Serve as a salad in its own right, or as an accompaniment to a main meal.

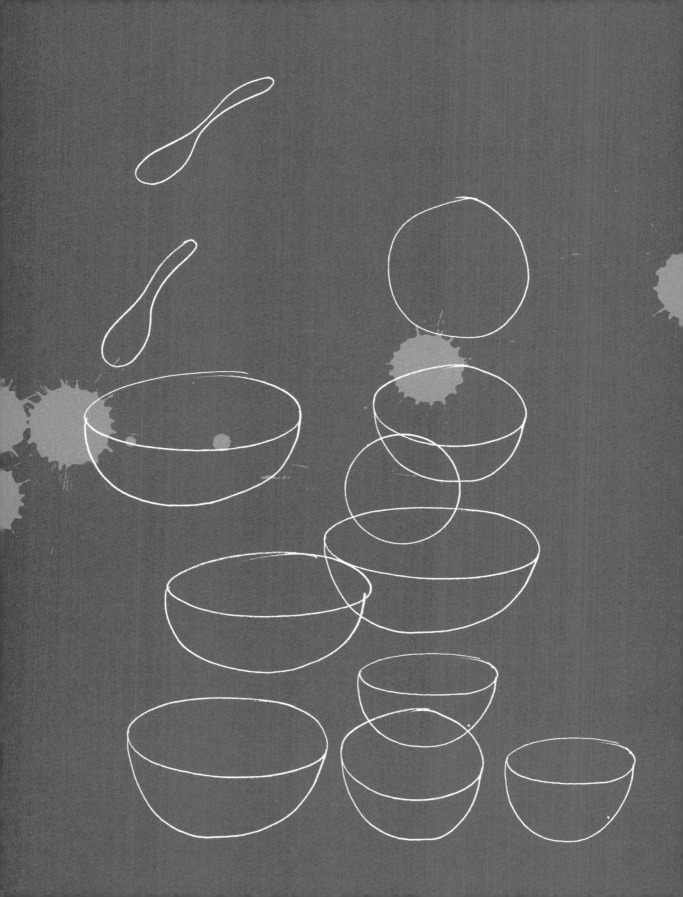

SOUPS

You might think cooking soup is a simple option, but actually I've realized that it's a real treat and quite brave and cool to make a soup for a dinner party or your family. Not only that, but it's cheap to make and virtually foolproof, even for the most inexperienced cook! For the last six months I've had a soup on the menu at Fifteen every day and it always sells well.

All the soups in this chapter will provide a good canvas for you to understand how diverse and great soups can be. Like breads, they are almost culinary signposts in the way they can sum up the place that they're from. I can imagine outdoor workers or farmers in Britain on a miserable day tucking into a thick leek and potato or oxtail soup; the Frenchman with so many onions that he makes an event out of a French onion soup; the clever Italian mum using up all her leftover broken bits of pasta to finish off her minestrone. And then in places like Kerala in Southern India, where it's humid and hot, the heat of the chillies in their soups actually helps you to perspire and cool down. These soups say so much about people and their cultures.

I had a conversation with a taxi driver recently. This guy liked his food, he cooked a fair bit, but he was desperately concerned about his teenage daughter, who refused to drink fruit juice or eat fruit and veg. Her skin was bad, she was moody and unhappy, and he was worried about her. I think there are probably a lot of parents out there who feel like that about their kids. I would say it's mainly to do with kids' lack of interest about what goes on in the kitchen, so use this to your advantage. You can put some great veg into their food without them knowing about it. The taxi driver's daughter did happen to like freshly squeezed orange juice, so I suggested that he buy a juicer and then, if he was to put a tiny bit of carrot or raw beetroot through the machine and top it up with orange juice, he could get away with saying it was a blood orange drink. She also loved tomato soup, so he tried spiking her soup with other puréed veg and it worked. At the end of the day, I do think that honesty is the best policy, but if you need to be a bit sneaky then things like fresh fruit juices, soups and stews are a wonderful way of using really wholesome ingredients that awkward eaters will unknowingly and gladly tuck into!

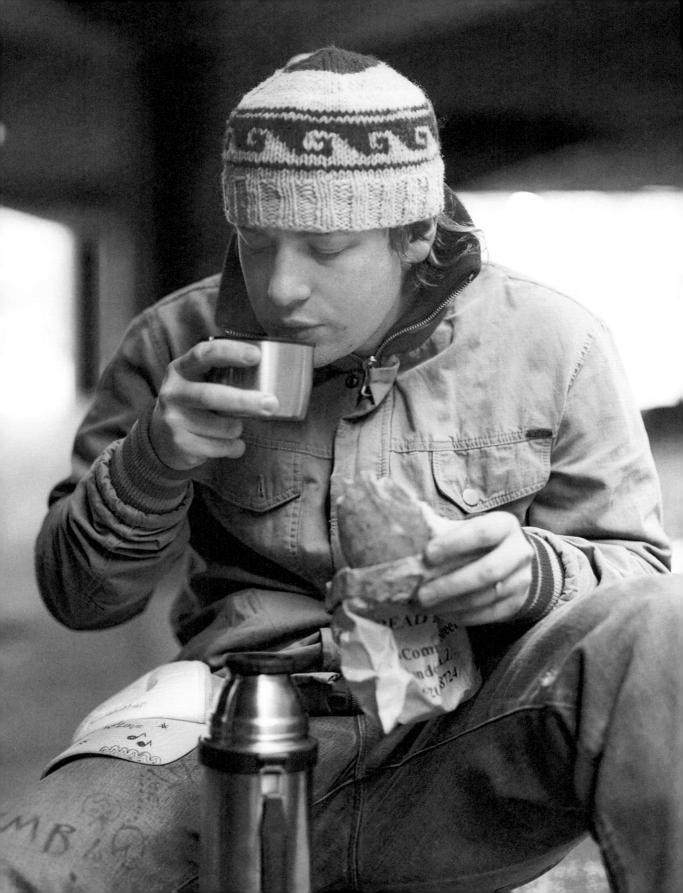

PUMPKIN RICE LAKSA SOUP

This is one of the best soups I've ever had. Laksa is a kind of brothy noodle stew, very often made with chicken and coconut milk. When I was coming up with the idea for this soup, I was thinking of the Anglo-Indian mulligatawny soup, which is made from rice, curry sauce and minced meat. If you're feeling a little bit theatrical, like I was, feel free to take the lid off the pumpkin, scoop out the flesh, and serve the soup in the pumpkin shell. Lovely!

PS If you have a Magimix food processor you can put it to good use for this recipe! If you don't have one then your pestle and mortar will come in handy instead.

SERVES 6

600g/1lb 6oz pumpkin, butternut squash, onion squash or acorn squash, halved, peeled and deseeded

a small handful of lime leaves

2–3 chillies, deseeded and finely sliced

2 cloves of garlic, peeled and finely sliced

2 thumb-sized pieces of fresh ginger, peeled

3 sticks of lemongrass, outer leaves removed

a large handful of fresh coriander, leaves picked, stalks chopped

1 heaped teaspoon five-spice

1 teaspoon ground cumin

olive oil

1 white onion, peeled and finely sliced

565ml/1 pint chicken or vegetable stock

200g/7oz basmati rice

2 x 400ml tins of coconut milk

sea salt and freshly ground black pepper

juice of 1 or 2 limes

optional: 1 fresh red chilli, sliced

optional: fresh coconut, grated

First of all you need to chop the pumpkin flesh into 5cm/2inch pieces. To make your fragrant soup base, first chop, then whizz or bash up the following in your food processor or pestle and mortar until you have a pulpy mix: the lime leaves, chillies, garlic, ginger, lemongrass, coriander stalks, five-spice and cumin. Remove any stringy bits that may remain in the pulp. Put this fragrant mixture into a high-sided pan with a little oil and your finely sliced onion and cook gently for about 10 minutes to release the flavours.

Add the pumpkin and the stock to the pan. Stir around, scraping all the goodness off the bottom of the pan. Bring to the boil, then reduce the heat and simmer with the lid on for about 15 minutes until the pumpkin is soft. At this point, add the rice and give it a really good stir. Some of the pumpkin will begin to mush up, but you'll also have some chunks. Continue to simmer with the lid on until the rice is cooked, then off comes the lid. Add the coconut milk, stir again, taste and season carefully with salt and pepper. To give it a bit of sharpness add the lime juice – the amount will depend on how juicy your limes are, but the idea is to give the soup a little twang.

Serve the soup in warmed bowls or pour it back into the pumpkin shell. If you're going to do this, put the pumpkin shell into the oven to warm it through first. It's a great show-stopper for dinner parties. Finish sprinkled with the coriander leaves, or some extra sliced fresh chilli, or grate over some fresh coconut if you have it.

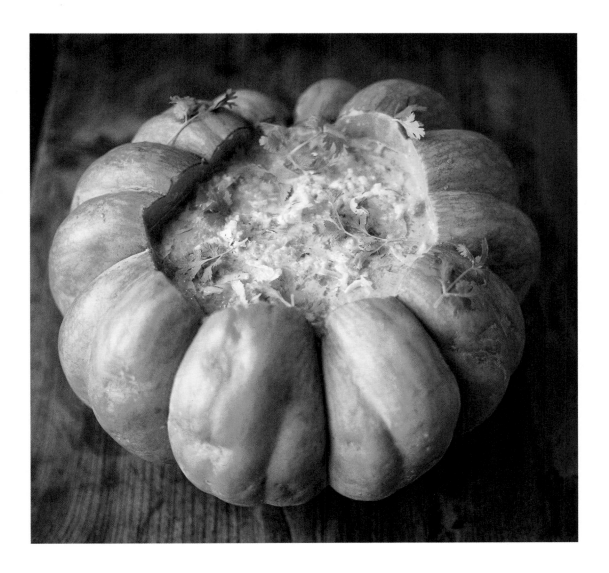

SCRUMPTIOUS SPANISH CHICKPEA AND CHORIZO SOUP

I first tasted this soup when I was in Barcelona. It may not look like the prettiest dish – it actually looks quite frumpy – but the flavours are amazing. The smoky spicy chorizo and Spanish ham are lovely with the creamy texture of the chickpeas and spinach. Definitely give this a go. You will always get good results with this soup, but you'll come up with something really special if you can get hold of the best quality chickpeas, chorizo and ham. There's a little bit of chopping to do in this recipe, but you can use a food processor if you don't have much time.

SERVES 4

olive oil
150g/5½oz chorizo sausage,
  finely chopped
1 onion, peeled and finely chopped
1 clove of garlic, peeled and finely
  chopped
2 sticks of celery, finely chopped
500g/1lb 2oz fresh spinach, washed
  and chopped
8 fresh tomatoes, deseeded and
  roughly chopped

1 x 410g tin or jar of good-quality
  cooked chickpeas, drained
1.3 litres/2 pints chicken stock
sea salt and freshly ground
  black pepper
55g/2oz pata negra, Spanish ham or
  prosciutto, finely chopped
extra virgin olive oil
2 hard-boiled eggs

Put a couple of tablespoons of olive oil into a large pot and add the chorizo. Allow to heat up and cook for a couple of minutes until the fat comes out of the chorizo, then add your onion, garlic and celery. Turn the heat down and cook slowly for 15 minutes with a lid on and without colouring the onions. Now take the lid off – the smell and colour will be fantastic. Stir it around and get some colour happening now. Add your spinach, tomatoes, chickpeas and chicken stock. Bring to the boil, then lower the heat and simmer for around 40 minutes.

At this point you can remove about a third of the mixture and purée it in a food processor. Pour it back into the pot, give it a good stir and season to taste with salt and pepper. Remove from the heat and stir in the pata negra or ham and 2 or 3 tablespoons of good Spanish extra virgin olive oil. Divide into bowls and grate some hard-boiled egg on top. The egg was a bit unexpected when I was given this in Barcelona, but it actually adds a lovely richness to it.

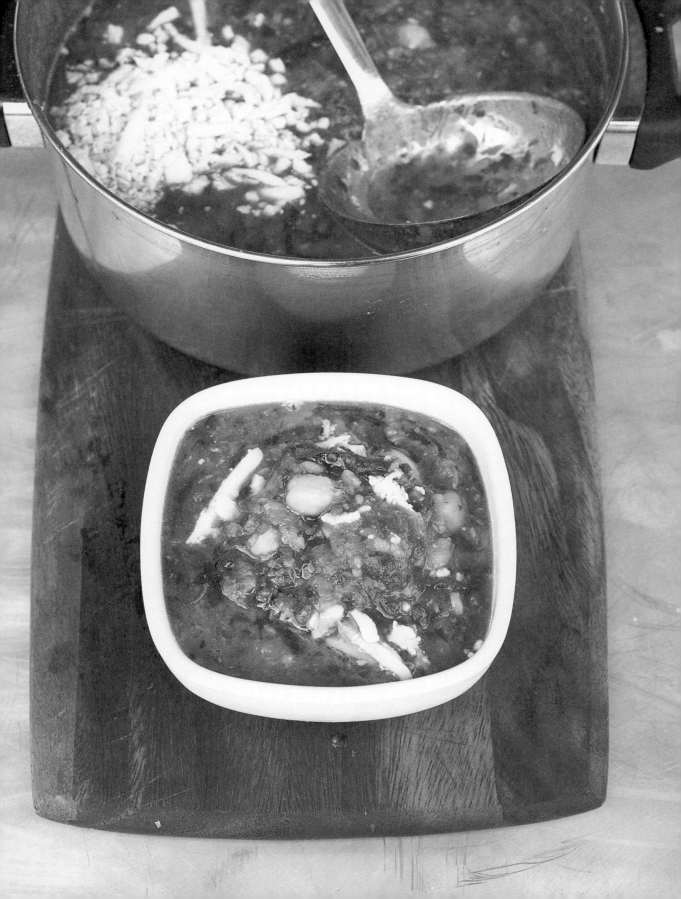

THE ULTIMATE ONION SOUP

The French often argue about where this soup originated – Lyon or Paris? Quite frankly I'd dispute whether it is actually from France and not Britain, as some of our onion soup recipes go back hundreds of years. However, most cultures and countries have a version of an onion-based or onion soup. In Italy there is a version called 'carabaccia' which is made from all different kinds of onion mixed together and slowly fried with chunks of potato and a little stick of cinnamon, which gives it the most incredible flavour. We only seem to get certain varieties of onion in our markets and supermarkets, but if you ever get down to a farmers' market you'll see that they come in all different shapes and sizes.

SERVES 4

1.1kg/2½lb onions,
   peeled and sliced
a handful of fresh thyme,
   leaves picked
6 cloves of garlic, peeled and
   finely sliced
1 bay leaf
olive oil

a good knob of butter
1.3 litres/2½ pints stock (beef, chicken
   or vegetable)
sea salt and freshly ground
   black pepper
1 baguette or ciabatta
115g/4oz Gruyère, or other melting
   cheese

In a thick-bottomed non-stick pan, slowly fry all the onions with the thyme, garlic and bay leaf in a good drizzle of olive oil and the butter. Place a lid on the pan and slowly cook them for about 15 minutes, without colouring, stirring occasionally so the onions don't catch on the bottom. The slower you can cook them, the better. Then remove the lid, turn up the heat and colour the onions until they are light golden. This will encourage a sweetness and a real depth of flavour. Add the stock, turn the heat down and then simmer for 20 minutes. You can skim any fat off, but I think it adds good flavour.

Correct the seasoning with salt and pepper. When it's perfect, pour into your serving bowls and place these on a baking tray. Now what I like to do, instead of slicing the bread all pretty and proper, is to tear it up. It's much more rustic and beautiful with all the knotty bits showing. Put the bread on top of the soup in each bowl, then drizzle over some olive oil and put the Gruyère on top. Place the baking tray in a preheated oven on a medium heat, or under the grill (be careful not to crack your bowls or burn the bread) to lightly toast the bread and melt the cheese.

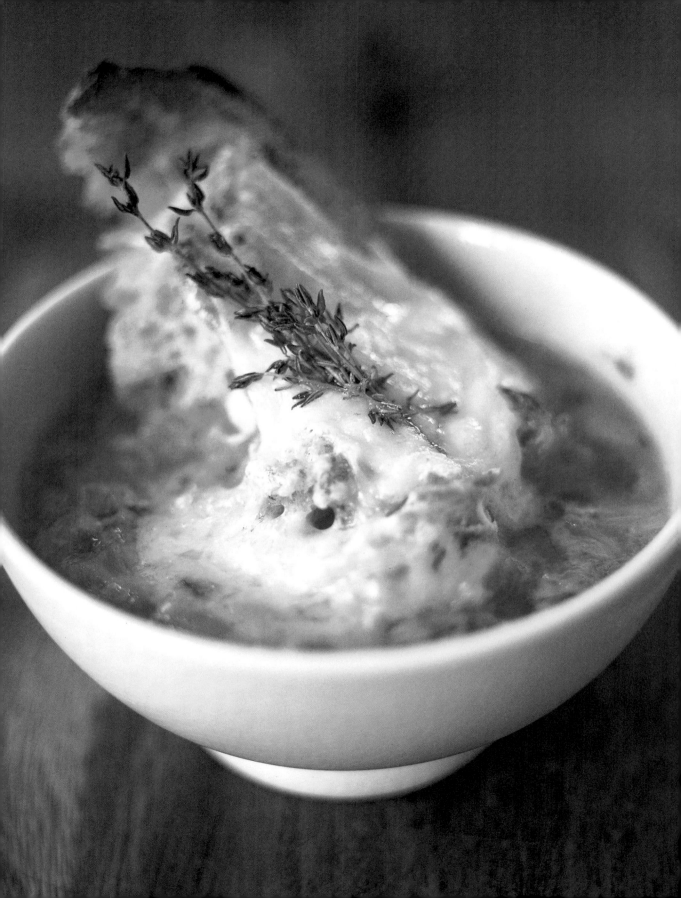

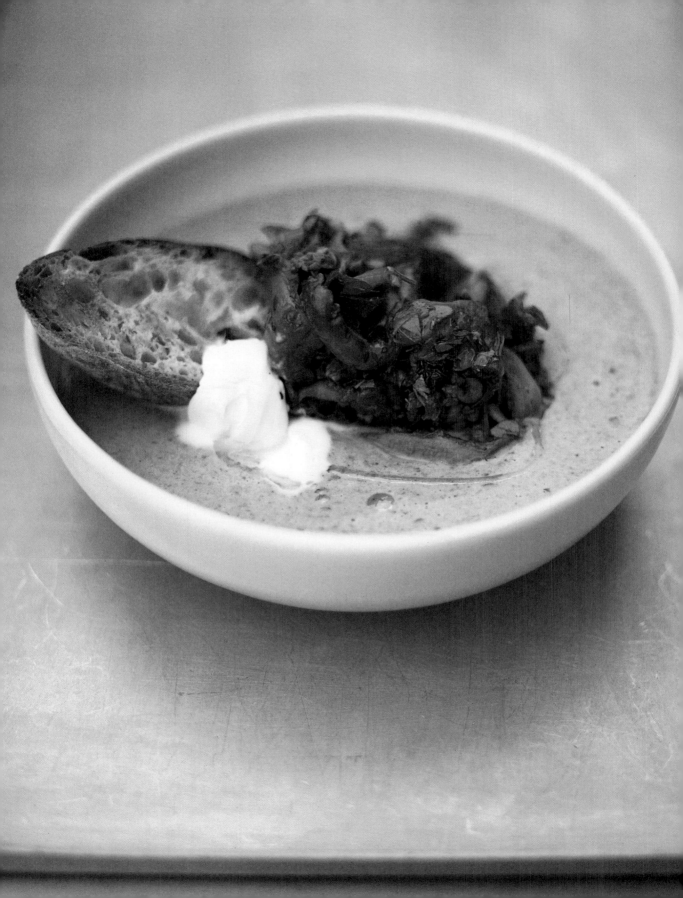

THE REAL MUSHROOM SOUP

When I first moved to London I worked in the Neal Street Restaurant in Covent Garden. It was famous for its wild mushrooms, and my mate Gennaro used to go out every day during mushroom season to find them. It was in this restaurant that I tasted a real mushroom soup for the first time. Those awful tins of mushroom soup that we've all tasted just became a distant memory!

The nice thing about nearly all mushrooms is that, if cooked correctly, they do have wonderful flavour. If you were to use a field of Portabello mushrooms to make a soup, just adding a tiny bit of dried porcini into the base would make the whole thing more luxurious.

SERVES 6

a small handful of dried porcini
olive oil
600g/1lb 6oz mixed fresh wild
    mushrooms (chanterelles, girolles,
    trompettes de la mort, shitake,
    oyster), cleaned and sliced
2 cloves of garlic, peeled and
    finely sliced
1 red onion, peeled and
    finely chopped
a knob of butter

a handful of fresh thyme,
    leaves picked
sea salt and freshly ground
    black pepper
1 litre/1¾ pints chicken or
    vegetable stock
a handful of fresh flat-leaf parsley,
    leaves picked and roughly chopped
2 tablespoons mascarpone cheese
1 lemon
optional: truffle oil

Place the porcini in a small dish, add boiling water just to cover, and leave to soak. Get a large casserole-type pan nice and hot, then add a good couple of lugs of olive oil and your fresh mushrooms. Stir around very quickly for a minute, then add your garlic, onion, butter and thyme and a small amount of seasoning. After about a minute you'll probably notice moisture cooking out of the mushrooms and at this point add half of your porcini, chopped up, and the rest left whole. Strain the soaking liquid to remove any grit, and add it to the pan. Carry on cooking for about 20 minutes until most of the moisture disappears.

Season to taste, and add your stock. Bring to the boil and simmer for around 20 minutes. I usually remove half the soup from the pan and whizz it up to a purée at this point, then pour it back in, adding the parsley and mascarpone, and seasoning carefully to taste.

You can serve this soup as you like, but there are a few things to remember when finishing it off. Mix together a pinch of salt and pepper with the zest of one lemon and the juice of half of it, then spoon a little of this into the middle of the soup. When you go to eat it, stir it in and it gives a wonderful flavour. Other things you can consider are little slices of grilled crostini put into the bottom of the bowls before the soup is poured over. Or you could even quickly fry some nice-looking mushrooms – like girolles, chanterelles or oysters – and sprinkle these on top of the soup. If I was going to use truffle oil, then I would use it on its own – a few drips on the top just before serving.

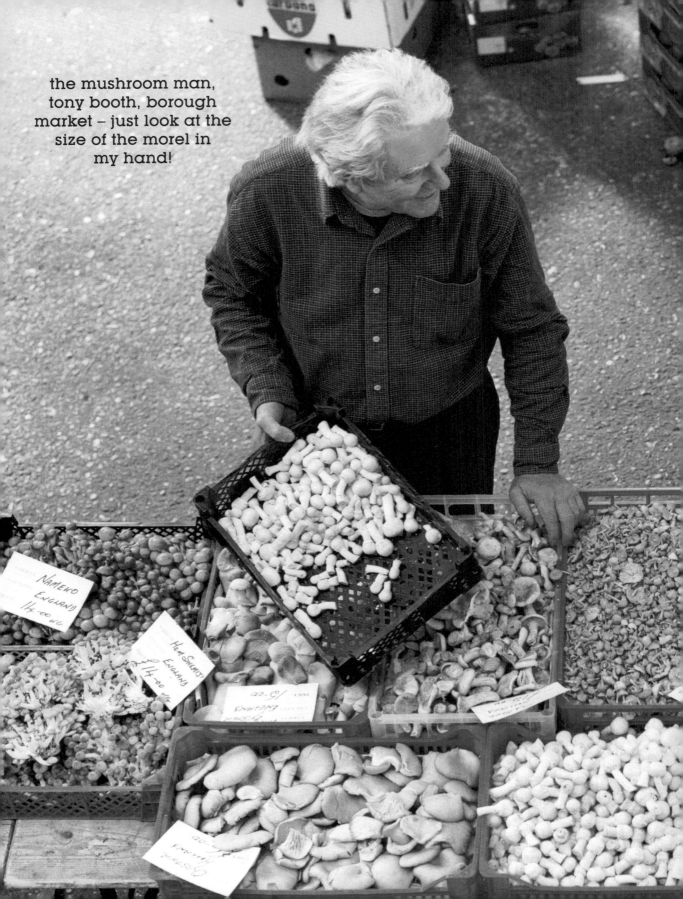

the mushroom man, tony booth, borough market – just look at the size of the morel in my hand!

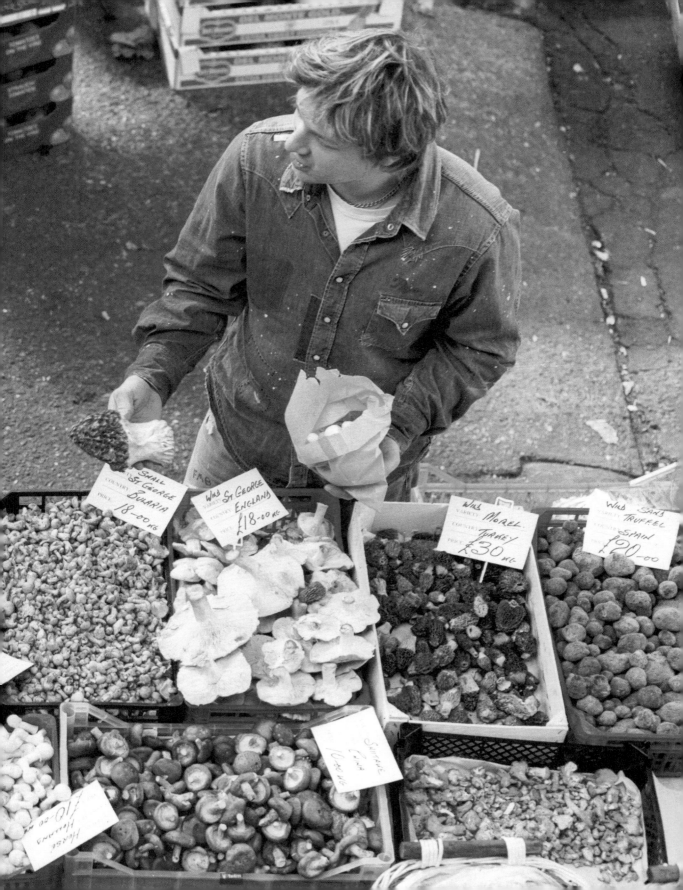

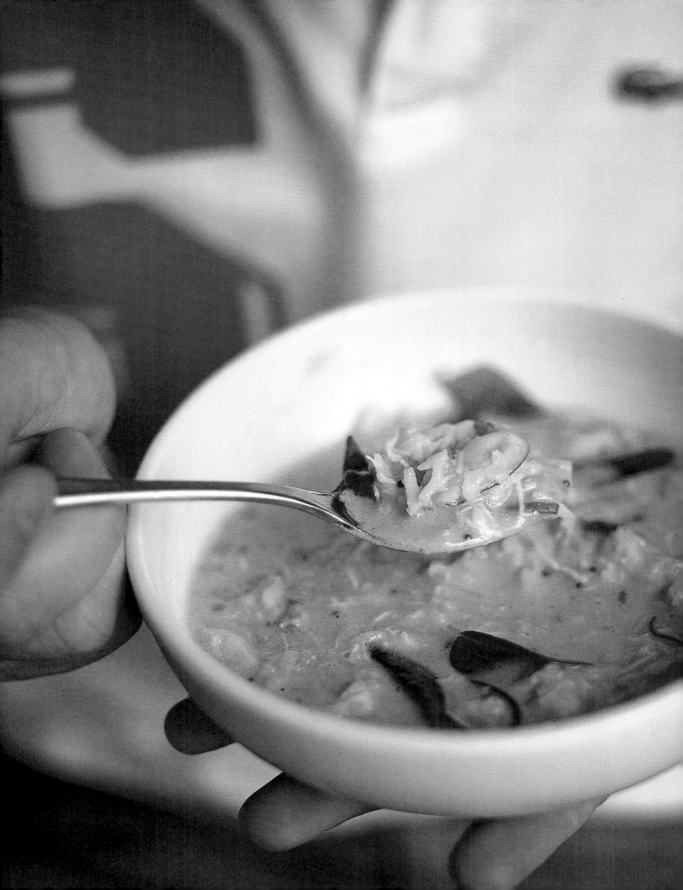

SOUTHERN INDIAN RICE AND SEAFOOD SOUP

This soup was first cooked for me by Das, my friend who runs the southern Indian restaurants in London called Rasa. I've based mine around his original recipe, and what's fantastic about it is that it's so easy to make. It only takes about 30 minutes, and the other great thing is that the ingredients are not particularly expensive, so it's economical. However, if you want to spend a little more and make it a bit luxurious using something like crab, then you can. The soup is just as good with frozen prawns and flaky white fish though. Use any selection of fish that you fancy – I like to use a good mixture of fresh-looking fish (John Dory, cod, haddock or red mullet all work well). Get it skinned and filleted, then all you have to do is chop it up. If you can find any coconut oil, use that, otherwise vegetable and sunflower oil are fine to use.

This really is one of my favourite soups. It's not too hot, but as you eat it you can pick out the individual flavours. And there's something about having rice in a soup that makes it really scrumptious.

SERVES 4

5 tablespoons vegetable or
    sunflower oil
3 tablespoons brown
    mustard seeds
a handful of fresh curry leaves,
    picked off stalks
2 teaspoons cumin seeds
1 teaspoon garam masala
1½ teaspoons chilli powder
2 teaspoons turmeric
3 red chillies, deseeded and
    finely sliced
2 large thumb-sized pieces of fresh
    ginger, peeled and grated
6 cloves of garlic, peeled and
    finely chopped

2 onions, peeled and finely chopped
2 handfuls of basmati rice
565ml/1 pint water
600g/1lb 6oz fish (see introduction),
    skinned, filleted and cut into
    5–8cm/2–3inch chunks
2 x 400ml tins of coconut milk
sea salt and freshly ground
    black pepper
juice of 2 limes
a handful of fresh coriander,
    roughly chopped
optional: 3 tablespoons freshly
    grated coconut

Get yourself a big pan and heat up your oil, then add the mustard seeds, curry leaves, cumin seeds, garam masala, chilli powder and turmeric. Cook for a few minutes and you'll get the most amazing smells filling the room from all these spices. Then add the chillies, the ginger, the garlic and the onions. Continue cooking slowly until the garlic and onions are soft. Then add the rice and the water. Bring to the boil then reduce the heat and simmer gently for 15 minutes. Add your fish and the coconut milk with a pinch of salt. Put the lid on the pan and simmer for a further 10 minutes, then stir well to break up the pieces of fish. Taste and correct the seasoning with salt and pepper, then just before you serve it squeeze in the lime juice and stir in half the coriander. Serve in warmed bowls, sprinkle over some freshly grated coconut, if you have it, and rip over the rest of the coriander.

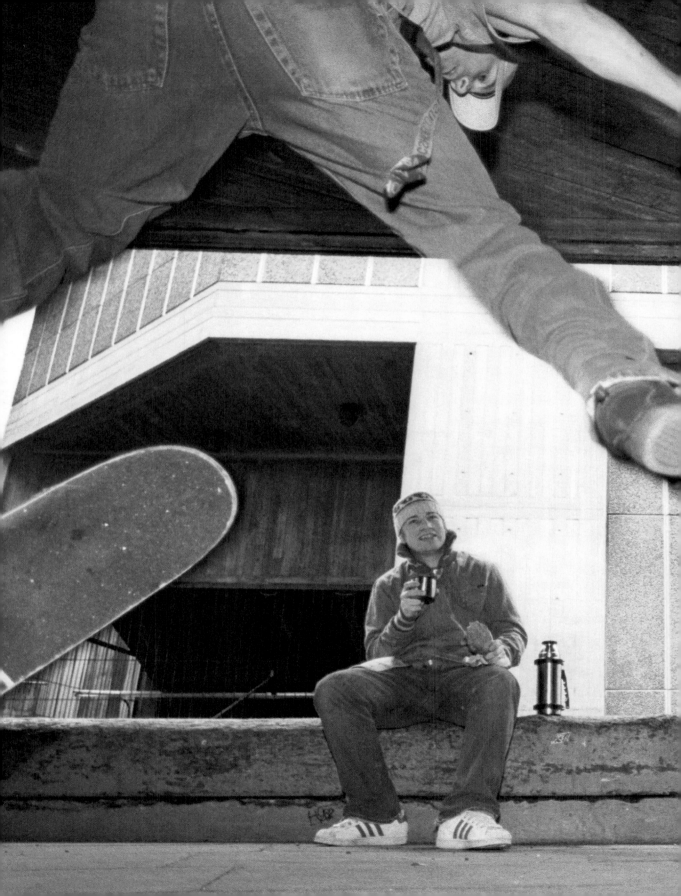

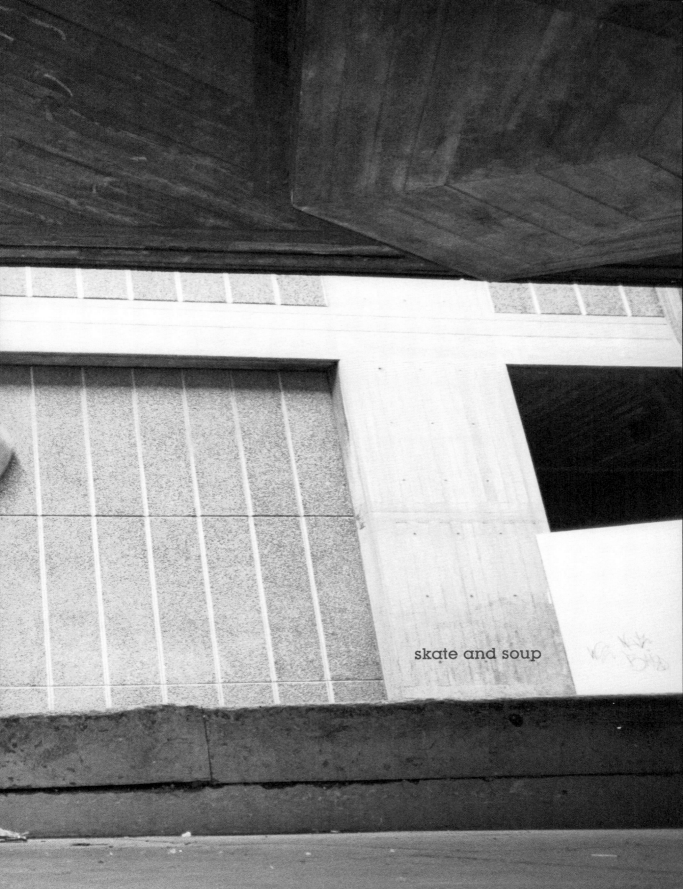

skate and soup

FEEL GOOD CHICKEN BROTH

When I was young and felt unwell with a cold or a headache, my mum would make this soup to help me feel better. It used to make me feel like a million dollars after I'd eaten it. It's probably one of the simplest soups to make because it just involves slowly boiling a whole chicken in a pot with a few roughly chopped root veg. The fat marbles on top during cooking, but underneath it is nice and clear, like a consommé. Like consommé, if you want to serve this at a dinner party or you want to vary its flavour, the actual soup will always stay the same but the garnish that you add can differ from mushrooms, to florets of cauliflower, to julienned veg. Another nice thing you can do is add a splash of sherry or port just before serving to give it a little twang. All these things are great to try, but I just really like my mum's simple chicken broth. Her secret ingredient was a rasher of smoked bacon, and sometimes she'd add a few sprigs of rosemary for the last ten minutes.

SERVES 6
1 x 1.5kg/3½lb free-range organic chicken
2 carrots, peeled and roughly chopped
2 sticks of celery, roughly chopped
1 rasher of smoked bacon
2–3 sprigs of fresh rosemary
a handful of shitake mushrooms
optional: a splash of sherry or port
sea salt
extra virgin olive oil

Put your chicken, carrot, celery and bacon in a large saucepan, cover with water and bring to the boil. Turn the heat down and simmer slowly for an hour and a quarter, skimming the white residue off the top every now and again. Add your rosemary sprigs, shitake mushrooms and sherry (if you are using it) for the last 10 minutes, then remove the chicken from the pan. It should be perfectly cooked, and will be great for salads or sandwiches or for tearing into slivers to put into the soup. Season the soup with salt and ladle it through a sieve into bowls, trying not to disrupt it too much as you want to keep it reasonably clear. Add the chicken slivers and a few mushrooms to each bowl and drizzle with a little extra virgin olive oil. The finished thing should be a kinda clear consommé.

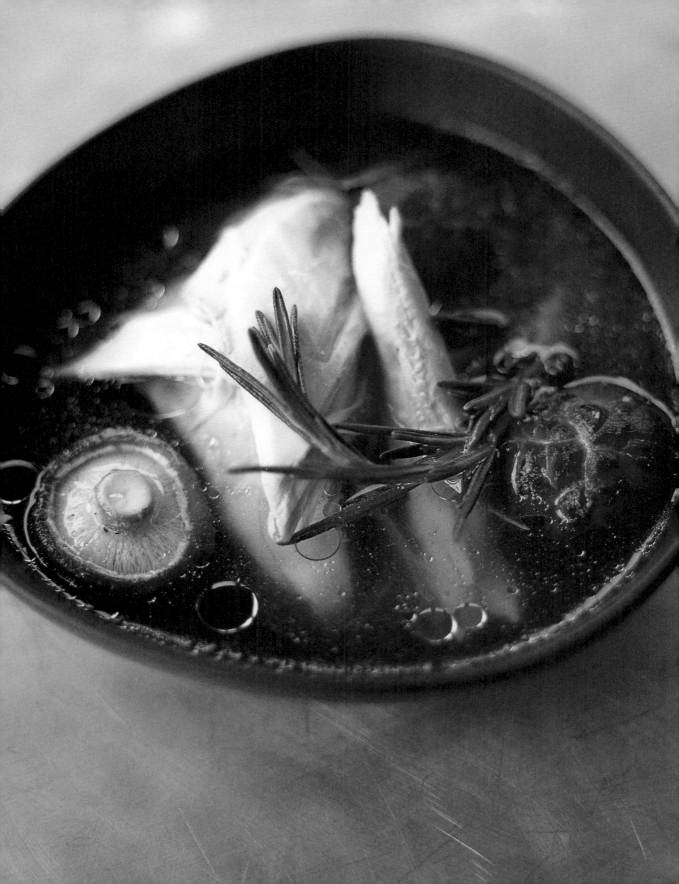

VEGET

ASLES

"CEBOLLA
TOMATE
LECHUGAS
ZANAHORIA

señora "

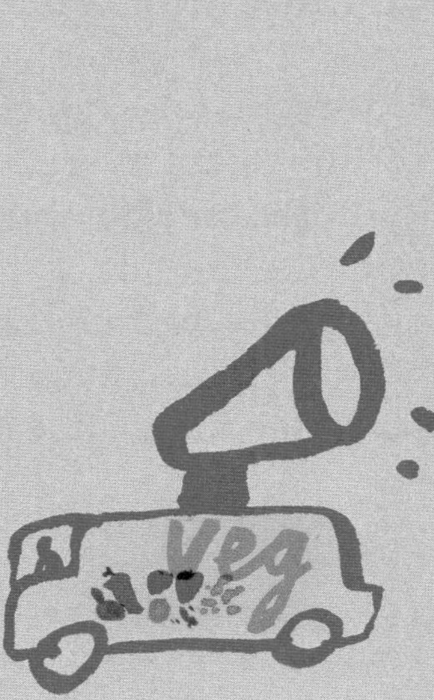

veg

A lot of people turn their noses up at vegetables and I think it's because, in general, the British are known for just boiling the hell out of them – whether they're using root veg or greens – and it's incredibly boring. However, I think that in the last five years people have been getting more into veg, and what I really wanted to put across in this chapter is that, actually, a good veg dish can completely set off a dinner when served alongside some simply cooked fish or meat.

Having now experienced a few trips abroad to America and Australia, as well as tours all round Britain, there's one thing that I've come to realize and that is that a lot of posh restaurants and many great chefs have a real lack of good veg on their menus. This is such a shame – I think we should be proud to have vegetables on our plates.

Seasonality is incredibly important when it comes to eating the best vegetables available to us. A lot of brilliant chefs think it's OK to use asparagus or broad beans four months out of season. And I know that supermarkets are guilty of supplying vegetables for twelve months of the year. But if you learn how to shop for veg when they are in season, you will benefit hugely. It's not just about the nutritional and flavour benefits of seasonal produce, it will also save you loadsa money! Farmers' markets are a great place to shop because the vegetables will probably have been harvested just hours before.

Experimenting with vegetables in cooking is easy, good fun and a great confidence builder when it comes to creating your own ideas. The main principle of this chapter is to show you ways of cooking a selection of my favourite veg, along with some of their best friends in terms of flavours. A combination such as carrots, butter, orange and rosemary or thyme pretty much always works well. Or take the turnip – a vegetable people really turn up their noses at – which can be truly brilliant when pan-roasted with a swig of white wine and herb vinegar. Vegetable dishes like this can really make eating any rich meats like lamb or beef or venison a real joy.

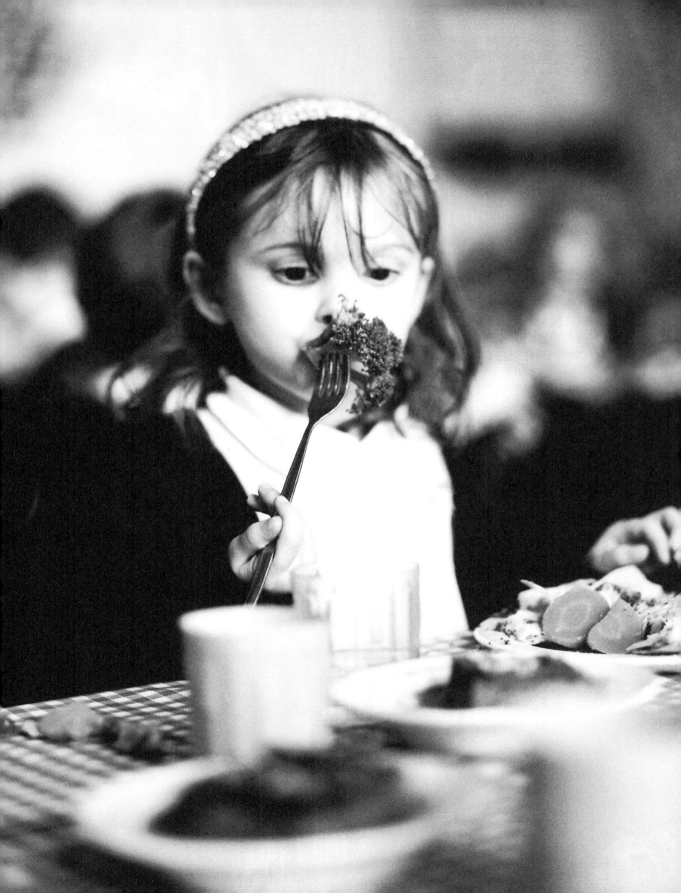

TURNIPS

You can pretty much buy baby turnips all year round – they are the size of a squashed golf ball and have little leaves on the stalky bit. I always tend to parboil my turnips for 5 minutes to soften them and take away the rawness. This also makes them more absorbent to flavours. Turnips love tarragon, rosemary, thyme, bay leaves, olive oil, radicchio and bitter leaves. These turnip dishes are great as part of an antipasti plate, eaten hot or cold with cured meats like bresaola or prosciutto. Also fantastic with all roasted meats, or with fish like salmon and trout.

BOILED TURNIPS WITH THYME BEURRE BLANC

SERVES 4
400g/14oz small turnips
3 tablespoons olive oil
55g/2oz butter, diced
6 tablespoons herb vinegar

1 wineglass of white wine
a small handful of fresh thyme, leaves
    picked and smashed
sea salt and freshly ground
    black pepper

Parboil the turnips, drain them, then put them back in the pan with the oil and half of the butter. Cook until the turnips are brown. Pour in the herb vinegar and scrape all the goodness off the bottom of the pan. Then add your wine, the rest of the butter and the thyme. Simmer until the wine and butter have reduced, giving you a creamy, emulsified sauce that coats the turnips. This normally takes a couple of minutes. Season carefully to taste and serve straight away.

THE BEST ROASTED TURNIPS

SERVES 4
400g/14oz small turnips
sea salt and freshly ground
    black pepper
a handful of fresh thyme or
    rosemary, leaves picked
6 tablespoons white wine or
    herb vinegar

2 tablespoons olive oil
a knob of butter
optional: 8 slices of prosciutto
optional: ½ a head of radicchio or other
    bitter leaves
optional: balsamic vinegar

Parboil the turnips, then drain them and put them into a large ovenproof frying pan with a pinch of salt and pepper, the herbs and the vinegar. Drizzle the oil over, dot them with butter, and cook in the oven at 220°C/425°F/gas 7 until golden. Give the pan a shake and serve straight away.

Or you can try something I did the other day which was superb. Simply lay some prosciutto slices, so they overlap, over the frying pan once the turnips are cooked. Dress some radicchio or bitter leaves with balsamic vinegar and place these over the prosciutto. Bake in the oven for about 5 minutes or until the prosciutto is crispy. Then remove the prosciutto on to plates and serve the turnips on top. A fabulous dish.

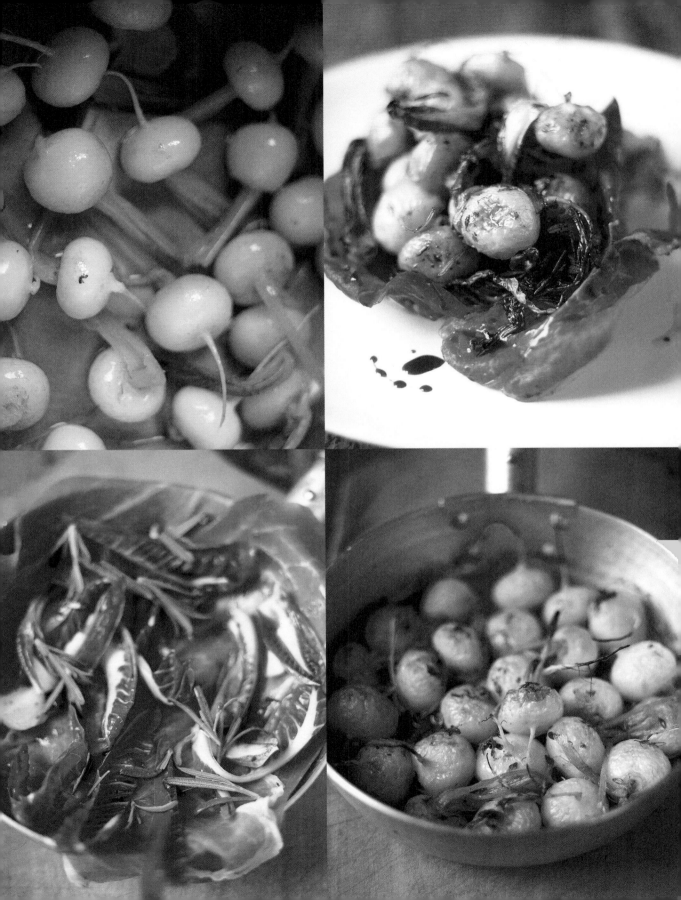

CARROTS

Carrots are brilliant – full of vitamins and extremely good for you. In the last year or so we've been lucky enough to have seen lots of different varieties of carrots available in the shops – long, round, peculiar-shaped, and even some purple ones. My favourite ways of cooking carrots all serve 4 people – for each recipe you will need 500g/1lb 2oz of carrots, either left whole if they are baby ones, or sliced into small erratic pieces – nothing too perfect.

CARROTS BOILED WITH ORANGE, GARLIC AND HERBS

Boil the carrots in salted boiling water with a tablespoon of sugar, a knob of butter and a little handful of fragrant herbs, tied up. Parsley, rosemary, thyme, bay – use just one or a mixture. Cut an orange into eighths and add them to the water, along with a few whole garlic cloves in their skins. If you really want to be a little tiger, add a pinch of cumin as well (seeds or ground) – it subtly cuts through with the most wonderful flavour. As soon as the carrots are cooked, drain them, discard the herbs and all but one of the orange pieces, squeeze the garlic out of its skin, chop the remaining orange piece finely and toss with the carrots, some seasoning and a little more butter. The flavour will be incredible. Another idea is to fry the chopped-up orange in a good tablespoon of sugar, so it almost jammifies, and serve this on top of the carrots. These two flavours together are one of the coolest things.

ROASTED CARROTS WITH ORANGE, GARLIC AND THYME

Or – just as easy – as soon as you drain the carrots you can throw them into a baking tray with the chopped-up orange and the garlic cloves and roast them at 200°C/400°F/gas 6 for 10 minutes – this will give you a slightly meatier flavour.

MASHED CARROTS

Or simply mash the carrots up with the orange and garlic, so you have some coarse and some smooth. Lovely.

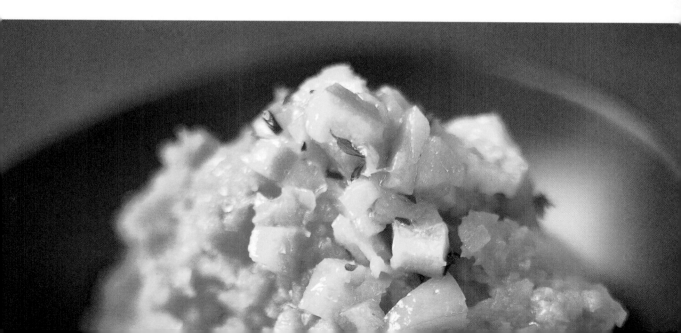

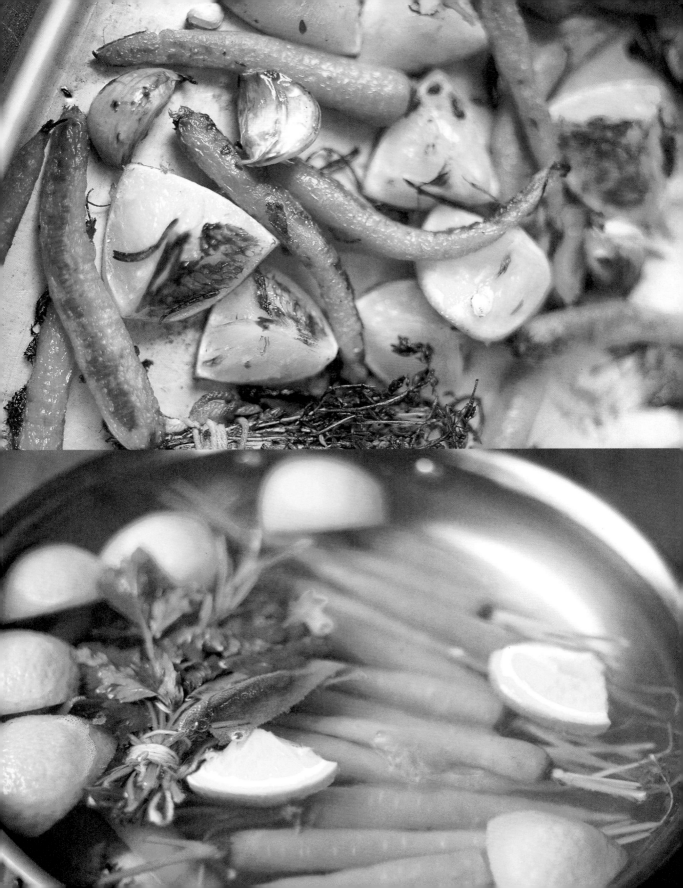

SWEETCORN

Sweetcorn is a great vegetable – most people love it. Full of Vitamins A and C, it is not only tasty but extremely good for you! I'm not averse to using a bit of tinned sweetcorn sometimes, as it does taste OK, but I'd like you to buy some corn on the cob and have a go at removing the kernels of corn yourself. It's very easy; just tear the husk off, then run a knife downwards to remove the kernels – it's definitely worth doing this to experience the sweetness and vibrancy of flavour. Sweetcorn is best served simply. It is massively in love with butter, has tendencies to flirt with the chilli family and loves a bit of bittersweet orange zest . . .

SWEETCORN WITH BUTTER, SALT AND PEPPER

The simplest way to cook sweetcorn is in a pan with a good knob of butter, salt and pepper. Place the lid on top and cook for around 8 to 10 minutes on a medium heat until you have beautiful tender sweetcorn, juicy and soft. A wonderful way to cook it.

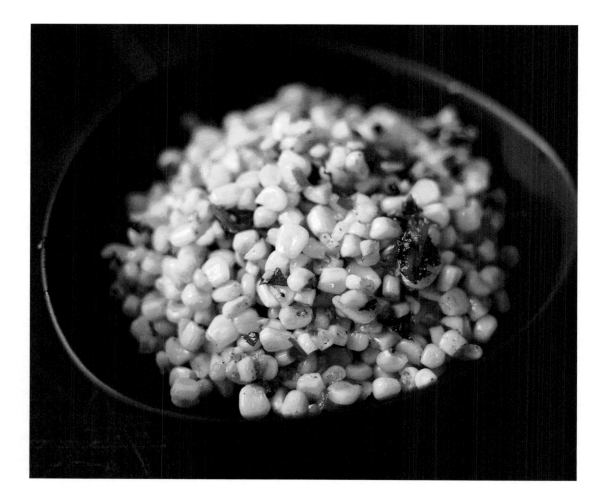

STIR-FRIED CORN WITH CHILLI, GINGER, GARLIC AND PARSLEY

One of the other things I love to do is to stir-fry the kernels in a hot wok or frying pan with 2 tablespoons of olive oil, a tablespoon of chopped ginger, a teaspoon of chopped chilli, a handful of chopped parsley and a couple of tablespoons of soy sauce. You can vary the flavours with different herbs, but this is a good base to start with.

CREAMED CORN

Another dish you should try is this creamed sweetcorn. It's delicious, and a great alternative to mashed potato or polenta. First of all, cook 400g/14oz of corn in a pan with a good knob of butter, a wineglass of water and some crumbled, dried chilli. Cook with the lid on, on a medium heat, until the corn is tender. Then place it in a food processor and blend until creamy and smooth. At this point you could add a little crème fraîche, but you may like it just as it is. Season to taste with salt and pepper and serve on a big plate, sprinkled with some baby mint leaves and orange zest.

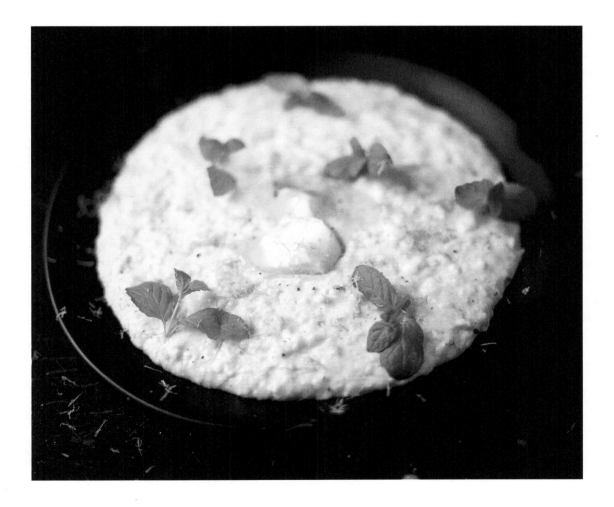

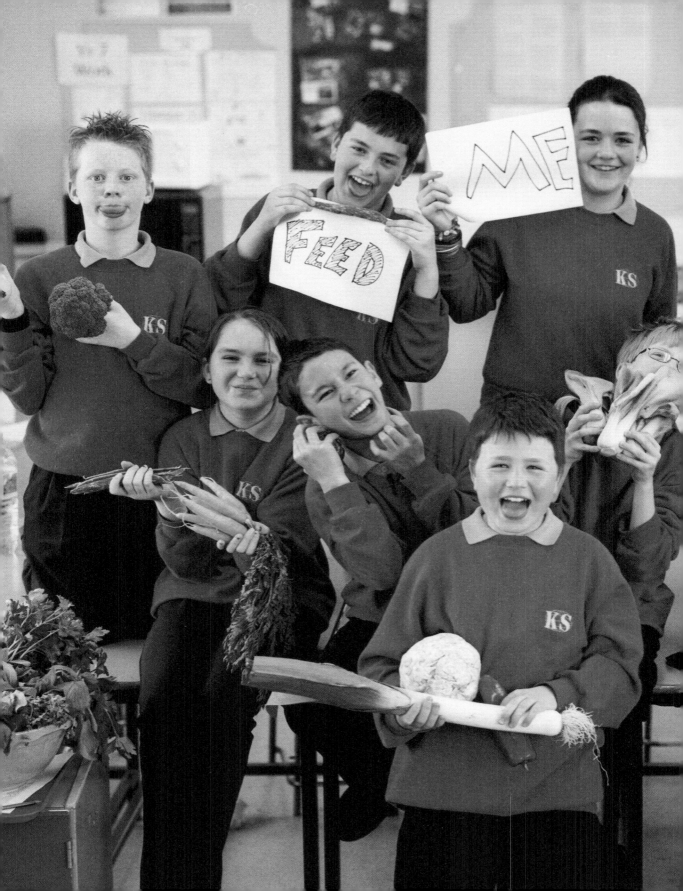

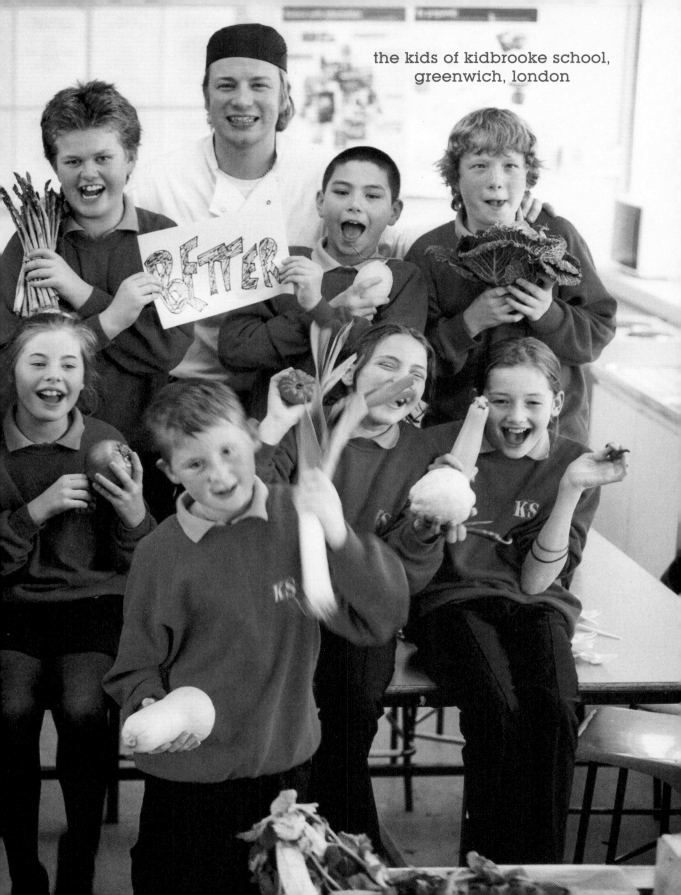

SPINACH

Spinach is a great leaf vegetable, whether you eat it cooked or use baby spinach raw in salads. It's worth remembering, though, that baby spinach doesn't have the depth of flavour that older spinach has. It is best friends with garlic, marjoram, nutmeg and cream. Spinach is an excellent source of Vitamins A and C, as well as antioxidants, and contains four times the beta-carotene of broccoli, so is very good for you! It also contains high levels of folic acid, and the nutrients within spinach can also help to lower blood cholesterol. One of the healthiest veggies around! It is one of the simplest vegetables in the world to cook as it literally takes a minute, but I'm still amazed that people will boil it for 5 minutes or more. This will leave the spinach grey, with all the green goodness left in the water. So make sure you don't do this – it's madness! Don't be fooled by spinach, though – by the time you've cooked it it will be a fraction of the size it started out as. So always use twice as much as you think you need. As a general guide I would suggest 150g/5½oz per person.

PERFECT BRAISED SPINACH

The simplest way to cook spinach is in a pan with a little olive oil, butter, a grating of nutmeg and a tiny squeeze of lemon juice with a lid on to let it steam. This will taste great, and it goes with just about anything – pasta, fish or meat. If there is any excess moisture when the spinach is cooked, just tilt the pan so it runs to the other side and pour it away. Let the spinach sit for a minute and then serve.

WONDERFUL CREAMED SPINACH

The second way I like to cook spinach is fairly similar to the braised method above. To serve 4 people, using a total of 600g/1lb 6oz of spinach, follow the recipe above but simply add a wine-glass of double cream and a handful of grated Parmesan cheese. Either stir, bring to the boil and serve, or pop in a dish and place in a hot oven at 200°C/400°F/gas 6 for 5 to 10 minutes, until just coloured on top, to gratinate.

CURRIED SPINACH

For this dish, all you need to do is melt 2 knobs of butter in a large pan and slowly fry ½ a teaspoon of ground coriander and ½ a teaspoon of garam masala. Add 2 cloves of garlic, finely sliced, a teaspoon of mustard seeds, 1 finely sliced red chilli, a pinch of ground cumin and a handful of fresh or dried curry leaves if you can get them. (Don't worry if you can't, but they are great.) Add the spinach and cook down until all the moisture has disappeared and the spinach is almost black. Indian chefs very often cook this to eat with paneer, which is an Indian cheese a bit like halloumi, but I've eaten it at home just with some boiled potatoes and finished with a tiny squeeze of lemon juice.

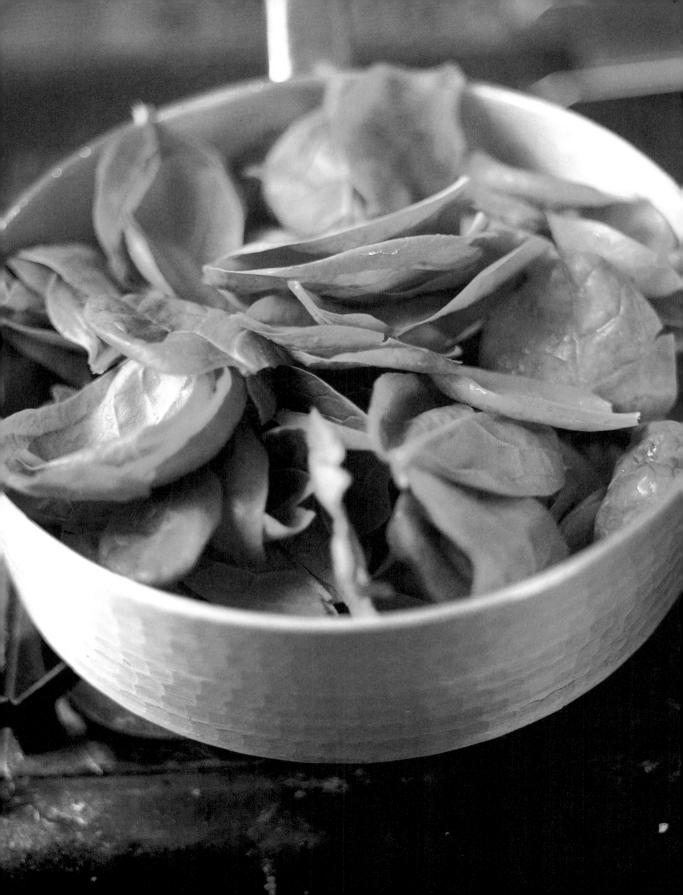

JERUSALEM ARTICHOKES

Jerusalem artichokes are sweet and almost garlicky and mushroomy and gorgeous. Although called artichokes they're actually tubers – like rough and ready potatoes. You can scrub and roast them whole like mini jacket potatoes and split them open, drizzled with a little chilli oil. You can even use them in a salad with smoky bacon. A Jerusalem artichoke's best friends are sage, thyme, butter, bacon, bay, cream, breadcrumbs, cheese and anything smoked.

SAUTÉD JERUSALEM ARTICHOKES WITH GARLIC AND BAY LEAVES

To serve 4, you will need 600g/1lb 6oz of Jerusalem artichokes. Peel them, then cut them into chunks. Place them in an oiled frying pan and fry on a medium heat until golden on both sides, then add a few bay leaves, 2 cloves of garlic, finely sliced, a splash of white wine vinegar, some salt and pepper, and place a lid on top. After about 20 to 25 minutes they will have softened up nicely and you can remove the lid and the bay leaves. Continue cooking for a couple of minutes to crisp the artichoke slices up one last time, then serve straight away. Personally, I think they go well with both meat and fish and are particularly good in a plate of antipasti, or in soups or warm salads.

SMASHED SAUTÉD JERUSALEM ARTICHOKES WITH PANCETTA AND SAGE

To cook them this way, follow the recipe above but once you've removed the lid and the bay leaves, push the Jerusalem artichokes to one side and fry 8–12 slices of chopped-up smoked bacon or pancetta with a handful of whole sage leaves until crispy. Then stir everything together until you have a wonderful mixture of chunky and mashed artichokes with crispy sage and bacon. Season to taste and serve.

GRATINATED ARTICHOKES

There are two ways in which you can do this. You can either cook the artichokes as in the first recipe above and add a little cream and grated Parmesan cheese to the pan at the end. Or you can boil the sliced artichokes until cooked and softened, then drain them and allow them to steam with the lid on for a few minutes. Get a pan hot and fry the artichokes in a little butter and some thyme until golden. Stir in a wineglass of cream and a little grated Parmesan. By this time the artichokes should be like a chunky mash. I then like to dress 2 handfuls of picked sage leaves with a little olive oil, and I sprinkle these over the top. Either way, you need to pop the pan into a hot oven at 200°C/400°F/gas 6 for 8–10 minutes until the sage is crispy.

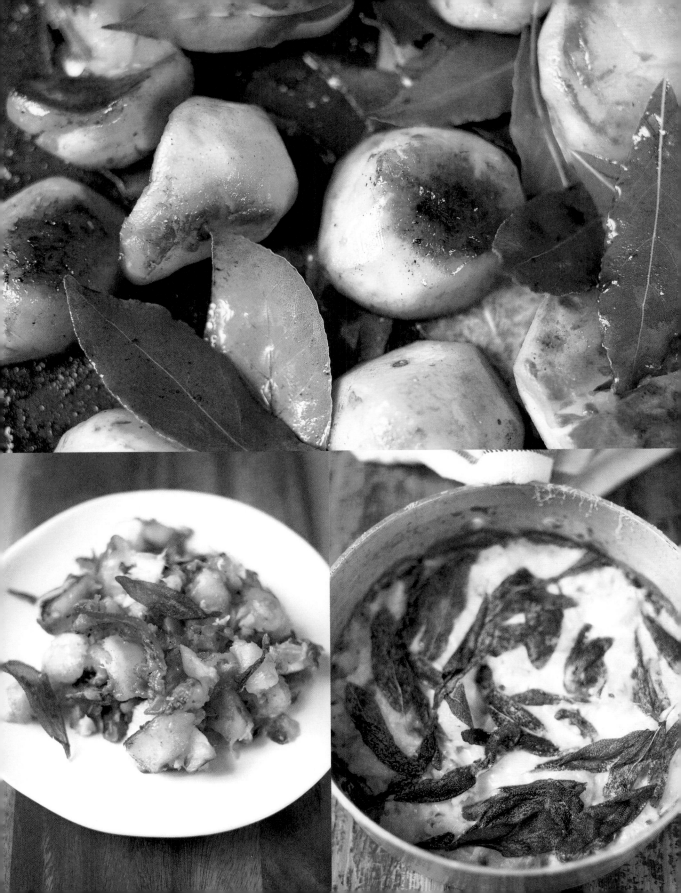

PEPPERS

Peppers are great. They make me feel summery and happy, and the thing I like most about them is their wonderful sweetness. The thing I hate about them, however, is their skin, which can sometimes be quite thick. The ultimate way to remove the skin is on a barbecue, or to hold the peppers with a pair of tongs directly over a flame on the stove until the skins are black. Place the peppers in a bowl with clingfilm on top, allow to sit and steam for 15 minutes, then simply peel the skin off. However, if you prick the peppers all over with a fork, put them in a jug covered with clingfilm and pop them into the microwave for a couple of minutes, after 10 minutes' cooling time you can normally remove the skins easily. Be very careful when you take them out, as the steam inside will be very hot. The peppers will still taste sweet doing it this way, but you won't get that lovely charred flavour from blackening them.

Peppers go well with loads of things, but their best friends are garlic, basil, tomatoes, onions, herbs, anchovies, capers, oils, balsamic or herb vinegars . . . basically peppers are right old tarts – they get round a bit! They are full of Vitamins A and C and they are also a good source of folic acid, so are good to eat if you are trying to get pregnant or in the early stages of pregnancy. They are extremely good for you as they are fat free, sodium free and cholesterol free, and can be treated as salads, tossed with pasta, stirred into risottos, used with rice, potatoes, most meats and most fish. Roasted, marinated peppers are lovely as part of an antipasti dish. You can get various colours of pepper, but the red ones, which have been left to mature for longer, are the sweetest.

MARINATED PEPPERS

Once you've peeled your red, yellow or green peppers, cut them in half, remove the seeds and cut them into 2.5cm/1 inch thick slices. Slowly fry in some olive oil with a couple of cloves of finely sliced garlic, one finely sliced red onion and a good handful of sliced basil. You don't have to brown the garlic or onions, you can just fry them for a couple of minutes to soften or you can give them just a little bit of colour, which is nice. Either way, put them in a bowl, correct the seasoning with salt and pepper, and then add a swig or two of wine or balsamic vinegar to give a marvellous twang. Serve sprinkled with a few whole basil leaves.

SPANISH STYLE PEPPERED POTATOES

Parboil 700g/1½lb of peeled and diced potatoes for 10 minutes in salted boiling water, then drain them and leave them to steam for a few minutes with a lid on. You will need the same amount of sliced marinated peppers (approx. 4 peppers, prepared as recipe above). While the potatoes are still steaming, dress them with the marinade from the peppers and pop them into a heatproof dish or baking tray. Sprinkle with salt, pepper, a teaspoon of smoked paprika and a teaspoon of finely sliced red chilli. Place the potatoes in the oven at 200°C/400°F/gas 6 until golden, then pour over your marinated peppers and give the potatoes a good shifty about so the peppers are well mixed in. Put back into the oven for 5-10 minutes until perfect and golden.

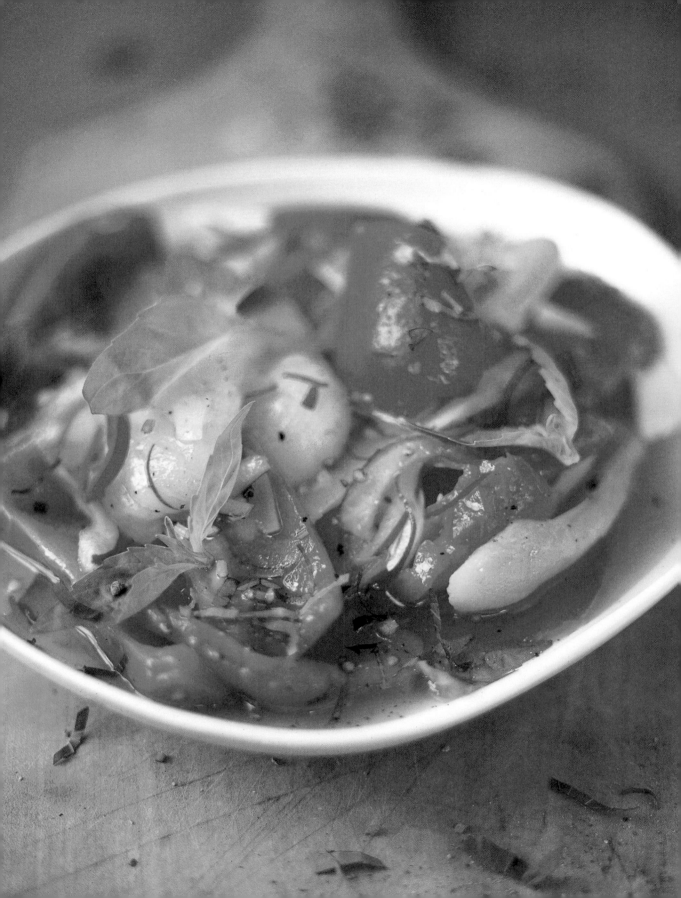

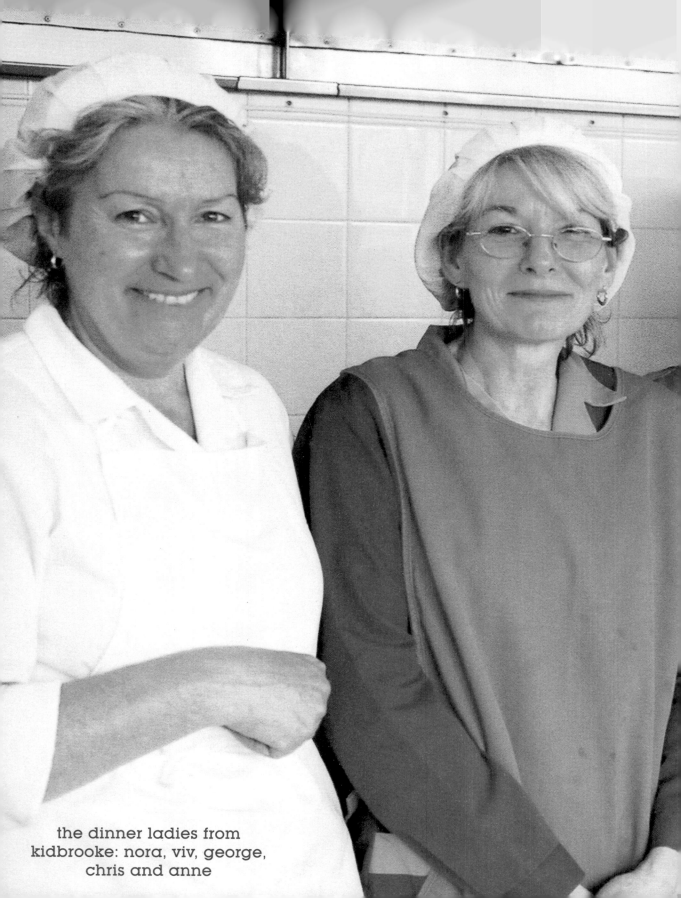

the dinner ladies from
kidbrooke: nora, viv, george,
chris and anne

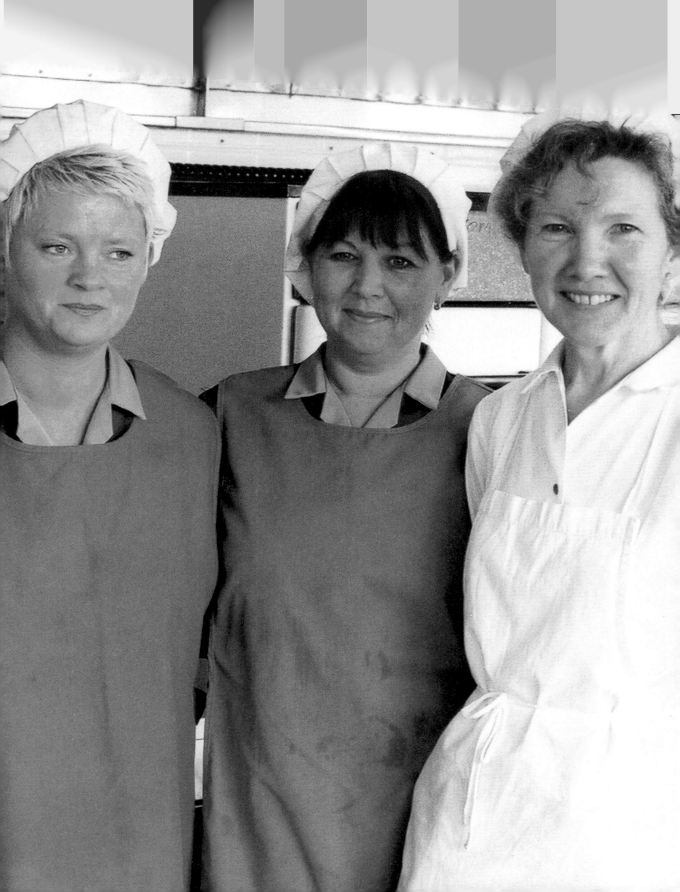

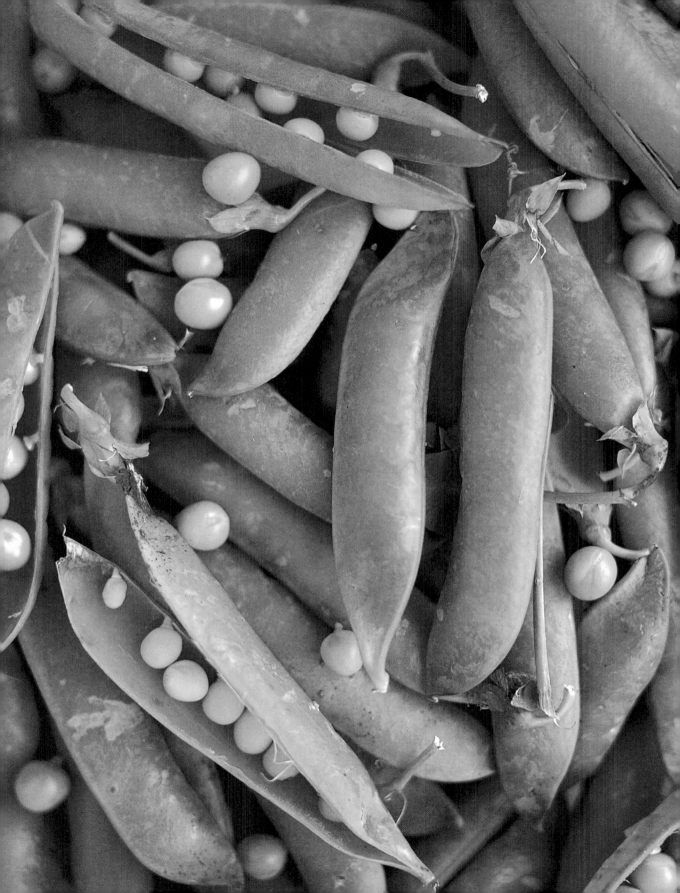

PEAS

Fresh peas are one of the real joys of the world – there is something wonderful about the taste of freshly podded peas served simply with a little butter. Unless you live in the countryside, and can grow your own, this opportunity has become rarer and rarer, but to the credit of commercialization, frozen peas still remain in the top ten of some of the things that we produce well in large quantities.

EASY PEAS

Whether you are using fresh or frozen peas, for 4 people you need to put 4 good handfuls of peas into a wide frying pan or casserole-type pan which has a lid (or you can use tinfoil), with ½ a wineglass of white wine, ½ a wineglass of water and 2 good knobs of butter. Place the lid on top and bring to the boil, then remove the lid and simmer for a minute or two while you finely slice a handful of mint leaves. With this reasonably small amount of liquid, the butter and wine should form a fantastically simple sauce. Throw in the mint at the last minute and serve straight away. Don't forget that it only takes a handful of grated Parmesan cheese and some cooked tagliatelle to turn these peas into a wonderful pasta dish. Or you can add them to a risotto, or whizz them up with some chicken stock to make a fine pea soup.

FRENCH STYLE PEAS

This isn't the classic French way of doing it, but peas and lettuce are wonderful together. People often think you can't cook lettuce, but it becomes wonderfully sweet. For 4 people, you will need 4 good handfuls of fresh or frozen peas, 6 rashers of smoked streaky bacon, 2 gem lettuces, 2 knobs of butter and some chicken or veg stock. First, finely slice the bacon and fry in a little oil until crisp and golden. Add the peas and the gem lettuce, finely sliced. Mix up well, cover with 140ml/½ pint of chicken stock, and then simmer for 15 minutes until tender, removing the lid for the last 5 minutes to let the liquid reduce a little. Remove from the heat and add the butter. This will make the juice really creamy and oozy. Check the seasoning and serve straight away.

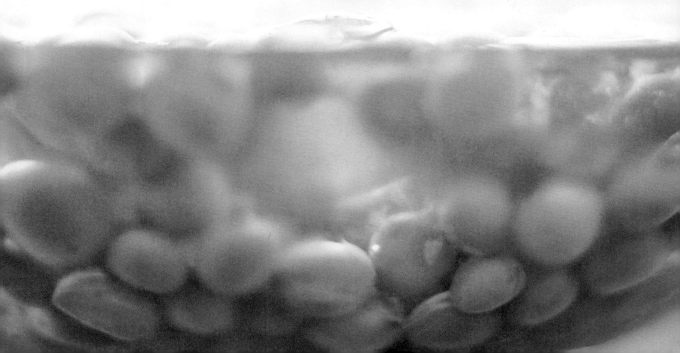

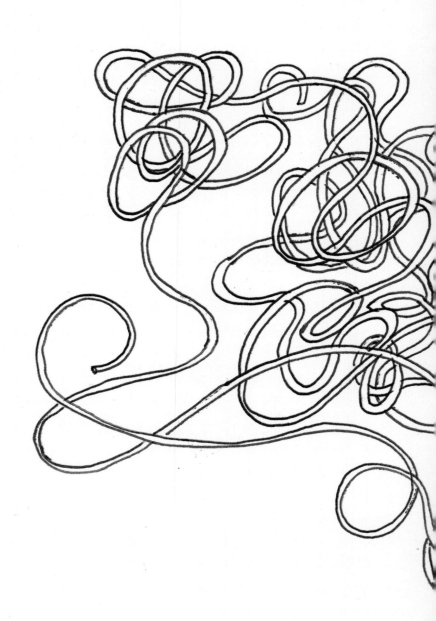

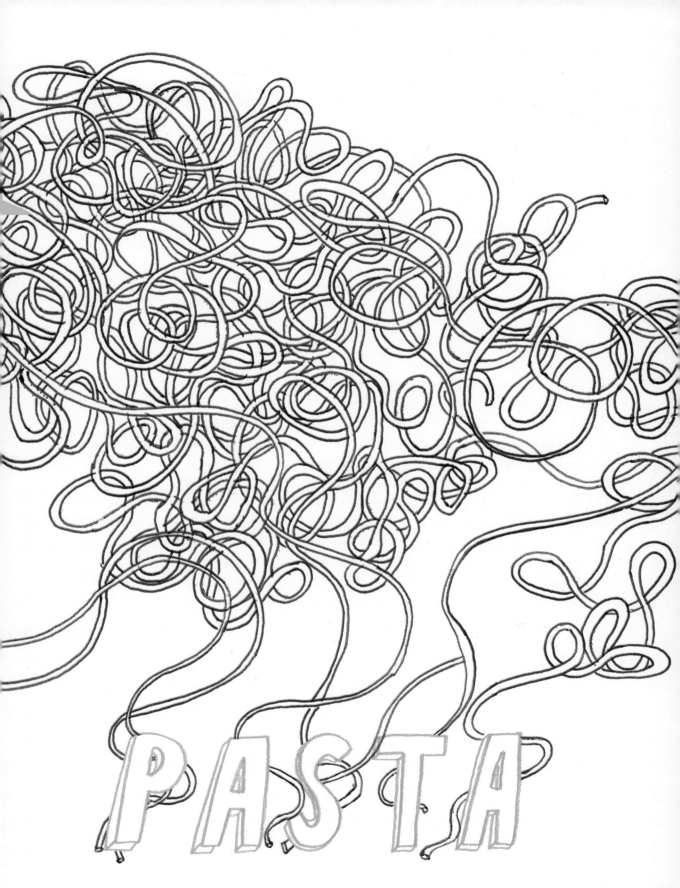

Pasta has always had a really important place in the kitchen, whether it's in a posh restaurant, in a school, or when you're living on a budget in your first place. That's the time when it was most important to me, because I wanted to eat well but economically too. So what I've done in this chapter is concentrate on all the cheap, accessible, hearty dishes that are great for making at home, or for large numbers of people. One thing I have noticed is that here in Britain people tend to use lots of sauce on their pasta, whereas in Italy only a small amount is used – just enough to lightly cover the 'star' of the dish: the pasta!

I've focused on dried pasta rather than fresh, as it's one of those store-cupboard items that's available all the time, just waiting to be used. There are some dishes included here that only take a few minutes to make, and others that can be baked in the oven and take a little longer. All are really comforting, easy to make and not particularly expensive, so have a go. I'm sure you'll love them all.

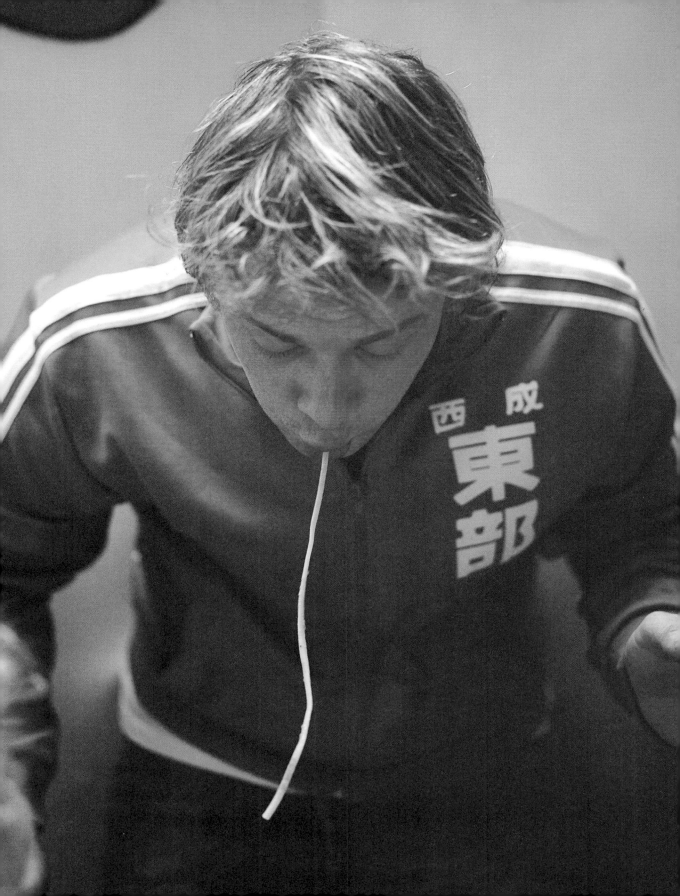

PASTA BIANCO

To kick this section off we're going to start with the most basic dish to make, using the simplest sauce – Pasta Bianco means 'white pasta'. When it comes to grating your garlic, I suggest you do this using a grater. The slices will almost turn into a paste when you fry them. You can use any kind of pasta, but classically it's made with fresh tagliatelle or tagliolini. This recipe gives you a really good feel for how to cook pasta properly – you want the sauce just to coat the pasta and not to be too claggy or sticky. If we ever have kids eating at the restaurant and they're a little fussy, they always tend to go for this, with a little bit of grated Parmesan cheese on the top.

This dish can also be quite luxurious. It's the key pasta dish that's made when white truffles are in season. The truffles are literally sliced over the top – I can't think of anything nicer to have with them than really cheesy, buttery pasta.

SERVES 4
2 cloves of garlic, peeled and finely grated
40g/1½oz butter
455g/1lb tagliatelle
2 or 3 handfuls of freshly grated Parmesan cheese
sea salt and freshly ground black pepper

In a small shallow pan, slowly fry the grated garlic in the butter without colouring for a couple of minutes. Bring a large pan of salted water to the boil, add the pasta, and cook according to the packet instructions. When it's done, drain it in a colander over a bowl so you save some of the starchy cooking water. Reserving this water and using it to finish off a pasta sauce is absolutely critical to getting any pasta sauce right, especially this one.

Get yourself a big warmed pasta or salad bowl and pour your melted garlic butter into it so that the whole surface is covered. Then toss in your cooked pasta with about 5 or 6 tablespoons of the reserved cooking water and the Parmesan cheese. Season to taste. With some tongs, or two forks, toss the pasta around. The butter, garlic, water and Parmesan will form a really creamy sauce.

What you need to do next is get everyone round the table. You may have to keep feeding the pasta with a little of the reserved cooking water, so the sauce stays silky and delicate and not too sticky. Once you get the consistency right, serve the pasta into bowls and pass round a big chunk of Parmesan cheese and a grater.

There are many ways of varying this sauce – you can lay some prosciutto over, or stir some chopped tomatoes into your garlic butter before removing from the heat, or you can incorporate different cheeses, but the key is to get simple, well-seasoned, delicate pasta coated in a butter cheese sauce. Once you get this pasta exactly right, try to make it with a bit more speed next time – the quicker you can do it and get it right, the better the pasta will be.

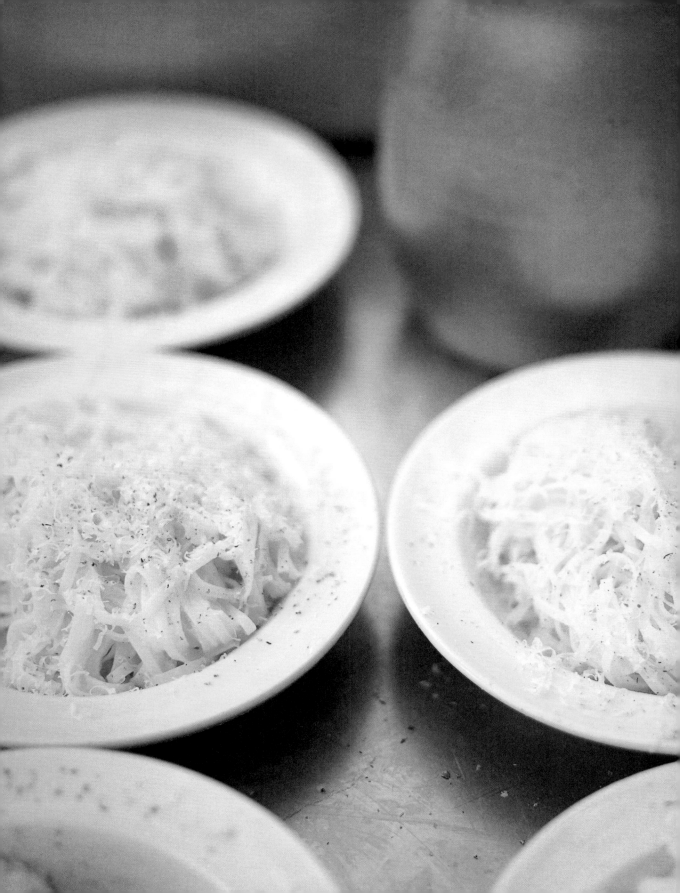

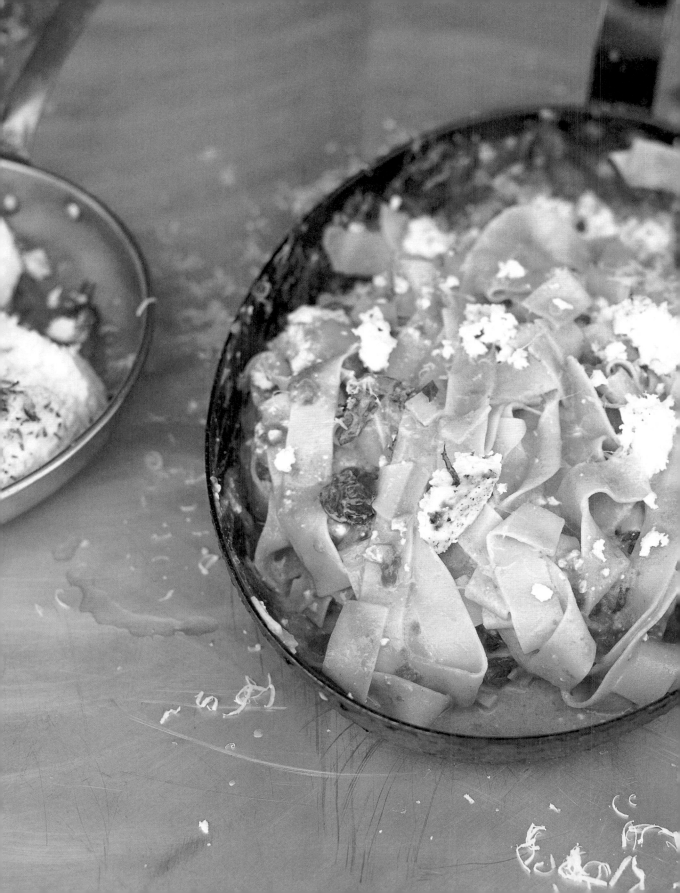

PASTA WITH SWEET TOMATO SAUCE AND BAKED RICOTTA

This pasta dish uses a basic tomato sauce. The sweetness of it will depend on the quality of your tinned tomatoes. If they are of the very best quality then you shouldn't need to add any sugar at all. You should also use whole tomatoes – don't buy pre-chopped ones, otherwise the seeds will add a bitterness to the sauce. The ricotta is baked separately with herbs and olive oil and is then crumbled over the top – it's a really good recipe.

SERVES 4

450g/1lb piece of ricotta cheese
extra virgin olive oil
sea salt and freshly ground
   black pepper
1 flat teaspoon dried oregano
½ a dried chilli, crumbled
1 onion, peeled and
   finely chopped
2 cloves of garlic, peeled and
   finely chopped

a knob of butter
2 x 400g tins of good-quality
   plum tomatoes
3 tablespoons balsamic vinegar
½ teaspoon sugar
455g/1lb pappardelle
a handful of fresh basil, leaves torn
2 handfuls of freshly grated
   Parmesan cheese

Preheat the oven to 200°C/400°F/gas 6. Rub the ricotta all over with the olive oil, salt, pepper, oregano and chilli, place on a baking tray, and cook in the oven for 20 minutes until golden and firm. In a pan, slowly fry the onion and garlic in the butter and a good drizzle of olive oil. Cook for 4 minutes until sweet and softened. Add the tomatoes, simmer gently for about 15 minutes, then break the tomatoes up with a spoon. Add the balsamic vinegar and the sugar and stir until you have a nice fine tomato sauce.

Meanwhile, bring a large pan of salted water to the boil and cook the pappardelle according to the packet instructions. When cooked, drain and reserve some of the cooking water. Toss the pasta with the tomato sauce and add a little of the reserved water to loosen, if necessary. Correct the seasoning carefully to taste, and then, working quickly, add most of the basil and Parmesan cheese. Place into a warmed bowl, rip over some extra basil, and grate over a little extra Parmesan. Either crumble the baked ricotta over the pasta, or serve it at the table with a spoon in it and let everyone crumble some over their plates.

TAGLIATELLE WITH SPINACH, MASCARPONE AND PARMESAN

Again, this is a really good dish for kids. Even though they may not eat spinach on its own, I've never had a problem feeding this to my two-year-old. The reason she likes it so much is because she can suck on the spaghetti, and the mascarpone and cooking water make a fantastic sauce.

SERVES 4
455g/1lb tagliatelle or spaghetti
olive oil
2 teaspoons butter
2 cloves of garlic, peeled and sliced
½ a nutmeg, freshly grated
400g/14oz fresh spinach, washed thoroughly and finely sliced
sea salt and freshly ground black pepper
120ml/4fl oz double cream
150g/5oz mascarpone cheese
2 handfuls of freshly grated Parmesan cheese

Bring a large pan of salted water to the boil, add the pasta, and cook according to the packet instructions. Meanwhile get a frying pan or wok warm, add a drizzle of olive oil, the butter, garlic and nutmeg. When the butter melts, add the spinach. After 5 minutes it will have wilted down and will be nice and dark. A lot of the liquid will have cooked away and you'll have wonderful intensely flavoured spinach. At this point season with salt and pepper until it tastes good, then add the cream, mascarpone and a little ladle of cooking water from the pasta. Let this come to a simmer and then season again.

Drain the pasta, reserving some of the cooking water, then stir it into the spinach sauce. Add the Parmesan and toss everything together. Loosen to a nice silky consistency with some of the reserved cooking water, so it doesn't become too claggy. Check once more for seasoning and serve straight away.

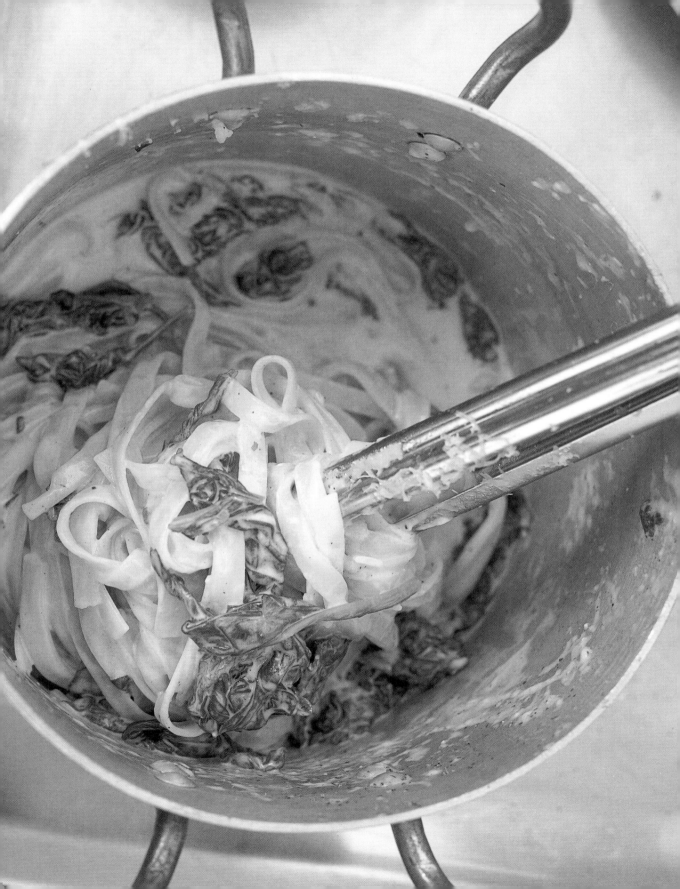

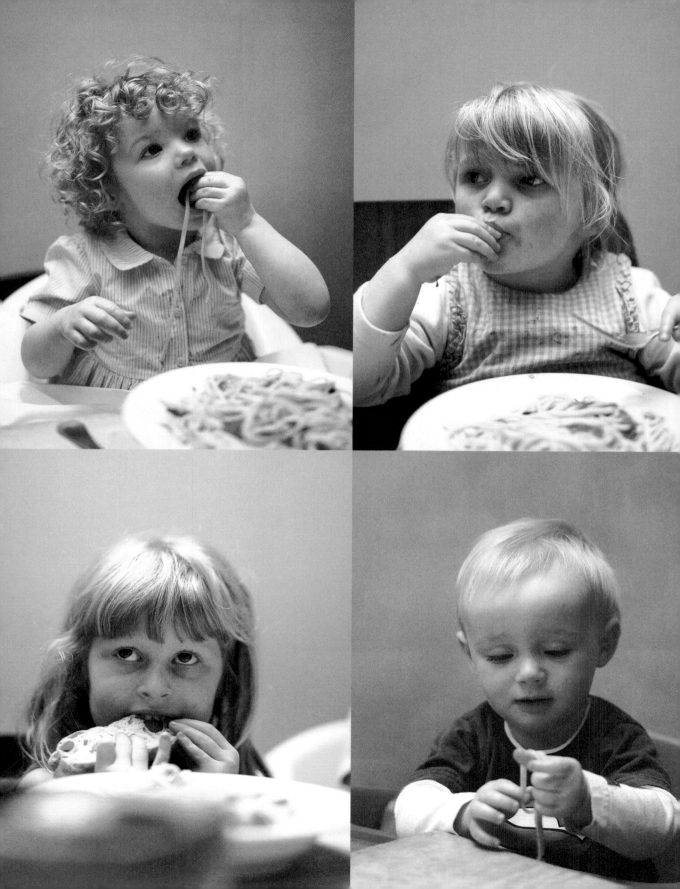

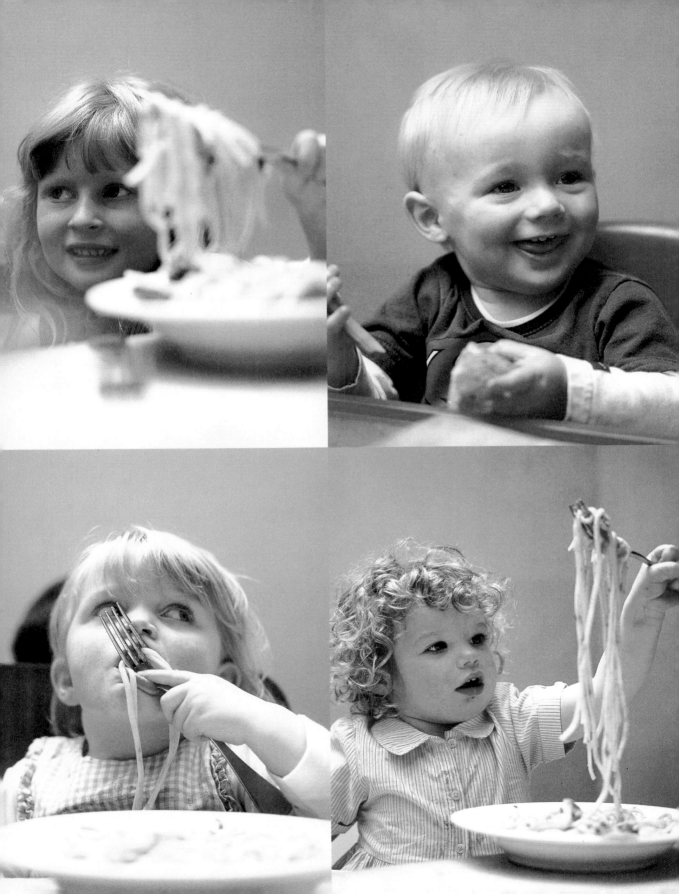

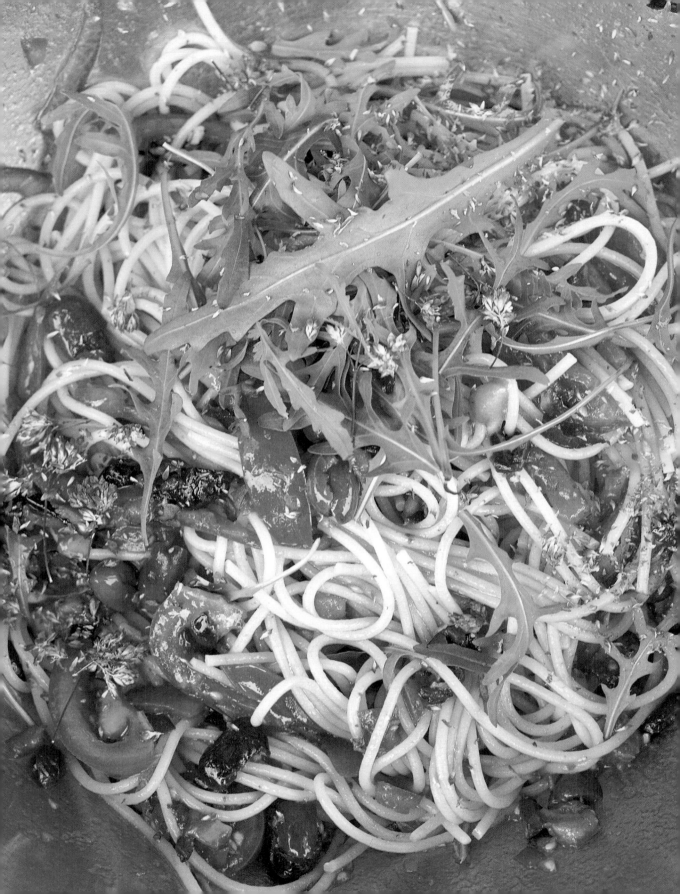

SPAGHETTI WITH UNCOOKED TOMATO, ROCKET AND OLIVE SAUCE

When you get home and you've got the munchies but no food planned, this is one of the quick things you can get done in ten minutes. The thing to remember is that you will get better results and a better flavour if your tomatoes are at room temperature before you begin, not used straight from the fridge.

SERVES 4
455g/1lb spaghetti
5 nice medium-sized ripe tomatoes
2 handfuls of fresh basil
a good handful of tasty black or green olives,
    stones removed
2 handfuls of fresh rocket, washed
1 flat teaspoon dried oregano, or a small handful of
    fresh oregano, chopped
2 tablespoons balsamic vinegar
6 tablespoons extra virgin olive oil
sea salt and freshly ground black pepper

Bring a pan of salted water to the boil, add your spaghetti and cook it according to the packet instructions. Gather your guests round the table and ask them to sort out drinks, plates and cutlery while you chop up the tomatoes and basil. You can do this any old way – little chunks, pulpy bits, just chop it all up. Chop the olives up a bit as well if you want to. Finely slice the stalky bits of the rocket and roughly chop the leaves. Put all these ingredients in a bowl with the oregano. Then add the balsamic vinegar and extra virgin olive oil, and season carefully with salt and pepper. Taste and season, taste and season, until you get it spot on.

By now your pasta should be cooked, so drain it, reserving some of the cooking water. Throw the pasta into the bowl with the tomatoes and toss well. You probably won't need to add any of the cooking water to this because the tomatoes are quite watery, but do add a little if you feel the sauce needs loosening slightly. Work quite fast, because it's the heat of the pasta that warms up the tomatoes and you don't want it to get cold. However, if it does get cold all is not lost, as it makes a great pasta salad! Serve with some wine and a green salad. Knowing Italians, they'd have some crusty bread as well. And a nice bit of Parmesan or pecorino to grate over the top is a joy.

RIGATONI WITH SWEET TOMATOES, AUBERGINE AND MOZZARELLA

This is a dish I've had many times in Italy, on the Amalfi coast. It's one of those dishes that tastes like home – it's comfort food and it makes you feel good. The interesting thing about it is that it uses the firmer cow's milk mozzarella, which is torn up and thrown in at the last minute so that when you dig your spoon in you get melted, stringy bits of cheese – a real joy to eat. You can serve this as soon as it's made, or you can put it all into a baking tray with a little cheese grated on top and reheat it as a baked pasta dish next day if you wish.

SERVES 4

1 firm ripe pink, black or
    white aubergine
extra virgin olive oil
2 cloves of garlic, peeled
    and sliced
1 onion, peeled and
    finely chopped
2 x 400g tins of good-quality
    plum tomatoes
1 tablespoon balsamic vinegar

sea salt and freshly ground
    black pepper
optional: 1–2 fresh or dried chillies,
    chopped or crumbled
a bunch of fresh basil, leaves ripped
    and stalks sliced
4 tablespoons double cream
455g/1lb rigatoni or penne
200g/7oz cow's milk mozzarella
1 piece of Parmesan cheese, for grating

Remove both ends of the aubergine and slice it into 1cm/½ inch slices, then slice these across and finely dice into 1cm/½ inch cubes. Some people prefer to season their aubergine with salt and let it sit for a while in a colander to draw out the bitterness, but I don't really do this unless I'm dealing with a seedy, bitter aubergine. This dish is really best made using a firm silky one.

Now put a large saucepan on the heat and drizzle in 4 to 5 tablespoons of extra virgin olive oil. When it's hot, add the cubes of aubergine, and as soon as they hit the pan stir them around with a spoon so they are delicately coated with the oil and not soaked on one side only. Cook for about 7 or 8 minutes on a medium heat. Then add the garlic and onion. When they have a little colour, add the tinned tomatoes and the balsamic vinegar. Stir around and season carefully with salt and pepper. At this point, if you wanted to give the dish a little heat you could add some chopped fresh or crumbled dried chilli, but that's down to you. Add the basil stalks, and simmer the sauce nice and gently for around 15 minutes, then add the cream.

While the sauce is simmering, bring a large pan of salted water to the boil and add the pasta. Cook according to the packet instructions until it is soft but still holding its shape, then drain it, saving a little of the cooking water. I like to put the pasta back into the pot it was cooked in with a tiny bit of the cooking water and a drizzle of olive oil and move it around so it becomes almost dressed with the water and oil.

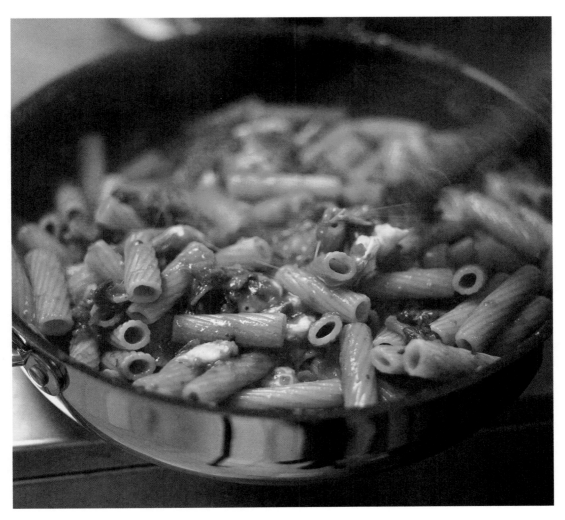

At this point add the lovely tomato sauce to the pasta. By now the aubergines will have cooked into a creamy tomatoey pulp, which is just yum yum yum! Season carefully to taste with salt and pepper. When all my guests are sitting round the table, I take the pan to the table, tear up the mozzarella and the fresh basil, and fold these in nicely for 30 seconds. Then very quickly serve into bowls. By the time your guests start to eat, the mozzarella will have started to melt and will be stringy and gorgeous and really milky-tasting. Just lovely with the tomatoes and aubergine. Serve at the table with a block of Parmesan cheese and a grater so that everyone can help themselves.

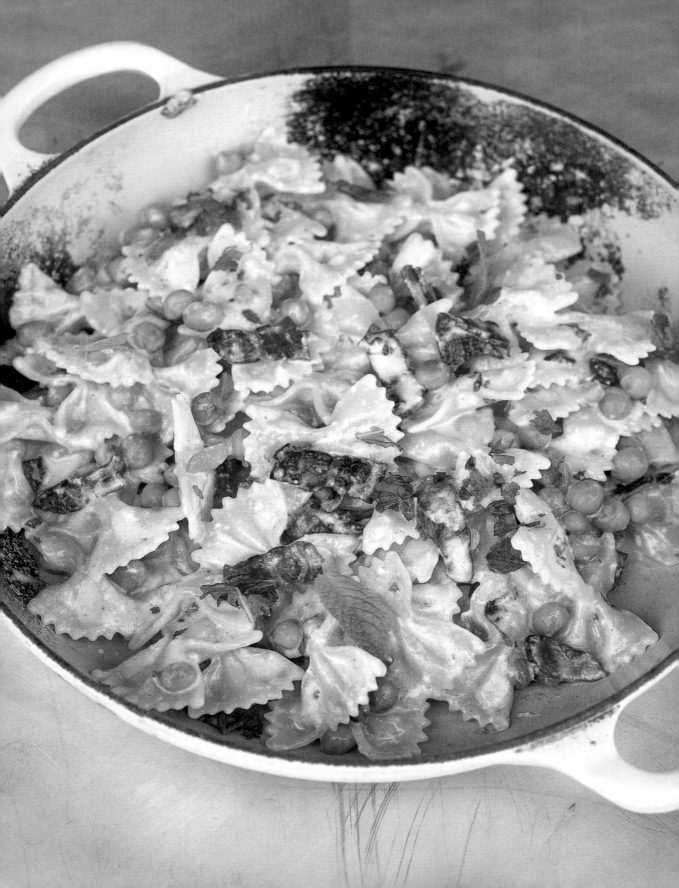

FARFALLE WITH CARBONARA AND SPRING PEAS

This is a twist on the classic carbonara, using spring peas and smoky bacon. A great combination and a great one for the kids. My girls just love it.

SERVES 4
455g/1lb farfalle
1 egg
100ml/3½fl oz double cream
sea salt and freshly ground black pepper
12 rashers of pancetta or smoked streaky bacon, roughly sliced
3 handfuls of fresh podded or frozen peas
2 sprigs of fresh mint, leaves picked
2 handfuls of freshly grated Parmesan cheese

First of all, bring a large pan of salted water to the boil, add the farfalle, and cook according to the packet instructions. Whisk the egg in a bowl with the cream, salt and pepper. Put your pancetta or bacon into a second pan and cook until crispy and golden.

When the farfalle is nearly cooked, add the peas for the last minute and a half. This way they will burst in your mouth and be lovely and sweet. When cooked, drain in a colander, saving a little of the cooking water. Add the pasta to the pancetta and stir in most of the mint, finely sliced – if the pan isn't big enough, mix it all together in a large warmed bowl.

Now you need to add the egg and cream mix to the pasta. What's important here is that you add it while the pasta is still steaming hot. This way, the residual heat of the pasta will cook the eggs, but not so that they resemble scrambled eggs, as I've seen in some dodgy old restaurants on the motorway! The pasta will actually cook the egg enough to give you a silky smooth sauce. Toss together and loosen with a little of the reserved cooking water if necessary. Season with salt and pepper, sprinkle with the Parmesan and the rest of the mint leaves, and serve as soon as possible.

PS Work quickly and eat straight away for best results.

AWESOME SPINACH AND RICOTTA CANNELLONI

This is such a wonderfully light and super-tasty cannelloni, and again I've avoided making the frustrating, painstaking béchamel sauce and given you a much tastier and simpler version. All you need to make sure of is that you fill the cannelloni well with the ricotta and spinach mix, so it's not all full of air. And the lovely thing about it is that it goes crispy and golden on top, but remains soft and moist at the bottom. You'll love it!

SERVES 4
2 knobs of butter
olive oil
2 cloves of garlic, peeled and
    finely sliced
a large handful of fresh marjoram
    or oregano, roughly chopped
¼ of a nutmeg, grated
8 large handfuls of spinach,
    thoroughly washed
a handful of fresh basil, stalks
    chopped, leaves ripped
2 x 400g tins of good-quality
    plum tomatoes, chopped

sea salt and freshly ground
    black pepper
a pinch of sugar
400g/14oz crumbly ricotta cheese
2 handfuls of freshly grated
    Parmesan cheese
16 cannelloni tubes
200g/7oz mozzarella, broken up

FOR THE WHITE SAUCE
1 x 500ml tub of crème fraîche
3 anchovies, finely chopped
2 handfuls of freshly grated
    Parmesan cheese

Preheat the oven to 180°C/350°F/gas 4. Then find a metal baking tray or ovenproof dish that will fit the cannelloni in one layer so it's nice and snug. This way you'll get the right cover of sauce and the right amount of crispiness on top. When I cook this at home I just use one pan to cut down on lots of washing up! Take your metal tray or a saucepan, put it on a high heat and add your butter, a drizzle of olive oil, one of the sliced garlic cloves, a handful of marjoram or oregano and the grated nutmeg. By the time the pan is hot the garlic should be soft. Put as much spinach as will fit into the pan. Keep turning it over; it will wilt quickly so you will be able to keep adding more spinach until it's all in. Moisture will cook out of the spinach, which is fine. By cooking it this way you don't lose any of the nutrients that you would if boiling it in water.

(Continued ➔)

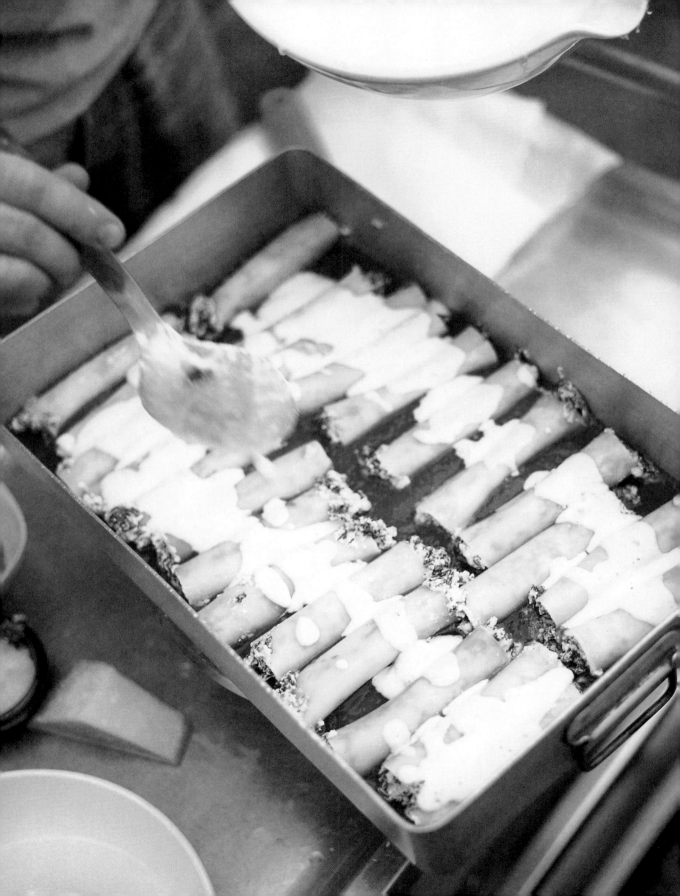

After 5 minutes, put the spinach into a large bowl and leave to cool. Place the pan back on the heat, add a little olive oil, the other clove of sliced garlic, your basil stalks and the tomatoes, then fill one of the empty tomato tins with cold water and add this too. Bring to the boil, then turn the heat down, add a pinch of salt and pepper and the sugar, and simmer for about 10 minutes, until you get a loose tomato sauce consistency. Then take the pan off the heat and add the basil leaves.

By now the spinach will have cooled down, so squeeze any excess liquid out of it and pour this back into the bowl. Finely chop the spinach and put it back into the bowl. Mix it with the liquid, add the ricotta and a handful of the Parmesan, and then use a piping bag to squeeze the mixture into the cannelloni. You can make your own piping bag by getting a sandwich bag and putting the spinach mix into the corner of it. Then twist the bag up and cut the corner off. Carefully squeeze the filling into the cannelloni tubes so each one is filled right up – really easy.

Lay the cannelloni over the tomato sauce in the pan. Or you can pour the tomato sauce into your ovenproof dish and lay the cannelloni on top. To make the white sauce, mix together the crème fraîche, anchovies and the 2 handfuls of Parmesan with a little salt and pepper, then loosen with a little water until you can spoon it over the cannelloni. Drizzle with olive oil, sprinkle with the remaining Parmesan and the mozzarella pieces, and bake for about 20 to 25 minutes until golden and bubbling.

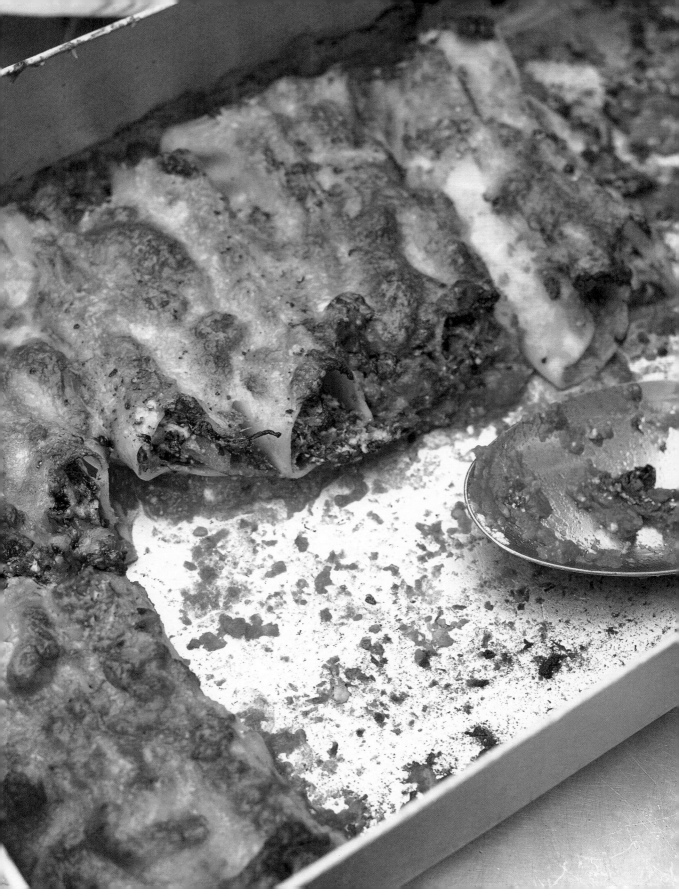

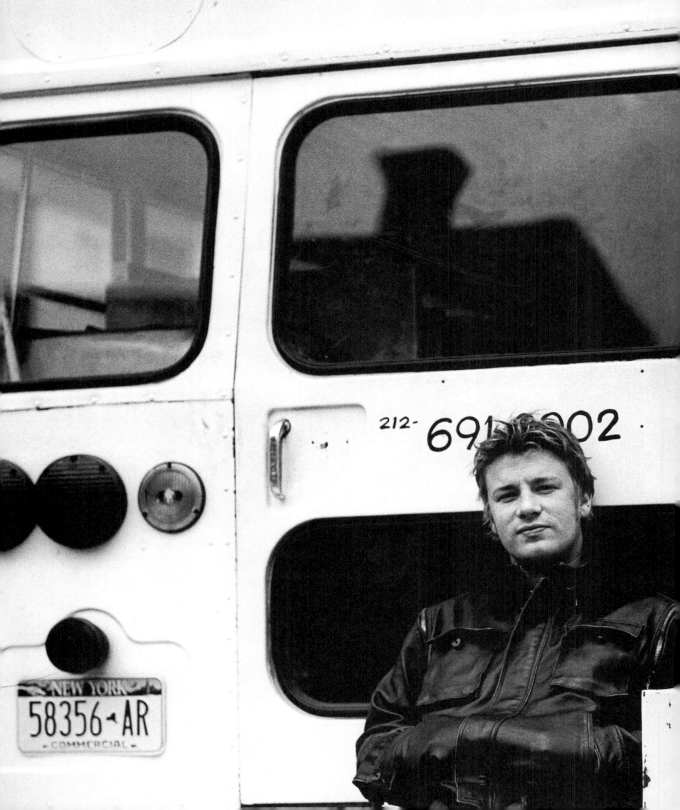

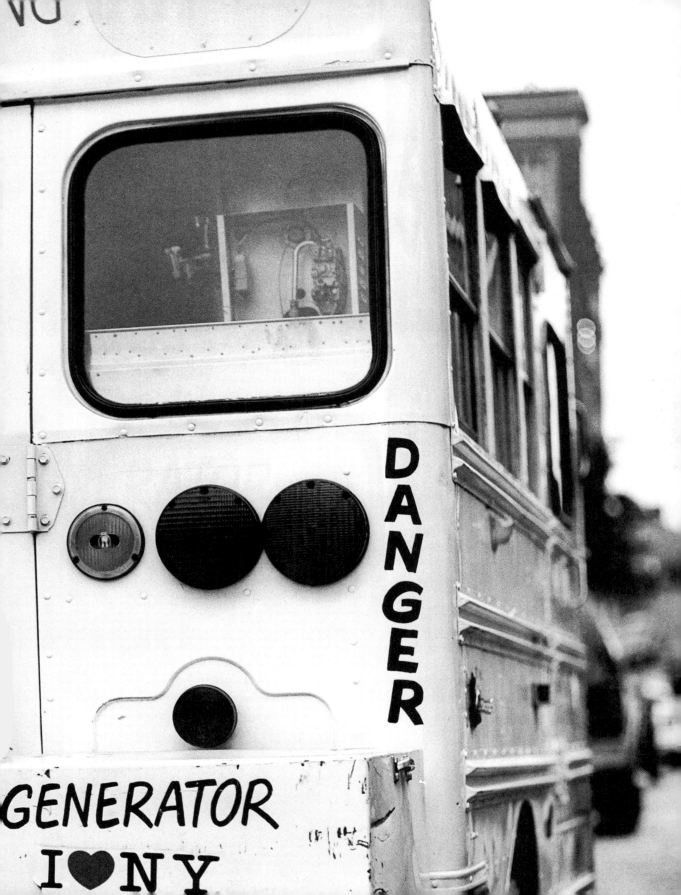

QUICK TOMATO MACARONI CHEESE

I think this is the best macaroni cheese recipe ever! This is a dish I make for the whole family, one that we all love to eat. I've used sweet tomatoes in my recipe as they really complement the cheese, and instead of béchamel sauce I've used single cream, as it's a lot lighter. I've also topped the dish off with cheesy breadcrumbs, which give it a wonderful crunch. I think you'll laugh when you see how easy it is to make. I put it together extremely quickly by using my Magimix food processor. Don't worry if you haven't got one – you can chop it all up by hand instead and then mix it in a bowl.

SERVES 4
340g/12oz macaroni
200g/7oz bread, preferably stale,
    for making breadcrumbs
800g/1¾lb super ripe tomatoes
1 clove of garlic, peeled
2 large handfuls of fresh basil
55g/2oz sun-dried tomatoes,
    chopped
2 anchovies
sea salt and freshly ground
    black pepper

3 handfuls of freshly grated
    Parmesan cheese
565ml/1 pint single cream
1 tablespoon red wine vinegar
½ a nutmeg, grated
400g/14oz cow's milk mozzarella,
    broken up
a handful of fresh thyme,
    leaves picked
extra virgin olive oil

Preheat your oven to 200°C/400°F/gas 6. Get a pan of salted boiling water going and cook your macaroni according to the packet instructions. Meanwhile, break your bread up, place it in the food processor and whizz up to form breadcrumbs. Set aside. Wash your tomatoes and place them in the food processor with the garlic, basil, sun-dried tomatoes, anchovies and a good pinch of salt and pepper. Whizz up for 30 seconds. Then add 2 handfuls of the Parmesan, the cream, vinegar and grated nutmeg. Whizz until smooth and season carefully to taste so it's really yummy!

By this time your macaroni will probably be cooked, so drain it in a colander, saving some of the cooking water. Place the pasta back into the pan and pour over every last bit of the cheesy sauce. You want it to be quite loose because you'll be surprised how quickly the sauce will disappear inside the macaroni and will look dry. So add a few spoonfuls of the reserved cooking water. Now you need to get yourself a baking dish about 8–10 cm/3 or 4 inches deep – this could be an earthenware dish or even a shallow ovenproof pan. Pour the pasta straight into your baking dish and break the mozzarella into little pieces over the top. Mix the last handful of Parmesan with the thyme leaves and breadcrumbs and sprinkle evenly over the top of the dish. Drizzle generously with good extra virgin olive oil – this will give you a lovely crunchy topping.

Place in the preheated oven for 20–25 minutes or until piping hot and golden on top. Serve straight away, sprinkled with a little extra Parmesan. Best eaten with a nice salad – and you'll love it.

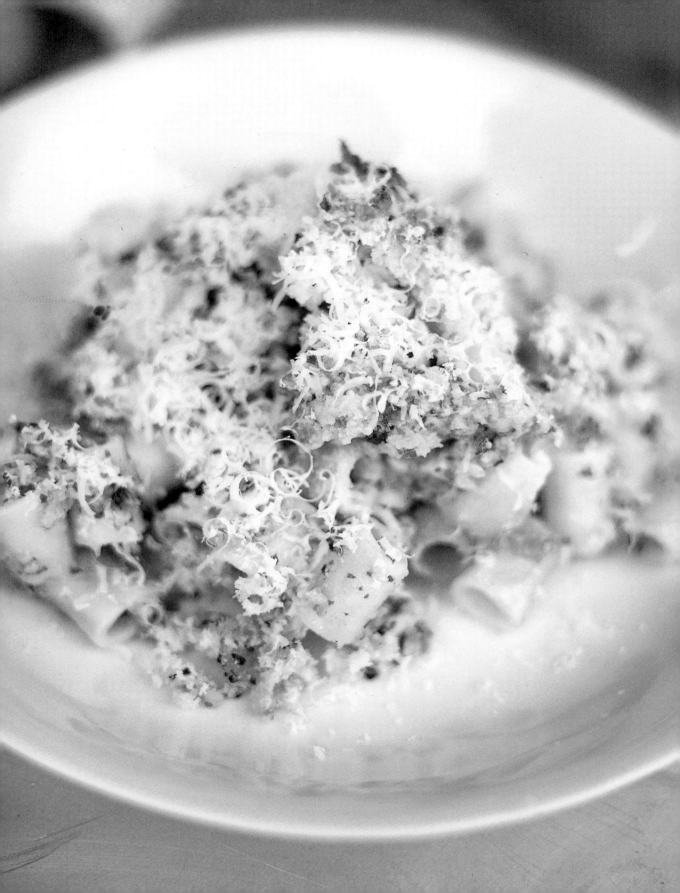

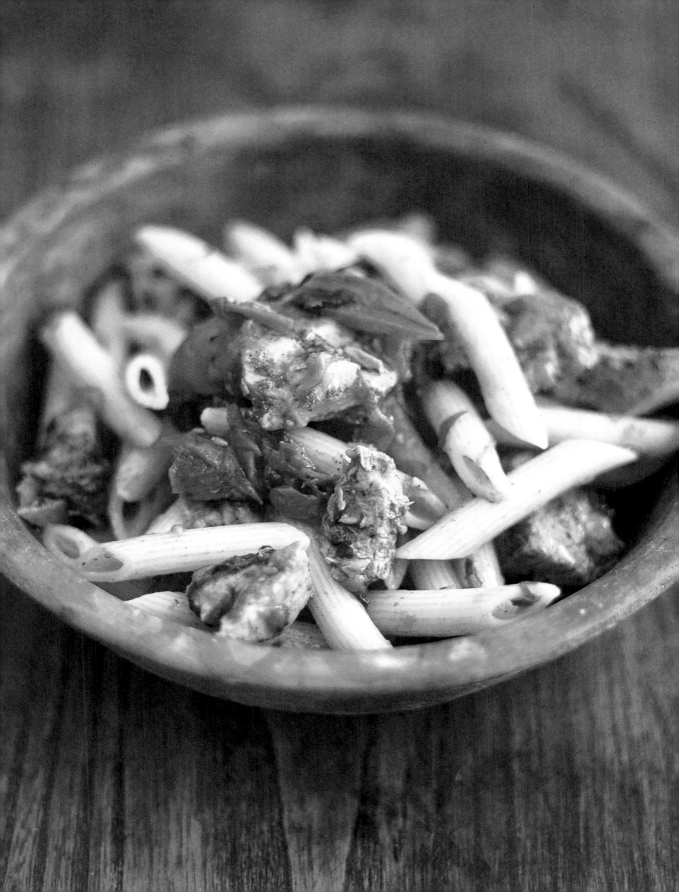

WORKING GIRL'S PASTA

This is a pasta dish that Gennaro Contaldo used to make for our staff dinners when we worked at the Neal Street Restaurant in Covent Garden. In Italian this is called 'pasta putana', which basically translates as 'whore's pasta'! I wanted to know why, as I'd never heard of this before. Maybe it's because the dish was cooked very quickly, with no effort involved, or maybe it's something the local prostitutes used to eat at home – who knows?!

But this is the way my darling Gennaro taught me to make it. He comes from the Amalfi coast, where fresh tuna would have been available. If you can get hold of some it will make the dish much more luxurious and an event to eat. But if you can't, then tinned will do.

SERVES 4

a handful of fresh basil
sea salt and freshly ground
    black pepper
zest and juice of 1 lemon
extra virgin olive oil
2 x 225g/8oz tuna steaks, chopped
    into bite-size chunks, or 2 tins
    of good-quality tuna, packed in
    oil, drained
400g/14oz penne or spaghetti
8 anchovy fillets
2 cloves of garlic, peeled and
    finely chopped

2 handfuls of soaked capers
a handful of black olives, stoned and
    roughly chopped
1–3 small dried chillies, crumbled to
    your taste, or 1 fresh red chilli,
    deseeded and finely sliced
2 handfuls of really ripe tomatoes,
    finely chopped
optional: a swig of white wine
a handful of fresh flat-leaf parsley,
    finely chopped

Smash the basil to a pulp with a pinch of salt and pepper. Add the lemon zest and juice and 2 good lugs of extra virgin olive oil. Mix this up and either rub over your chopped-up fresh tuna or mix with your broken-up tinned tuna and allow to marinate.

Get a large pan of salted boiling water on and cook the pasta according to the packet instructions. As soon as you put the pasta on, put 3 or 4 good lugs of extra virgin olive oil into a large frying pan and put on the heat. As the pan starts to get warm, add your anchovy fillets and allow them to fry and melt. At this point add your garlic, capers, olives and chilli and stir around for a couple of minutes. If you have used fresh tuna, add it to the pan now with all of the marinating juices and sear it on both sides. When done, add the tomatoes and a little swig of white wine if you have some. If you have used tinned tuna, add it to the pan at the same time as the tomatoes. Bring to the boil, then simmer for around 5 minutes, stirring regularly with a spoon, breaking the tuna up into smaller pieces. What you don't want to do is overcook the tuna so it goes tough. You want it to be soft and silky. Correct the seasoning carefully with salt and pepper.

The pasta should now be ready, so drain it in a colander, reserving some of the cooking liquid. Toss the hot pasta with the hot tuna sauce, add the parsley and mix well. You may need a few more lugs of olive oil and a spoonful of cooking water to make the sauce nice and loose.

PASTA PEPERONATA

This is a great pasta dish using rigatoni, which is quite robust. It makes a really nice lunchtime snack. The mascarpone or crème fraîche is a lovely addition, but you can leave it out if you prefer. It will give you a wonderful mottled sauce, but try it without first and see how you go.

SERVES 4

2 red peppers, deseeded
  and sliced
2 yellow peppers, deseeded
  and sliced
extra virgin olive oil
sea salt and freshly ground
  black pepper
2 red onions, peeled and
  finely sliced
2 cloves of garlic, peeled
  and grated

2 handfuls of fresh flat-leaf parsley,
  leaves finely chopped, stalks reserved
2 tablespoons red wine vinegar or
  balsamic vinegar
2 handfuls of grated Parmesan cheese
optional: 2 heaped tablespoons
  mascarpone cheese or crème fraîche
455g/1lb rigatoni, penne or spaghetti

Put all the peppers in a large frying pan over a medium heat with a little olive oil and a pinch of salt and pepper. Place a lid on, and cook slowly for 15 minutes until softened. Don't rush this too much, as cooking the peppers slowly like this really helps to bring out the flavour. Add the onion and cook for a further 20 minutes. Then add the garlic and parsley stalks and toss around, keeping everything moving in the pan. Cook for about 3 minutes more. Have a little taste, and season with a bit more salt and pepper. Add the vinegar – it will sizzle away, so give everything a good toss. Then add one handful of the grated Parmesan and the mascarpone or crème fraîche if you are using it and turn the heat down to minimum while you cook the pasta.

Meanwhile put a large pot of salted water on to boil. Add the pasta to the boiling water and cook according to the packet instructions. When cooked, drain in a colander, reserving some of the cooking water. Put the peppers, pasta and parsley leaves into a large warmed bowl. Give them a good toss together, then add a little of the pasta cooking water and a few good lugs of extra virgin olive oil to coat the pasta nicely. Serve straight away, sprinkled with the rest of the Parmesan.

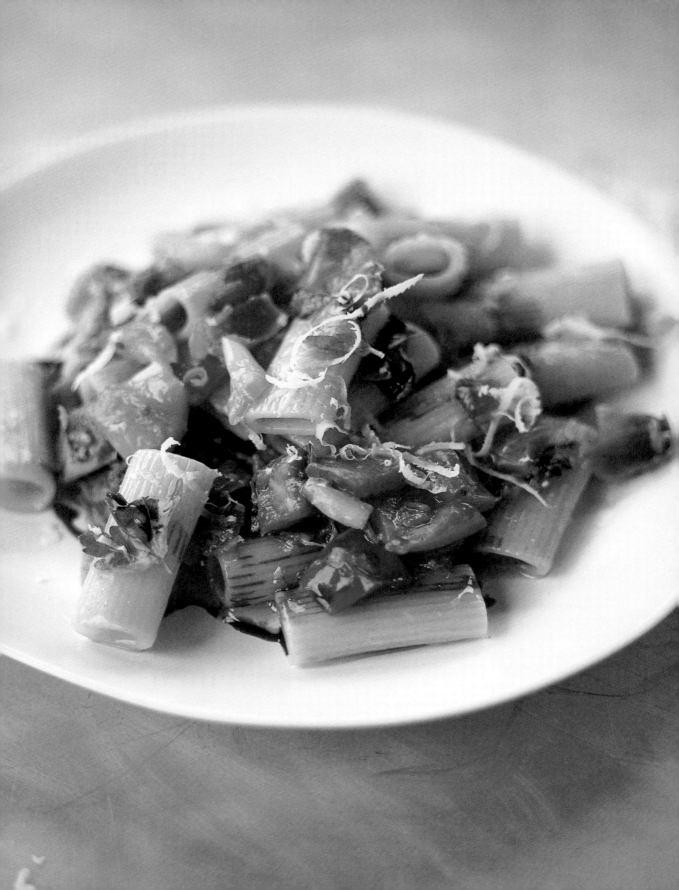

SWEET RED ONION PASTA

I was inspired to make this after hearing of a soup called 'carabaccia' that is flavoured with a stick of cinnamon. One of my students brought the recipe back from his work experience in Tuscany and it tastes amazing. So, on the same vibe, here's a pasta dish which I've made a little brothy – unusual but very nice. I would suggest using as many different varieties of onion as you can find.

SERVES 4

olive oil
2 large knobs of butter
2 white onions, peeled and sliced
3 red onions, peeled and sliced
1 clove of garlic, peeled and
    finely sliced
1 red chilli, finely sliced
200g/7oz potatoes, finely sliced
½ a stick of cinnamon
a small handful of fresh thyme,
    leaves picked

sea salt and freshly ground
    black pepper
a grating of nutmeg
455g/1lb fusilli or spaghetti
250ml/9fl oz chicken or vegetable stock
2–3 handfuls of freshly grated
    Parmesan cheese
a handful of fresh flat-leaf parsley,
    finely chopped

Put a drizzle of olive oil and both knobs of butter into a casserole-type pan and slowly fry your onions, garlic, chilli and potatoes with the cinnamon stick. Cook slowly for 5 minutes, then put the lid on and continue cooking for another 5 to 8 minutes until lightly golden. Add the thyme leaves and season carefully with salt, pepper and a light grating of nutmeg.

Bring a separate pan of salted water to the boil, add the pasta and cook according to the packet instructions. Try one of the potatoes to check that it is soft (if not, you've made the slices too thick, but no worries – just add a little water to the pan and continue cooking until softened). Drain the pasta, reserving some of the cooking water. Add the stock to the onions and mush up about half of the potatoes. Discard the cinnamon stick and season to taste. Working quickly, toss the pasta with the onions and potatoes, loosening if necessary with a little of the reserved cooking water and add one or two handfuls of Parmesan and the parsley. When it's all nicely mixed together, serve in warmed bowls.

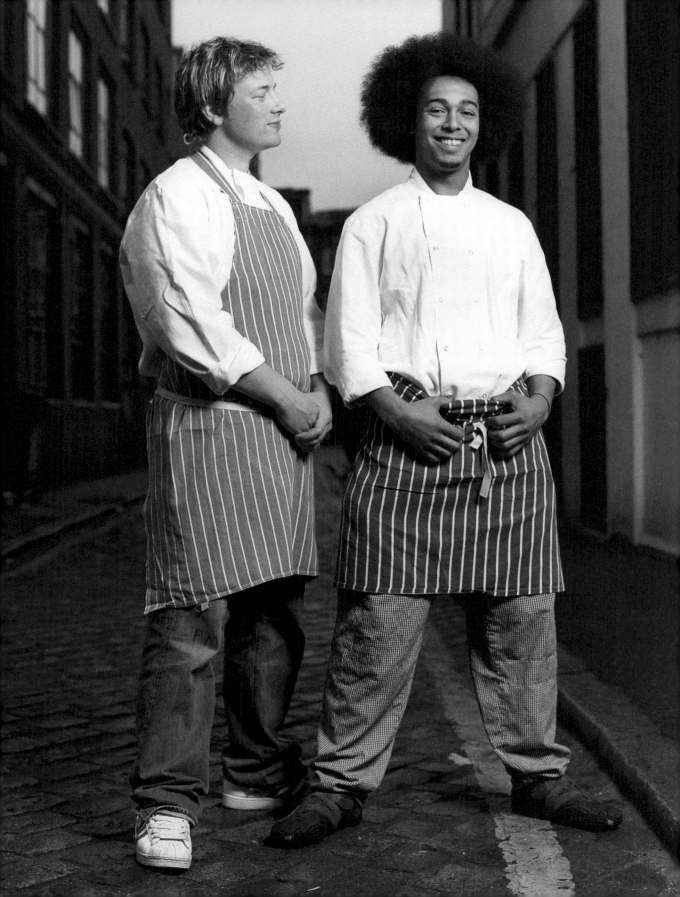

WING

NECK

MEAT

FRONT
QUARTER

BACK

WISHBONE

THIGH

HIND
QUARTER

DRUMSTICK

LEG

BREAST

HU

BRISK

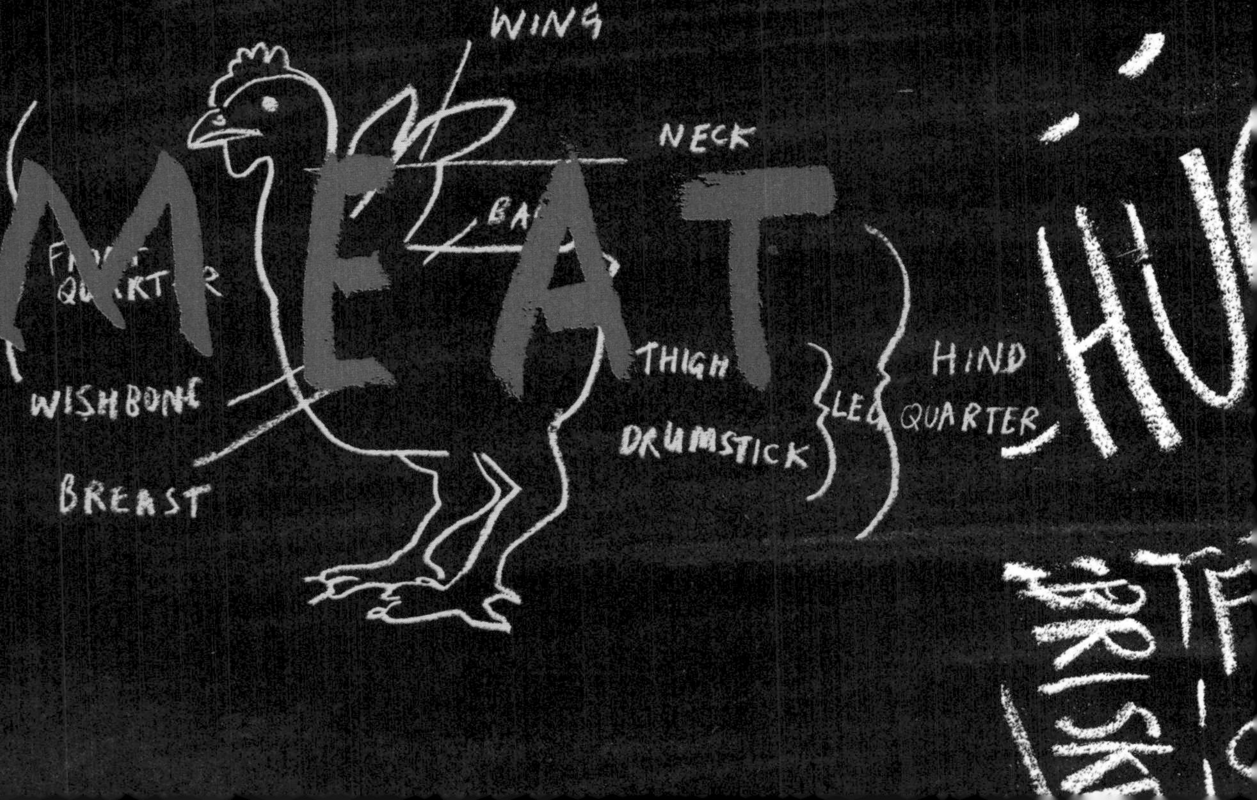

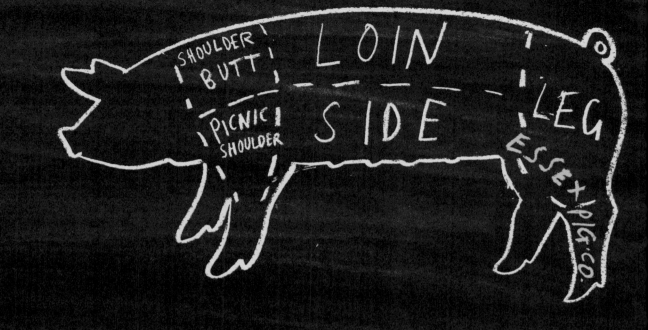

SHOULDER
BUTT

LOIN

LEG

PICNIC
SHOULDER

SIDE

ESSEX PIG CO.

RIB

LOIN

SHORT
RIB

SIRLOIN

RUN

RO

FEED ME FOOD - NOT MY FAMILY

ORGANIC FREE RANGE

When it comes to meat, always try to get the best you can afford. Although it's not always practical, it's great to know where your meat has come from, how it was raised, how long it was hung for and how it was butchered – try to build a relationship with your butcher and don't be afraid to ask him these things. Pale and pink meat, although it looks prettier than when it's a darker brown, just means that it has not been hung for very long, and it will always be far less tasty and far less tender. Also, don't be afraid of meat that is marbled with fat – it will have much more flavour.

Even though I try not to preach too hard about it, I'm a great believer in using organic or free-range meat. I'd much rather eat a slow-cooked cheaper cut of organic meat that's been properly raised than have a more expensive fillet or sirloin steak from God-knows-where, which will be tough with no flavour. If meat is organic it means that the animal has been reared without the routine use of drugs and antibiotics, which are common in intensive livestock farming. My friend Patrick Holden, Director of the Soil Association, told me that all organic livestock products – from eggs to sausages to milk – are automatically free-range as this is a required standard. Free-range basically means that the animals aren't kept cooped up, but are allowed to roam freely. I've come across quite a few skint students who have been cooking this way in their halls of residence really successfully. They have come to realize that they would rather spend their money on organic meat, so they choose cheaper cuts like brisket, shin, skirt and flank of beef, to name just a few.

Another thing to remember is that meat should be taken from the fridge in advance and allowed to reach room temperature before it's cooked – this will give you even cooking, and for the same reason it should also be allowed to rest for a while out of the oven, after cooking, before carving or serving.

What I like about this chapter is that a lot of the dishes are very easy to prepare. I've taken a few cheap, ultra-accessible meats and with a little bit of imagination and a twist have created some fantastically economical dishes – which is what family food and home cooking are all about.

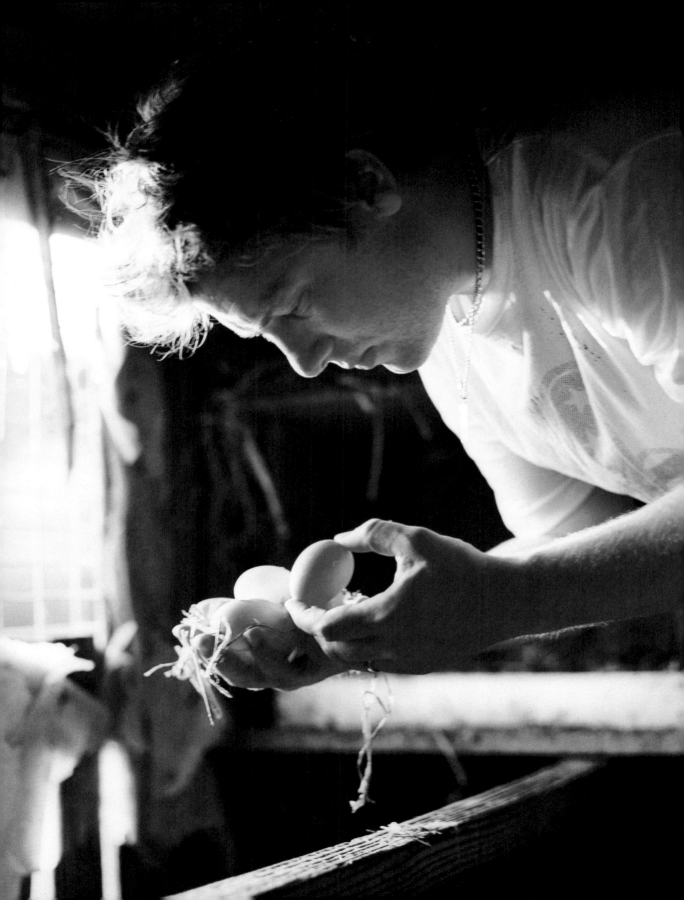

SUPER TASTY SPANISH ROAST CHICKEN

This is a cracker of a dish to cook at home. It will really get your taste buds going as it fills the house with the most fantastic smells.

SERVES 4
1kg/2lb 3oz potatoes, peeled and cut into 2.5cm/1 inch dice
4 lemons
a handful of fresh flat-leaf parsley, finely chopped
1 x 2kg/4½lb free-range organic chicken
sea salt and freshly ground black pepper
300g/11oz good chorizo sausage
olive oil
2 cloves of garlic, peeled and finely chopped

First preheat your oven to 220°C/425°F/gas 7, then place your potatoes with 2 of your lemons into a small pan of water and boil for 5 minutes. Drain, and then prick the lemons all over with a knife. (The reason for doing this is that you are going to put them inside the chicken and their wonderful juices will be released while cooking. They will burst with flavour and fragrance, and the heat from the lemons will help the chicken to cook quicker from the inside as well as making it taste and smell amazing.) Remove the parsley leaves from the stalks and put to one side. Stuff the chicken with your hot lemons and the parsley stalks. Then season the chicken and the potatoes with a little salt and freshly ground black pepper, and slice your chorizo at an angle, 0.5cm/¼ inch thick.

Get yourself an appropriately sized baking tray. Take a piece of greaseproof paper and wet it under a tap so it becomes flexible, then shake it out and lay it into the baking tray. Place the potatoes into the centre of the greaseproof paper, then place the chicken on top and sprinkle with the chorizo and a little of your chopped parsley. Drizzle with a little olive oil. Cook in the preheated oven for around 1 hour 20 minutes.

While the chicken and potatoes are cooking you can make what the Italians call gremolata, by finely chopping the zest of your 2 remaining lemons and mixing it with the chopped parsley and garlic. Season lightly and toss together to create a really fragrant seasoning-type garnish. Remove the tray from the oven, take the chicken out and put to one side to rest. Give the potatoes a shake about and put them back in the oven for a few minutes to crisp up.

Carve the chicken and divide between 4 plates, with the potatoes. The potatoes will have taken on the smoky paprika flavour from the chorizo, so if there is any juice left over in the tray, pour every last drop over the plates. When you sprinkle over the gremolata it will hit the hot juice and smell fantastic. You're going to love this one! A rocket salad goes really well with it.

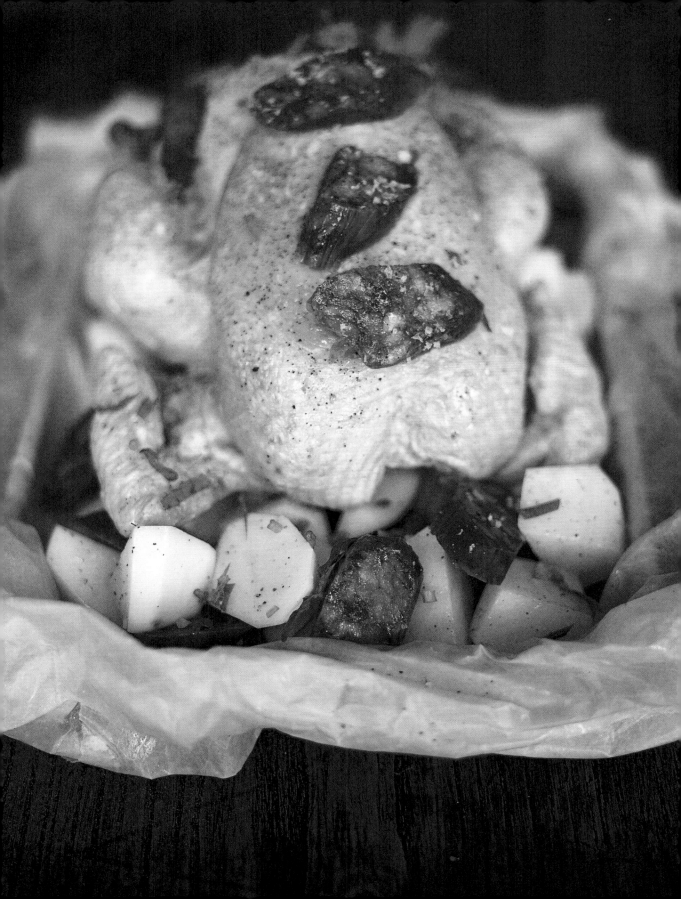

BEST LAMB CUTLETS WITH SPECIAL BASIL SAUCE

This dish is fantastic and you can literally have it ready in just over 5 minutes. Use either wild mushrooms that are in season, like girolles, trompettes de la mort and pieds de mouton, or more readily available farmed mushrooms like field, chestnut or oyster, as these are really tasty when cooked properly.

SERVES 4
12 lamb cutlets
a small handful of fresh thyme,
    leaves picked
extra virgin olive oil
sea salt and freshly ground
    black pepper

400g/14oz mushrooms, brushed
    clean and torn
a small handful of fresh flat-leaf parsley
1 lemon
2 handfuls of pine nuts
2 large handfuls of fresh basil
3–5 tablespoons balsamic vinegar

These lamb cutlets are best cooked on a hot barbecue with wood or charcoal, to give you a wonderful smoky flavour. Otherwise use a preheated ridged griddle pan. Slap the cutlets with the heel of your hand to flatten them slightly. Then bash up your thyme in a pestle and mortar and add a little olive oil. Mix together, then rub the oil over the cutlets and season both sides of them. Put to one side.

Cook the mushrooms dry on the bars of your hot griddle pan. This is quite an unusual way to do it, but it gives you a nutty flavour that you wouldn't get otherwise. Just grill them on both sides to mark them and put them into a large bowl. Once the mushrooms are done you can put the lamb on the barbecue or griddle pan. If the cutlets are about 1.5cm/¾ inch thick, just give them 3 or 4 minutes on each side until they're really golden. This should cook them medium. (To be honest, I'm not really into rare lamb cutlets, but if you prefer them like that then cook for a little less time.)

When cooked, put the lamb cutlets into the bowl with the mushrooms and drizzle with a little olive oil. Tear over the parsley, in quite large pieces, and add a good squeeze of lemon juice. Season lightly and toss around. Place to one side to rest, to allow all the lovely juices to get sucked up by the mushrooms.

Meanwhile you can make a really quick sauce. It looks a bit like pesto, but although it contains basil and pine nuts it has no similarity in flavour. In a pestle and mortar pound up the pine nuts until you have a mushy pulp – this will give the sauce a creamy flavour and texture. Remove the mixture to a bowl, then use the pestle and mortar to bash the basil up into a pulp. Add this to the pine nuts and loosen with extra virgin olive oil so that the sauce easily drops off the end of a spoon. Now you need to balance it with quite a lot of balsamic vinegar to give it a good zing, almost like a mint sauce, but add it to taste. Give the lamb and mushrooms a final toss. I like to serve this up on a big platter and let everyone help themselves. Have the sauce and a simple watercress salad on the side.

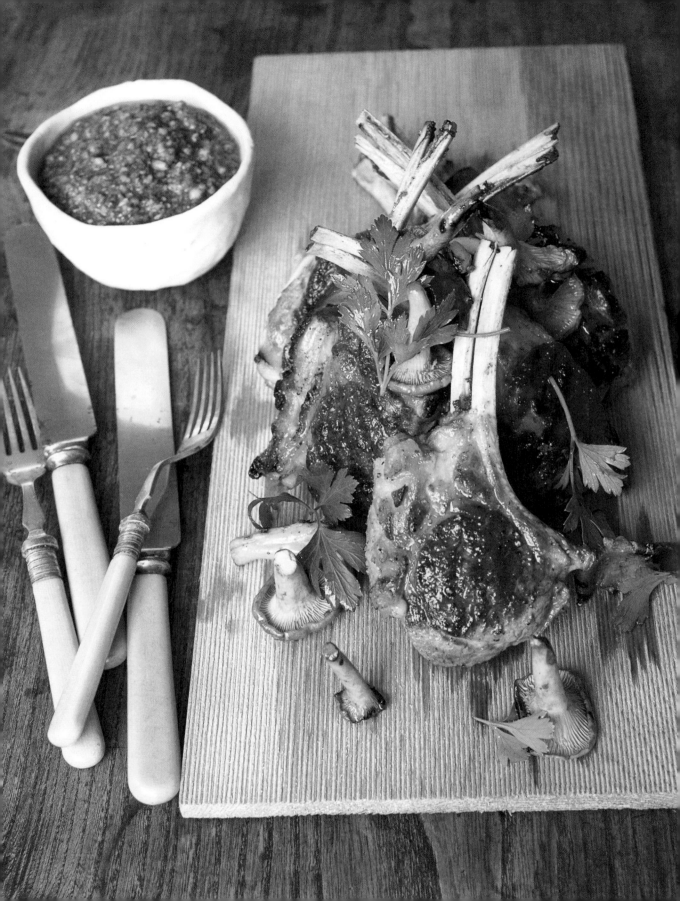

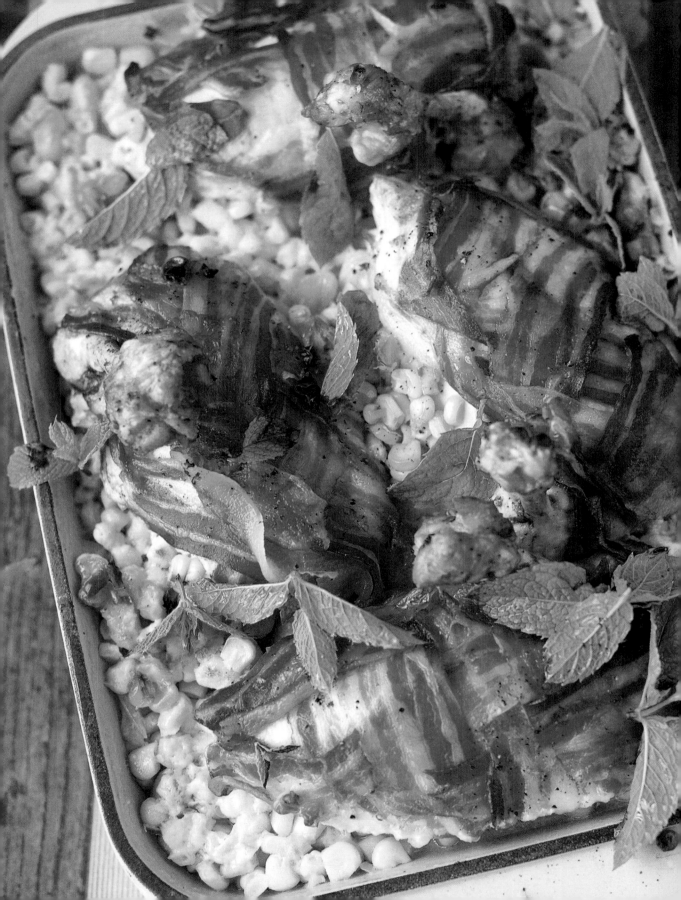

TRAY-BAKED CHICKEN MARYLAND

This is a really quick and convenient dinner to make – great for Saturday nights with your family. Everyone I've cooked it for has loved it, including the kids. It's kinda like an easy and healthy version of the southern American Maryland or, as many call it, 'sunshine' cooking. Although the idea of cooking chicken with sweetcorn and banana may sound grotesque to you, it really does work! Anyway, I've taken a few liberties in order to move this dish on to another level. You can use tinned sweetcorn, but remember that the flavour won't be anything near as good as fresh.

SERVES 4
4 chicken breasts, skin removed
4 fresh corn on the cobs
1 x 410g tin of cannellini or butter beans, drained
2 bananas, peeled
sea salt and freshly ground black pepper
1 large wineglass of white wine
300ml/10fl oz double cream
55g/2oz butter
12 rashers of smoked streaky bacon or pancetta
a handful of fresh mint, leaves picked

Preheat your oven to 220°C/425°F/gas 7 and get yourself an appropriately sized roasting tray in which you can snugly fit the chicken breasts side by side. Run a knife down the length of the raw corn cobs to remove the lovely sweet bits of corn. It takes literally no time at all to do this. Once done, add the corn to the tray and discard the cobs. Using a fork (or your fingers!), squash up half your cannellini or butter beans until you have a pulp and add these, with the unsquashed half of the beans, to the tray.

Next thing to do is to put the chicken breasts on a chopping board. You will notice that each breast has a little strip or flap of meat on one side. If you fold that back using a knife and make a cut you can carefully form a little pocket inside the chicken breast. Once you have done this to all 4 chicken breasts, squash half a banana into each pocket. Then fold the flap back over to cover the banana up and season with salt and freshly ground black pepper.

Turn the fillets the other way up and carefully place them on top of the corn and beans. Add your wine and double cream, then divide the butter into little knobs and scatter these all around the tray. Drape the bacon or pancetta slices over the chicken breasts and bake in the oven for 35 to 40 minutes, until the bacon is crisp. The smoky flavour from the bacon and the smooth flavour of the bananas will have really cooked into the corn and the chicken. A lovely combination of flavours. Taste and correct the seasoning if it needs it. I usually serve this in the dish at the table, with a handful of fresh mint thrown over, and let people help themselves.

EVERYDAY CRISPY CHICKEN WITH SWEET TOMATOES

This recipe takes literally minutes to put together but then requires slow, gentle cooking. However, in return for your patience, what happens in the pan from just a couple of ingredients is an absolute joy and never fails, so it's a good one to serve if you have guests. Basically the skin of the chicken goes beautifully crisp and the meat becomes sticky and tender and falls away from the bone, while the tomatoes are slow-roasting and creating the most fabulous broth. The finished dish can be flaked into warm salads, tossed with some cooked and drained pappardelle or simply eaten as it is. A great recipe.

SERVES 4
4 chicken legs, jointed
sea salt and freshly ground black pepper
a big bunch of fresh basil, leaves picked, stalks finely chopped
2 big handfuls of red and yellow cherry tomatoes, halved,
    and ripe plum tomatoes, quartered
1 whole bulb of garlic, broken up into cloves
1 fresh red chilli, finely chopped
olive oil
optional: 1 x 410g tin of cannellini beans, drained
optional: 2 handfuls of new potatoes, scrubbed

Preheat your oven to 180°C/350°F/gas 4. Season your chicken pieces all over and put them into a snug-fitting pan in one layer. Throw in all the basil leaves and stalks, then chuck in your tomatoes. Scatter the garlic cloves into the pan with the chopped chilli and drizzle over some olive oil. Mix around a bit, pushing the tomatoes underneath. Place in the oven for 1½ hours, turning the tomatoes halfway through, until the chicken skin is crisp and the meat falls off the bone. If you fancy, you can add some drained cannellini beans or some sliced new potatoes to the pan and cook them with the chicken. Or you can serve the chicken with some simple mashed potato. Squeeze the garlic out of the skins before serving. You could even make it part of a pasta dish – remove the chicken meat from the bone and shred it, then toss into a bowl of linguini or spaghetti and serve at once.

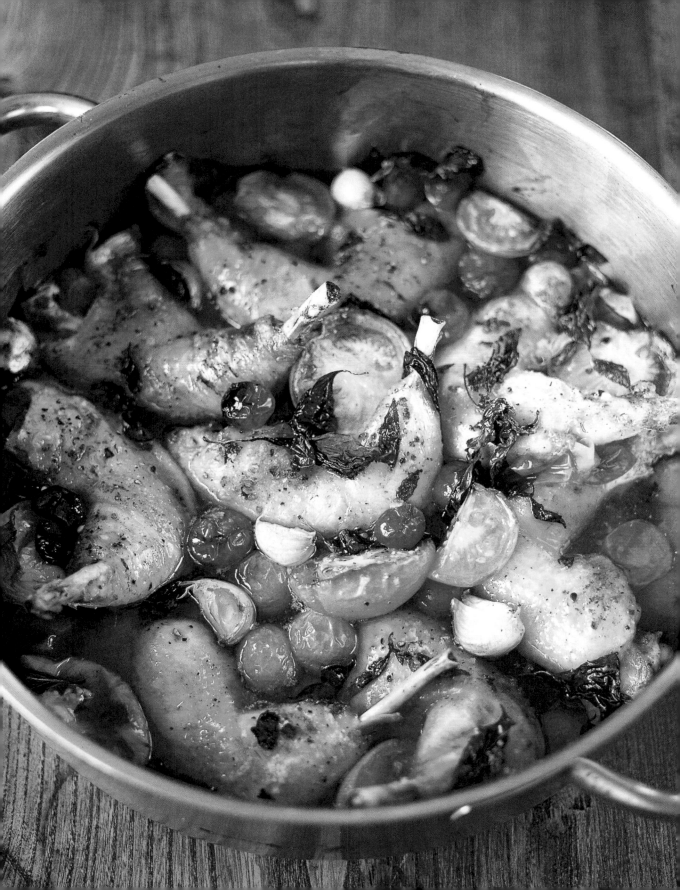

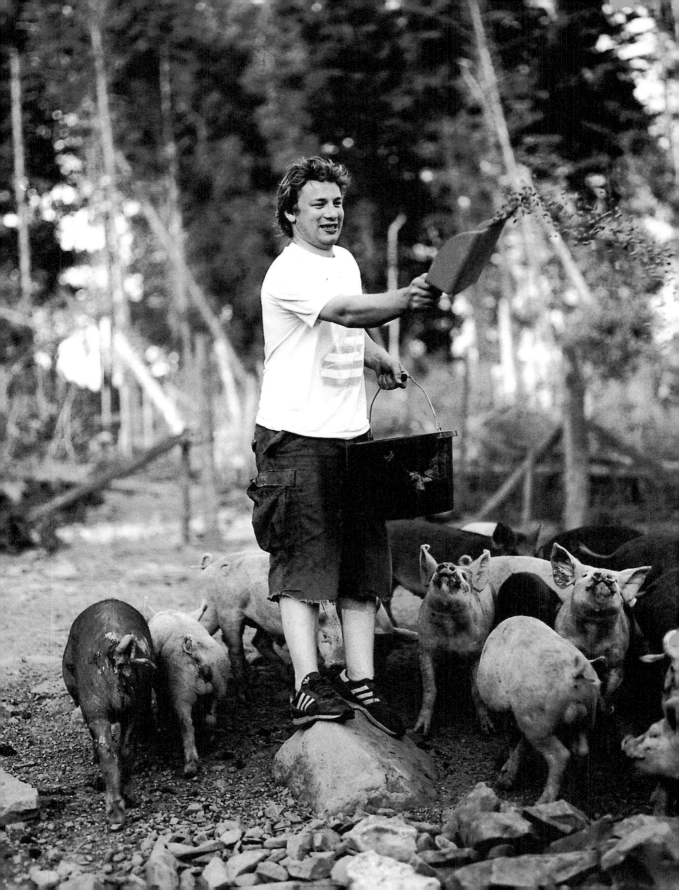

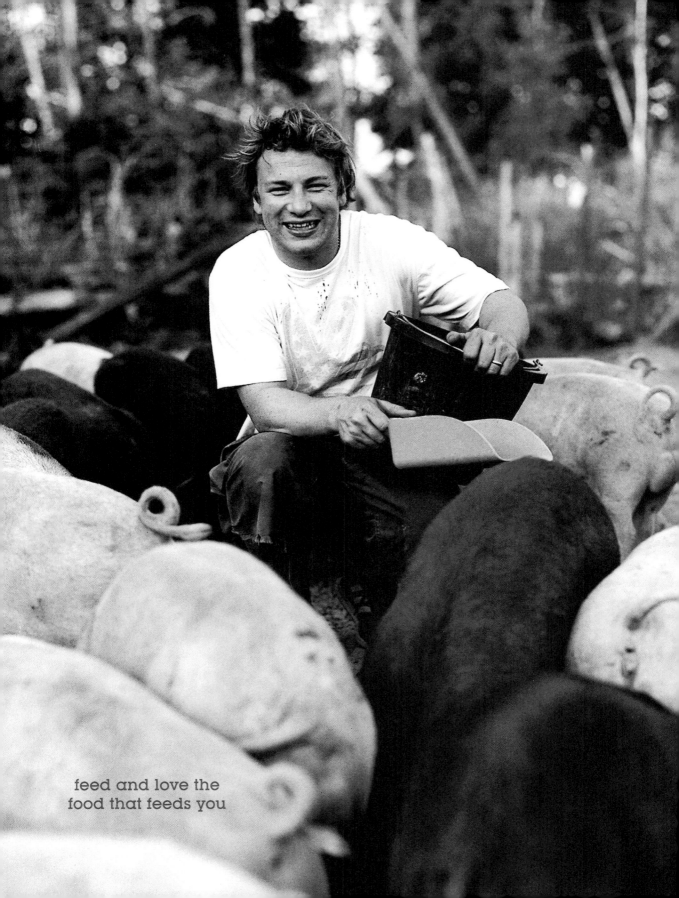

feed and love the
food that feeds you

ROASTED MARMALADE HAM

If you've got a family dinner or a party coming up, or you want to reinvent the Sunday roast, there's nothing outrageous about buying a ham and cooking it this way. You can feed loads of people and still have some left over for sarnies. There is something quite old English about this dish. It almost feels like something that would have been eaten at a royal banquet, it looks so sumptuous! But forgetting the romantic notions, the reason this combination is so genius is because through careful poaching you will get juicy moist meat, by sprinkling the meat generously with black pepper you will get a wonderful heat, and by smearing the whole thing in marmalade you will get a beautiful tart sweetness. It really does make the most wonderful roast dinner, and the left-overs can be sliced into a crusty baguette the next day with some hot mustard and a little rocket.

SERVES 10 PLUS

3–4kg/7–8½lb middle cut gammon with the knuckle left on
2 carrots, roughly chopped
2 sticks of celery, roughly chopped
2 bay leaves
16 black peppercorns
1 bouquet garni (a piece of leek, celery, a bay leaf, a sprig of fresh thyme)

2 oranges
2 tablespoons sea salt
3 tablespoons freshly ground black pepper
1 jar of best thin-rind marmalade
a handful of fresh rosemary, leaves picked

First of all you want to place the gammon in a large but snug-fitting pot. Cover it with water, then throw in your veg, bay leaves, peppercorns and bouquet garni. Peel the zest from the oranges and add to the water, then squeeze the juice in and add the salt. Bring to the boil, then turn the heat down and simmer for an hour and a quarter with a lid on, skimming when need be. Remove from the heat and allow to cool for half an hour in the broth. This will allow the flavours to really penetrate the meat. Discard the vegetables from the broth, but keep the broth for making minestrone-type soups – it will freeze well for use another day.

Preheat the oven to 170°C/325°F/gas 3. Carefully remove the meat to a board and, using a knife, take off the skin. Depending on the breed and quality of the pig, you should have a nice layer of fat. Remove some of the fat as well, to leave you with about 1cm/½ inch. The extra fat can be kept in the freezer for roasting with potatoes another time. Score the fat left on the meat in a criss-cross fashion, and while it's moist, season it generously with the ground black pepper. Place the meat in a roasting tray and roast for 20 minutes until the fat renders and becomes slightly crispy. Remove from the oven, stir up the marmalade to loosen, then smear and rub it all over the meat with the rosemary. Place back in the oven for about 1 hour and baste frequently until beautifully golden and crisp. Serve as you would a roast dinner or as part of a picnic.

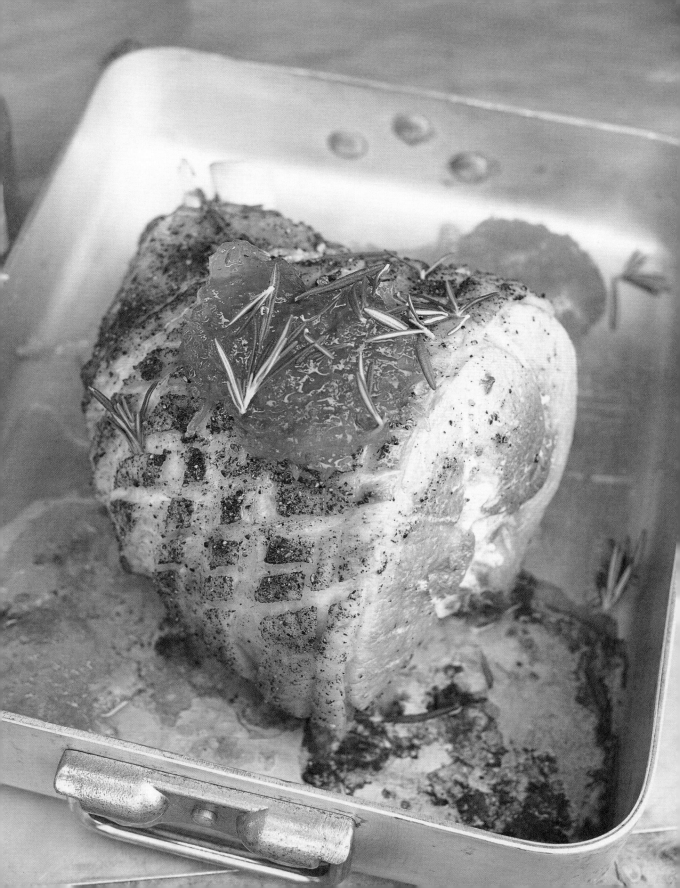

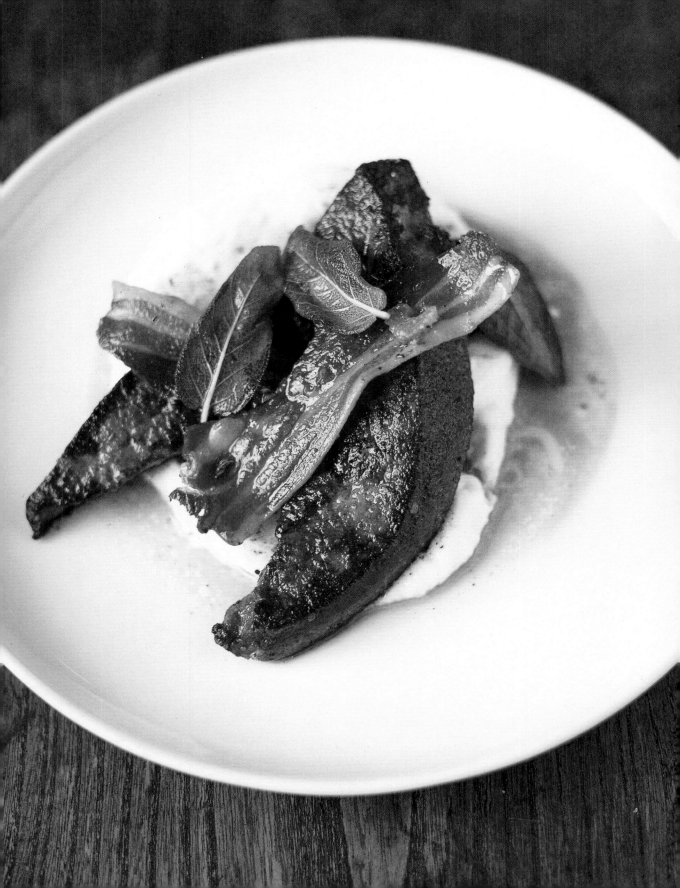

GOOD OLD LIVER AND BACON WITH A TWIST

Anything with liver in it always reminds me of my childhood. There were two things Dad wouldn't eat – one was rabbit, and the other was liver. And when it came to having liver for dinner, God bless my mum! She always used to cook the hell out of it and it would be quite chewy. And like all good food, dinner cooked by mothers is dinner cooked with a lot of love, so if it's not eaten it can cause some upset. Mum would lecture Dad about how he should set an example to us and eat it. One day, it wasn't me or my sister who got told off for not eating our dinner – it was my poor old dad this time who refused to eat the liver she'd cooked. I don't remember what was said exactly, but I do remember, to our amusement, Mum picking up the *Royal Horticultural Society Gardeners' Encyclopaedia of Plants and Flowers* (not relevant, just handy and big) and chasing him round the kitchen with it. To which my dad very calmly sat down, 'tutted' and rolled his eyes. I've started doing this myself over the last five years – aargh – I'm turning into my dad! So, Mum and Dad, I dedicate this recipe to you and all heavy books.

SERVES 4
12 rashers of smoky bacon
olive oil
a small handful of fresh sage leaves
600g/1lb 6oz calf's or lamb's liver, trimmed
    of sinews and cut into strips
flour, to dust
2 medium onions, peeled and finely sliced
sea salt and freshly ground black pepper
4 tablespoons red or white wine vinegar
4 heaped tablespoons butter

Get your biggest frying pan nice and hot. Add your bacon, cook until nice and crispy on both sides, then remove to a plate. Add a little olive oil to the bacon fat left in the pan, sprinkle in your sage leaves, and cook for 30 seconds. When crispy they give the most fantastic flavour and texture. Remove from the pan and put to one side with the bacon.

Dust your liver in a little flour, shaking off the excess, and put to one side. Add your onions to the pan with a good pinch of salt. Cook for a few minutes, then remove the onions when they've softened. Allow the pan to heat up once more with a drizzle of olive oil, then add the liver and cook in two batches over a really high heat for a minute on each side to caramelize and seal in the flavour – don't overcook the liver as it's nice to leave it a little pink. Then put the onion, sage and bacon back into the pan with the vinegar, butter and all the liver. It will sizzle and spit, becoming creamy and saucy. Season to taste, and serve with buttery mashed potato mixed with loads of jarred, creamed or grated fresh horseradish. If you fancy, you can add a little double cream or crème fraîche to make the mash nice and oozy.

STIR-FRIED DUCK WITH SUGAR SNAP PEAS AND ASPARAGUS

Lots of people have woks, but so many people get it wrong because they don't really understand the principle of stir-frying – i.e. you get a pan really hot and you don't overcrowd it with veg so that it starts boiling and not stir-frying. You could make this with breast of chicken instead, if that takes your fancy, or slices of pork. There are many ways you can vary this using different vegetables – try beansprouts, water chestnuts, spinach, courgettes or baby corn.

SERVES 4

4 x 200g/7oz duck breasts
2 teaspoons five-spice
sea salt and freshly ground black pepper
2 tablespoons sunflower or groundnut oil
2 large handfuls of thin asparagus, trimmed
2 large handfuls of sugar snap peas or mangetouts

4 cloves of garlic, finely sliced
1–3 fresh red chillies, deseeded and finely sliced
2 thumb-sized pieces of fresh ginger, peeled and grated
4 oranges, zested and segmented
1 tablespoon honey
a handful of fresh mint, leaves picked
4 tablespoons soy sauce

First of all, score the skin of the duck with a sharp knife. Then dust the breasts all over with the five-spice and a good pinch of salt. Put the duck breasts skin side down in a cold wok, then bring it slowly up to a medium low temperature so the white fat turns into wonderful thin, crispy, golden crackling. Cook for around 12 minutes, then turn the breasts over and cook for a further 5 minutes.

By which time they will be cooked medium, so remove them to a plate and pour away the duck fat. Get all your veggies and flavourings ready to go and wipe your wok. Now you want to get it really hot – if you want to open the window (and cover the fire alarm – joke!), then do. You may need to cook it all in smallish batches depending on the size of your wok.

Add a couple of tablespoons of sunflower or groundnut oil to your hot wok. Carefully swill the oil around so that it covers the whole pan. Add your asparagus and sugar snap peas or mangetouts and toss around, then add the garlic, chilli and ginger. Continue stir-frying on the highest heat for a couple of minutes, until the asparagus has softened a little but still has a nice crunch. By all means have a taste. Remove the veg to a plate. Slice up your duck breasts into little slivers and put these back into the wok with any resting juices and maybe an extra pinch of five-spice. Cook until nice and crispy.

Put all your vegetables back into the wok, and turn down the heat. Add the oranges, honey, half the mint and the soy sauce, and serve straight away on a large plate, sprinkled with the rest of the mint. Serve with rice or noodles, as a starter or main course.

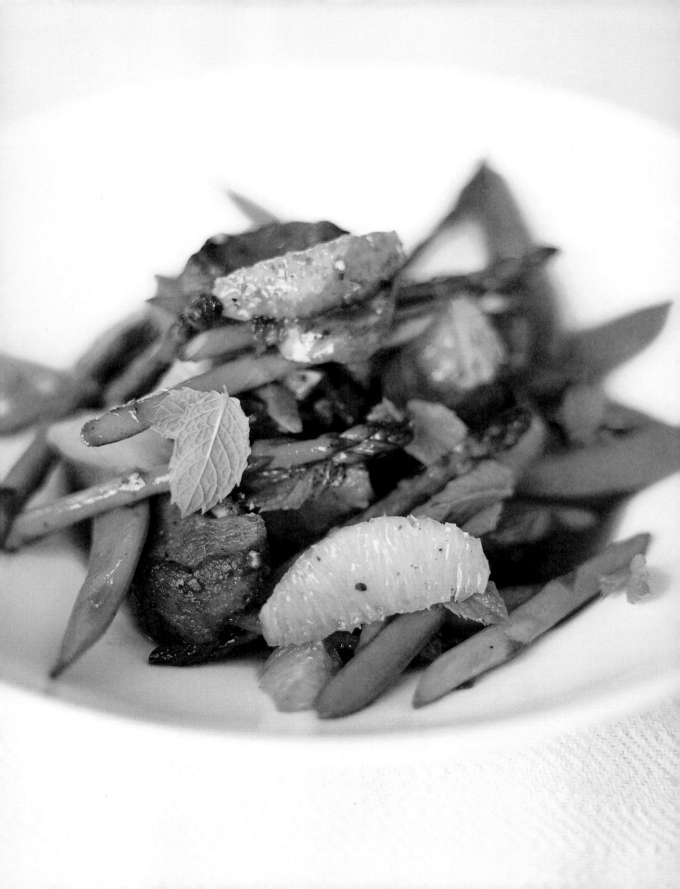

SPRING POACHED CHICKEN

To be honest, I think this has got to be one of my favourite meals, but at the same time none of my friends would even think about having poached chicken for dinner. It sounds boring, doesn't seem like much fun and it might even sound a bit healthy (which it is!). But do you know what, this is one of the most truly brilliant meals. People I've fed it to have been gobsmacked and I'm sure you will be too. So please, trust me, I won't stitch you up. Have a go!

SERVES 4

1 x 2kg/4½lb free-range
   organic chicken
a handful of fresh flat-leaf parsley
4 bay leaves
sea salt and freshly ground
   black pepper
2 handfuls of new potatoes,
   scrubbed
2 handfuls of baby carrots
2 handfuls of baby turnips or
   radishes

1 bulb of fennel, quartered, herby tops
   removed and reserved
freshly grated horseradish
optional: 1 jar hot creamed horseradish
285ml/10fl oz of crème fraîche
2 handfuls of fresh peas
2 handfuls of broad beans
1 colanderful of spinach or Swiss chard
olive oil
optional: small handful of inner celery
   leaves

You will need a large casserole or stock pot to fit your chicken in so that you can cover it with water by about 2.5cm/1 inch. Stuff the chicken with the parsley and bay leaves, then add your chicken to the pot, cover with water and add a good teaspoon of salt. Scatter in the potatoes, bring to the boil, then turn down, place a lid on top and simmer for about 20 minutes. At this point you can add your baby carrots, turnips or radishes and fennel. Carry on simmering for 30 to 40 minutes.

When you can easily pull the leg bone away from the chicken, you know that it's cooked to perfection. By that time the other veg will certainly be cooked, but don't break them up. Now . . . while this is all cooking, you can prepare your horseradish cream – the most joyous thing to have with the chicken. In your supermarket you will be able to find creamed or hot grated horseradish in a jar, which is OK to use, but if you're really lucky you'll be able to get hold of some fresh horse-radish which you can simply peel and grate, season with salt and mix with the crème fraîche. (I'm lucky because my local Sainsbury's sells them whole – just ask at yours if there are none in stock.)

All you have to do now is carefully remove the chicken to a bowl and add the peas, broad beans and spinach to the broth. Allow them to cook for one minute, then season carefully to taste. You can get all your guests to help themselves if that's easier, but if you want to serve it up, divide a nice mixture of veg between 4 bowls, put some shredded chicken on top, then ladle over some of the wonderful, comforting broth. Sprinkle over some of the chopped reserved fennel tops or some celery leaves, with a healthy dollop of horseradish crème fraîche on top and a drizzle of nice peppery olive oil – it will look and taste brilliant.

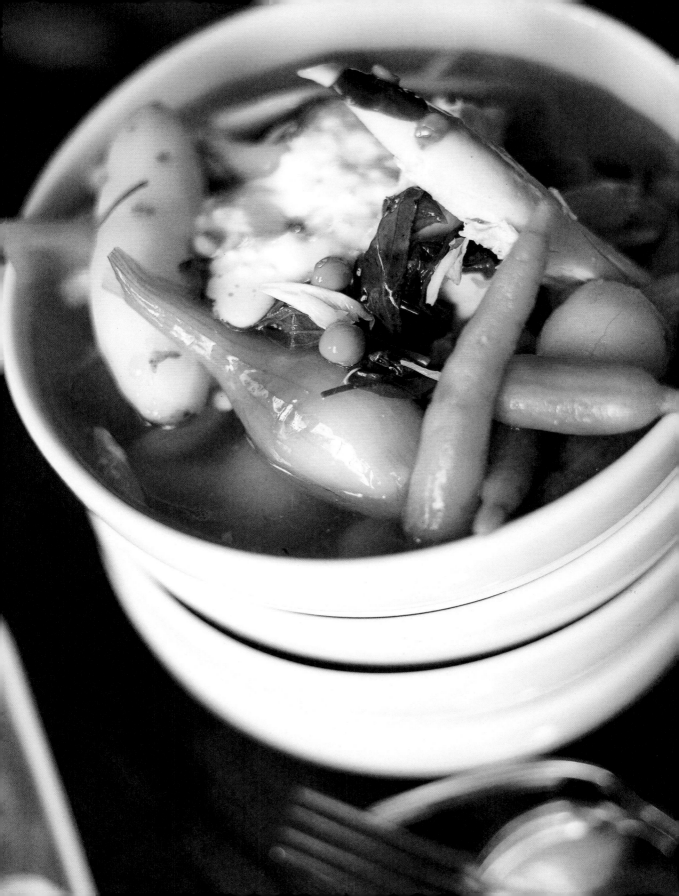

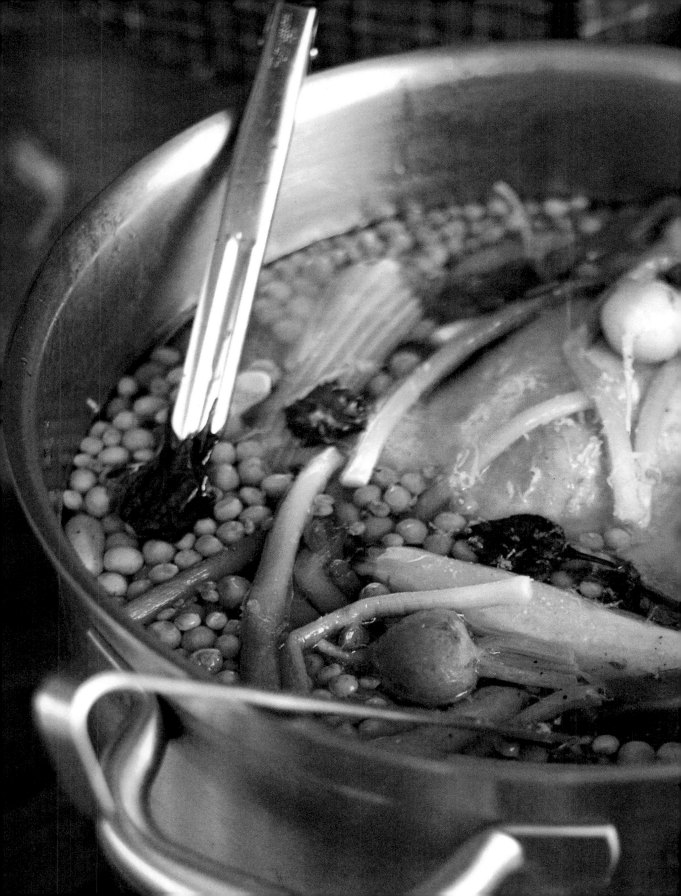

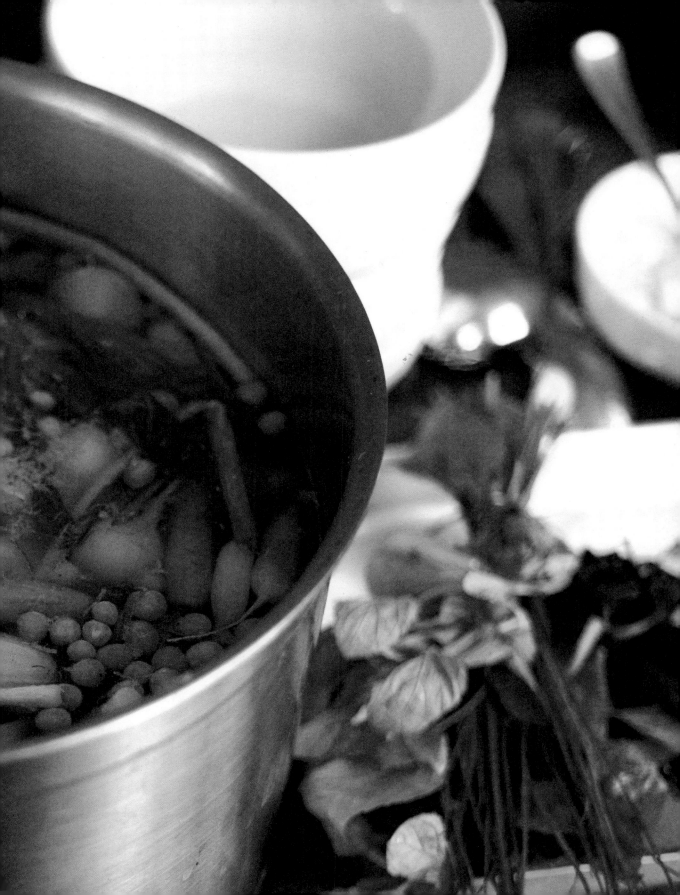

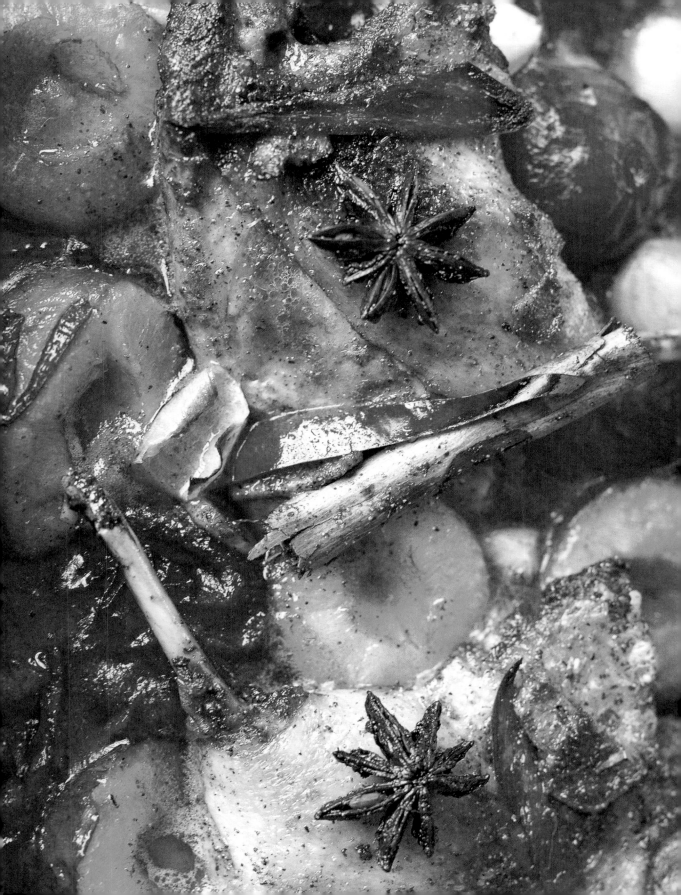

SWEET DUCK LEGS COOKED WITH PLUMS AND STAR ANISE

If you are the type of person who goes into a supermarket and buys prepacked chicken or duck breasts, thighs or drumsticks, then I really want to start you thinking along the lines of buying a whole chicken or duck. It's far better to buy the whole bird and then remove the breasts or legs. I've also noticed that duck legs aren't as popular, because the packs of duck legs never seem to shift from the supermarket shelves like the chicken ones do – which is strange, because all they need is some slow cooking and you'll get thin crispy skin and beautiful melt-in-your-mouth meat. Check out this recipe, which works a real treat.

SERVES 4
4 fat legs of duck
4 tablespoons soy sauce
3 teaspoons five-spice
a handful of star anise
½ a stick of cinnamon
1 tablespoon olive oil
1–2 fresh chillies, deseeded and sliced
16 plums, halved and destoned
2 tablespoons Demerara sugar

Place the duck legs in a sandwich bag with the soy sauce, five-spice, star anise, cinnamon stick and olive oil and let them marinate for a minimum of 2 hours. To really get the flavours going, you could keep this in your fridge to marinate for up to a day. Then get yourself a pan, casserole or high-sided roasting tray that snugly fits the duck legs. Place the chillies, plums and sugar in the bottom of the tray and then pour the marinade from the bag over the top. Mix it all up using your fingers, and place the duck legs on top.

Place the tray in a preheated oven at 170°C/325°F/gas 3 for 2 to 2½ hours until the meat falls away from the bone. Remove the star anise and cinnamon stick, then taste the sauce to see if it needs to be seasoned with a little more soy sauce. It's now down to you how you would like to serve it. You could have it as a starter with some of the little Chinese pancakes that you can buy, or served simply with rice or noodles and the chunky, jammy plum sauce that the duck has cooked in.

JOOLS'S FAVOURITE BEEF STEW

Jools goes mad for this stew in the colder months of the year, and the kids love it too. It's a straightforward beef stew to which all sorts of root veg can be added. I really like making it with squash and Jerusalem artichokes, which partly cook into the sauce, making it really sumptuous with an unusual and wonderful flavour.

The great thing about this stew is that it gets put together very quickly, and this is partly to do with the fact that no time is spent browning the meat. Even though this goes against all my training, I experimented with two batches of meat – I browned one and put the other straight into the pot. The latter turned out to be the sweeter and cleaner-tasting, so I've stopped browning the meat for most of my stews these days.

SERVES 4

olive oil
a knob of butter
1 onion, peeled and chopped
a handful of fresh sage leaves
800g/1¾lb stewing steak or beef
   skirt, cut into 5cm/2 inch pieces
sea salt and freshly ground
   black pepper
flour, to dust
2 parsnips, peeled and quartered
4 carrots, peeled and halved
½ a butternut squash, halved,
   deseeded and roughly diced

optional: a handful of Jerusalem
   artichokes, peeled and halved
500g/1lb 2oz small potatoes
2 tablespoons tomato purée
½ a bottle of red wine
285ml/½ pint beef or vegetable stock
zest of 1 lemon, finely grated
a handful of rosemary, leaves picked
1 clove of garlic, peeled and finely
   chopped

Preheat the oven to 160°C/300°F/gas 2. Put a little oil and your knob of butter into an appropriately sized pot or casserole pan. Add your onion and all the sage leaves and fry for 3 or 4 minutes. Toss the meat in a little seasoned flour, then add it to the pan with all the vegetables, the tomato purée, wine and stock, and gently stir together. Season generously with freshly ground black pepper and just a little salt. Bring to the boil, place a lid on top, then cook in the preheated oven until the meat is tender. Sometimes this takes 3 hours, sometimes 4 – it depends on what cut of meat you're using and how fresh it is. The only way to test is to mash up a piece of meat and if it falls apart easily it's ready. Once it's cooked, you can turn the oven down to about 110°C/225°F/gas ¼ and just hold it there until you're ready to eat.

The best way to serve this is by ladling big spoonfuls into bowls, accompanied by a glass of French red wine and some really fresh, warmed bread – lovely when torn up and shared. Mix the lemon zest, chopped rosemary and garlic together and sprinkle over the stew before eating. Just the smallest amount will make a world of difference – as soon as it hits the hot stew it will release an amazing fragrance.

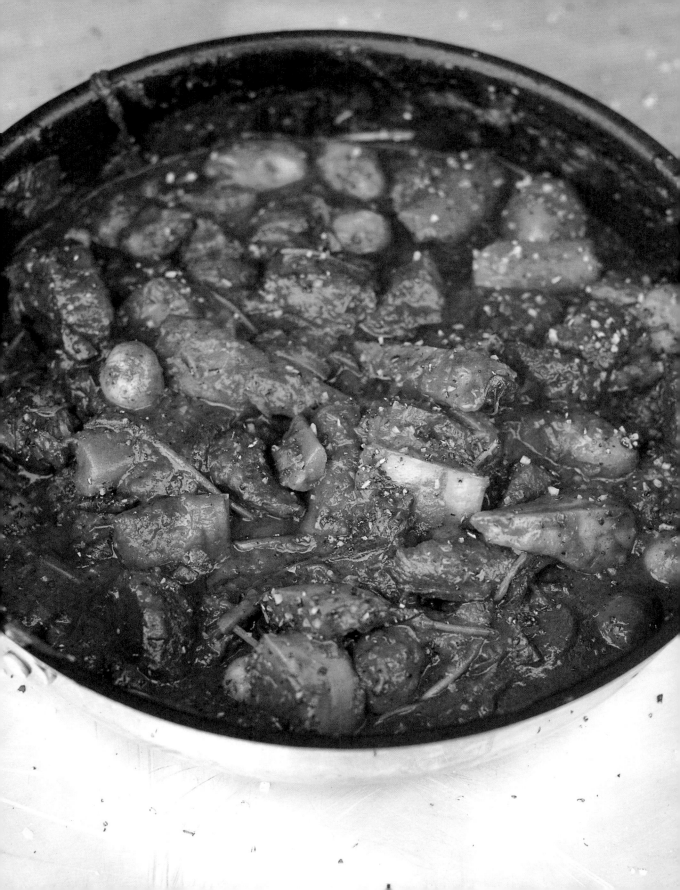

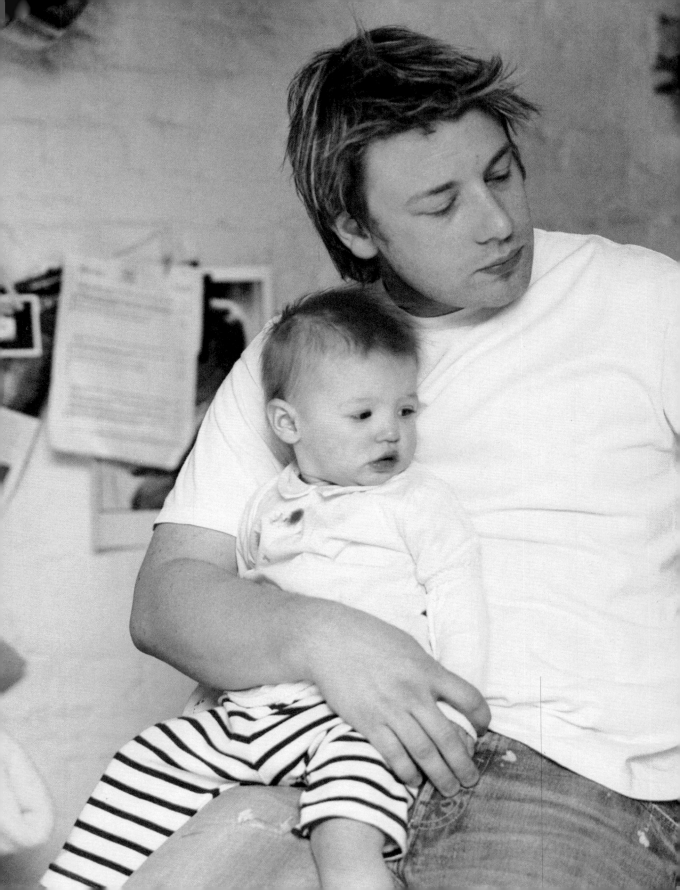

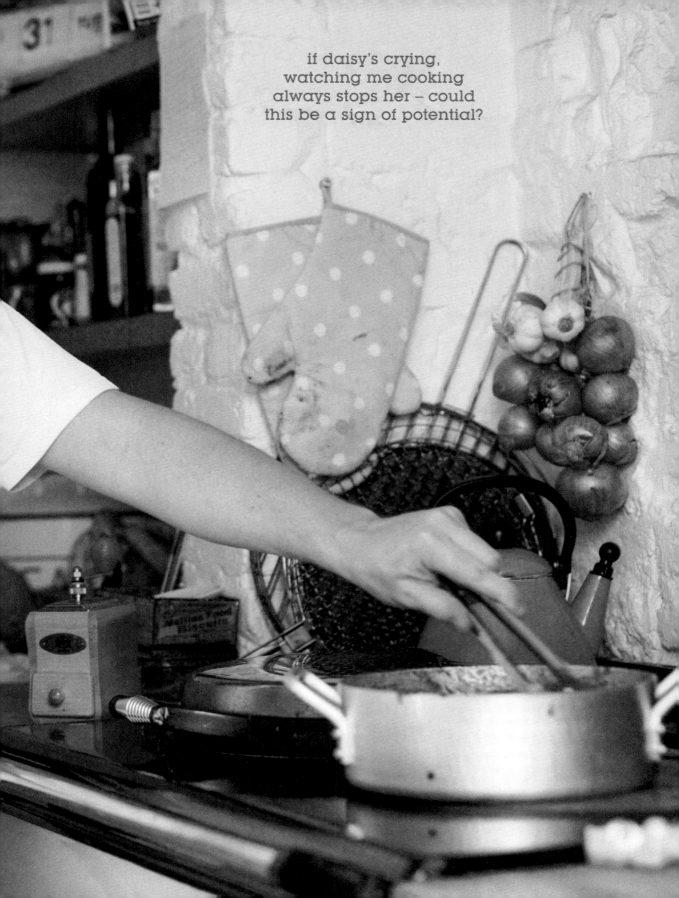

if daisy's crying,
watching me cooking
always stops her – could
this be a sign of potential?

LAMB WITH CHICKPEAS, YOGHURT AND TRAY-ROASTED VEG

Leg of lamb is a real favourite in British households, but I want to give you a totally different take on it. When buying your leg of lamb from the butcher, ask him to remove all the bones and butterfly the whole leg to open it out. This gives you a piece of meat that can be fried or grilled or cooked on the barbecue, because it's tender enough. It also allows it to be wonderfully marinated so it can take on great flavours, and it cooks much quicker than a normal leg of lamb. The flavours in this recipe are Moroccan-based. It's not an authentic Moroccan recipe, but it does taste really good and that's enough for me.

SERVES 4–6

1 leg of lamb, butterflied and opened up like a book
2 teaspoons coriander seeds
3 cloves of garlic, peeled and finely chopped
a large bunch of fresh coriander, chopped
a large bunch of fresh mint, chopped
1 x 410g tin of chickpeas, drained
sea salt and freshly ground black pepper

juice of ½ a lemon
1 x 500ml tub of natural yoghurt
12 baby turnips, scrubbed
a bunch of baby carrots, scrubbed, tops left on
1 butternut squash, unpeeled, cut into 8 wedges
2 red onions, peeled and quartered
1 whole bulb of garlic, broken into cloves
2 teaspoons ground cumin
extra virgin olive oil

Score the lamb on both sides. Using either a pestle and mortar or a food processor, grind or whizz up the coriander seeds with the garlic, fresh coriander, mint and half the chickpeas until you have a paste. Season this paste or 'marinade' with salt and freshly ground black pepper, then add the lemon juice and yoghurt. Place half of this flavoured yoghurt in a large plastic bag and add the lamb. Put the other half of the flavoured yoghurt in the fridge. Tie the bag up to seal it and turn it around to allow the yoghurt to coat all the lamb. Leave to marinate for at least an hour but up to 24 hours in the fridge.

Preheat the oven to 200°C/400°F/gas 6. Place the turnips and carrots in a roasting tray with the squash, onions, garlic and remaining chickpeas, then sprinkle with the cumin, salt and pepper. Drizzle with olive oil and toss together to coat.

Remove the lamb from the marinade, then place the meat directly on the oven rack with the tray of vegetables on the shelf below. Cook for about 1 hour, tossing the vegetables halfway through. Serve the lamb well cooked with the veg and flavoured yoghurt on the side.

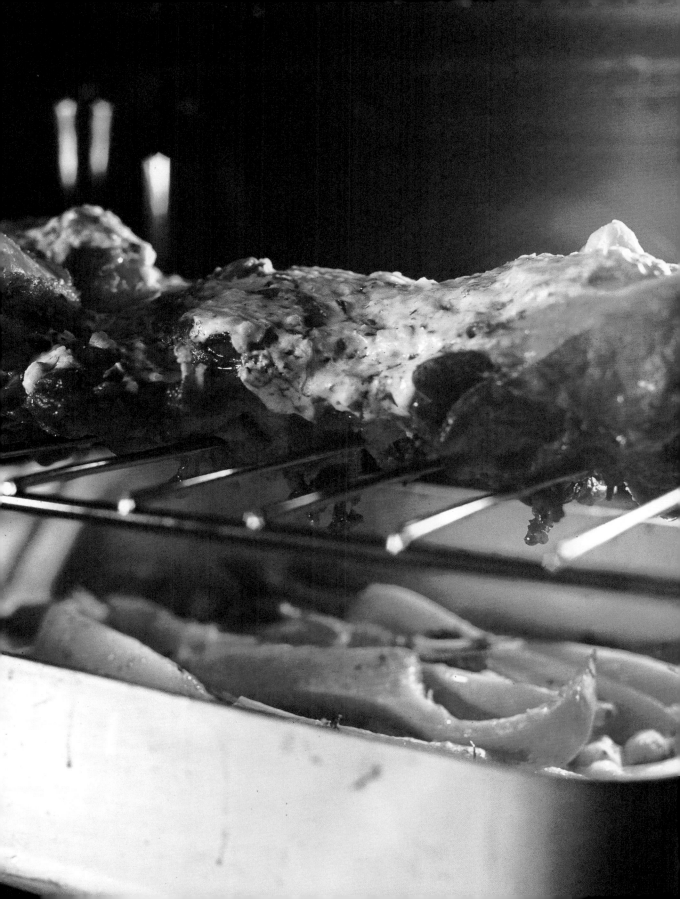

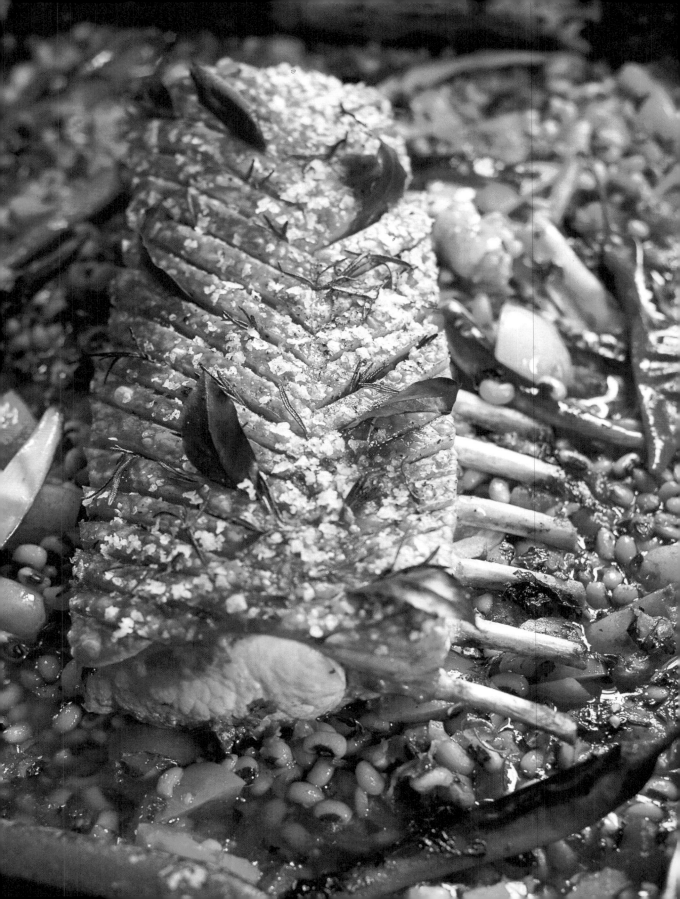

SLOW-ROASTED SPICED PORK LOIN WITH BLACK-EYED BEANS AND TOMATOES

This dish works as described here, but you can also stuff it into hot flour tortillas or pitta breads to be eaten like a kind of fajita or burrito – superb. Spanish smoked paprika is now widely available, and your butcher can do the trimming and scoring of the pork loin for you to save you some time.

SERVES 8

3kg/7lb rib-end loin of pork with skin on, French-trimmed
sea salt and freshly ground black pepper
5 teaspoons smoked paprika
juice of 1 lemon
olive oil
3 red onions, finely sliced
6–8 fresh red, yellow and green chillies
200g/7oz small whole chorizo sausages, thickly sliced
6 bay leaves
2 sprigs of fresh rosemary, finely chopped
3 x 400g tins of good-quality plum tomatoes, roughly chopped
2 handfuls of fresh ripe tomatoes, halved
4 x 410g tins of black-eyed beans, drained
5 cloves of garlic, peeled and finely chopped
a handful of fresh flat-leaf parsley, chopped
red wine vinegar
soured cream, to serve

Preheat your oven to 240°C/475°F/gas 9. First, score the skin of the pork in a criss-cross pattern every 1cm/½ inch with a sharp knife, trying not to cut into the meat itself. Mix a little salt with a teaspoon of paprika, the lemon juice and a little olive oil, then rub this over the meat and into the score lines. Put the meat in a high-sided roasting tray and cook in the preheated oven for 30 minutes to start the skin crisping up.

Remove the meat from the oven, turning the heat down to 180°C/350°F/gas 4. Take the pork out of the tray and put it to one side, then spoon out half the fat and discard it. Place the tray on the hob, add the onions, whole chillies, chorizo, bay leaves and rosemary with the remaining paprika, and fry gently until the onions are soft. Add all the tomatoes, the beans, garlic, parsley and a wineglass of water to the tray, stirring and scraping up all the lovely sticky bits from the bottom. Place the pork on top, return to the oven and cook for another hour or so or until the skin is crispy and the meat is meltingly tender.

When cooked, remove the pork from the tray and allow to rest. Taste the sauce and season with salt, pepper and a few swigs of red wine vinegar to give it a twang. Then remove the chillies and control the heat by chopping up as much chilli as you like and stirring it back into the sauce. Lovely served with soured cream.

ANDY THE GASMAN'S STEW

You might have heard me talking about my mate Andy the Gasman – he's the one who didn't ever want to use his oven as he thought it might devalue the price of his house, so he left it in its cellophane wrapper! Five years on and nothing's changed, but I wanted to get him cooking, so this is something I invented for him to try out. It's so easy to make because all it involves is throwing a few things into the pot and leaving it in the oven for a while. In Andy's case he'll go to a football match while it's cooking so it's ready as soon as he gets home. You can serve it as a stew or in tortillas with crunchy salad and guacamole. The other great thing about it is that you can bulk it out with different types of roughly chopped root veg, or butternut squash, or even with different types of beans (try cannellini, flageolet or butter beans), and if you want a bit of heat, feel free to add a couple of crumbled dried chillies. PS Andy is a strapping lad currently looking for a wife if any of you can help – just look out for him out on the town in Saffron Walden at the weekend!

SERVES 4
olive oil
700g/1½lb potatoes, peeled and
    cut into 2.5cm/1 inch dice
2 red onions, peeled and roughly
    chopped
2 carrots, peeled and roughly
    chopped
2 sticks of celery, trimmed and
    roughly chopped
2 sprigs of fresh rosemary,
    leaves picked
1 level teaspoon ground cumin

1 heaped tablespoon smoked paprika
zest and juice of 1 orange
800g/1¾lb stewing steak, lamb
    or pork, cubed
1 x 410g jar or tin of good-quality
    cooked chickpeas, drained
2 x 400g tins of good-quality plum
    tomatoes, chopped
sea salt and freshly ground
    black pepper
1 tub of fresh live yoghurt
a handful of fresh coriander, leaves
    picked

First of all you need to preheat your oven, but the temperature will depend on how long you want to cook the stew for. If you want it ready in 3 hours, preheat it to 180°C/350°F/gas 4, but if you want to cook it for 6 hours then you need the oven on at 140°C/275°F/gas 1.

Put a large casserole-type pan on the hob on a high heat and add a couple of good lugs of olive oil. Let this heat up, then add your potatoes, onions, carrots, celery, rosemary, cumin, paprika, and orange zest and juice, and stir together. Cook for 1 minute, then mix around again before adding the meat, the chickpeas and the tomatoes. Season lightly with salt and pepper and pour over enough water to cover everything. Bring to the boil and put into the oven. You are now free to go out for a few hours (for the whole day if you want to!). Serve the stew in bowls with a dollop of yoghurt and a sprinkle of coriander leaves.

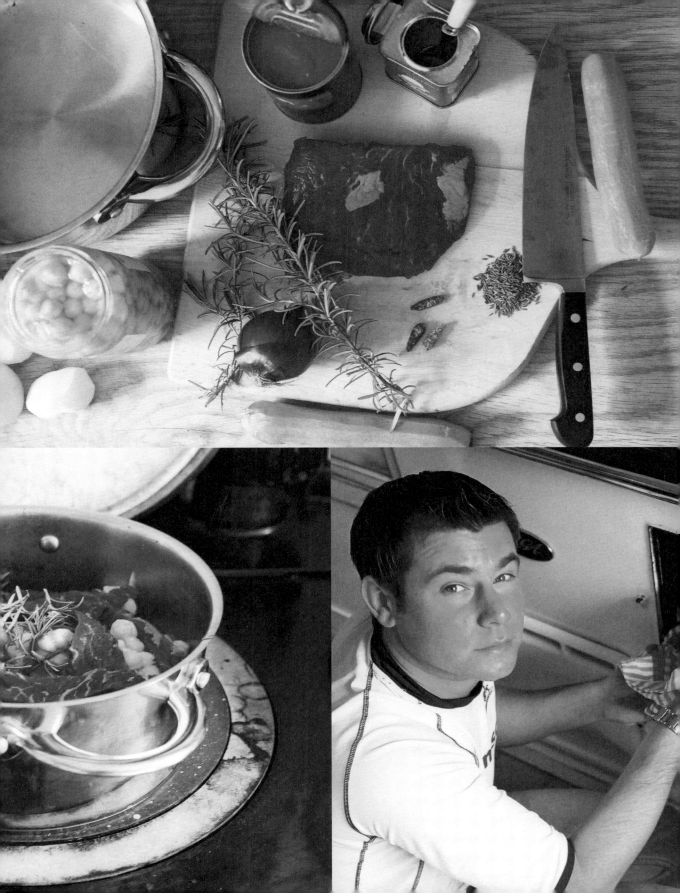

MY FISHy FRIENDS

PLAICE
TURBOT
HALIBUT
COD
SARDINE
HADDOCK
WHITING
MACKEREL
SEA BREAM
SALMON
TROUT
MULLET
SWORDFISH

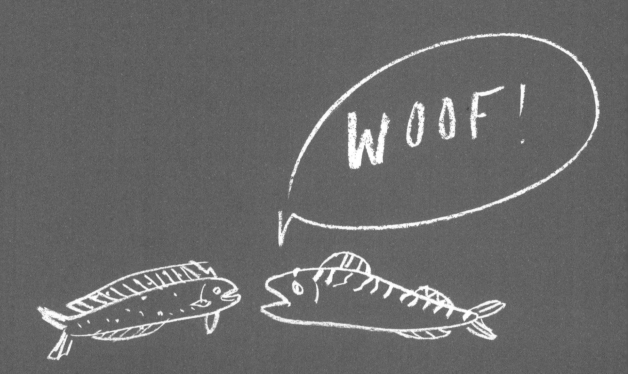

Some of the most healthy nations in the world consume a huge amount of fish. In Britain, though, I don't think we eat enough fish or do enough to promote it, especially when you consider that we live on an island. I think there are two major factors: the first is that people can often be too scared to have a go at cooking fish, and the second is that fish isn't sold fresh enough. When it comes to buying fish it's very simple: if it smells of the sea and looks nice and shiny and beautiful, then you should want to buy it.

I really want to encourage you all to eat more oily fish as it's so good for you. My mate Jane Clarke, who's a fantastic nutritionist, was telling me that oily fish (like salmon, fresh tuna, herrings, kippers, mackerel and sardines) provide a rich source of a polyunsaturated oil called omega 3 fatty acids. These omega oils are crucial for keeping us healthy – they not only help to protect our hearts, but they also help to prevent strokes and some forms of cancer, as well as helping to relieve the symptoms of arthritis. Some research even suggests that omega 3 can improve kids' concentration, moods and behaviour. So, what's stopping you … get down to the shops, buy some oily fish and serve it to the family this week! If you can eat a portion twice a week, even better.

And please don't think that non-oily fish without the omega oils, such as plaice and haddock, are off the menu. They contain high levels of protein, vitamins and minerals, and are very good for you. So let's all eat fish!

In this chapter I've used the tray-baking method several times because I've received so many letters and emails from people who have had success with this way of cooking. It's great because it means you have your vegetables and fish cooking at the same time in the same tray and they flavour each other.

If you don't feel confident about cooking fish, have a go at tray-baking first. Then, if you find you're enjoying it and you want to do more, have a look at other books on the subject, such as *Fresh* by Mitchell Tonks, or any of Rick Stein's books.

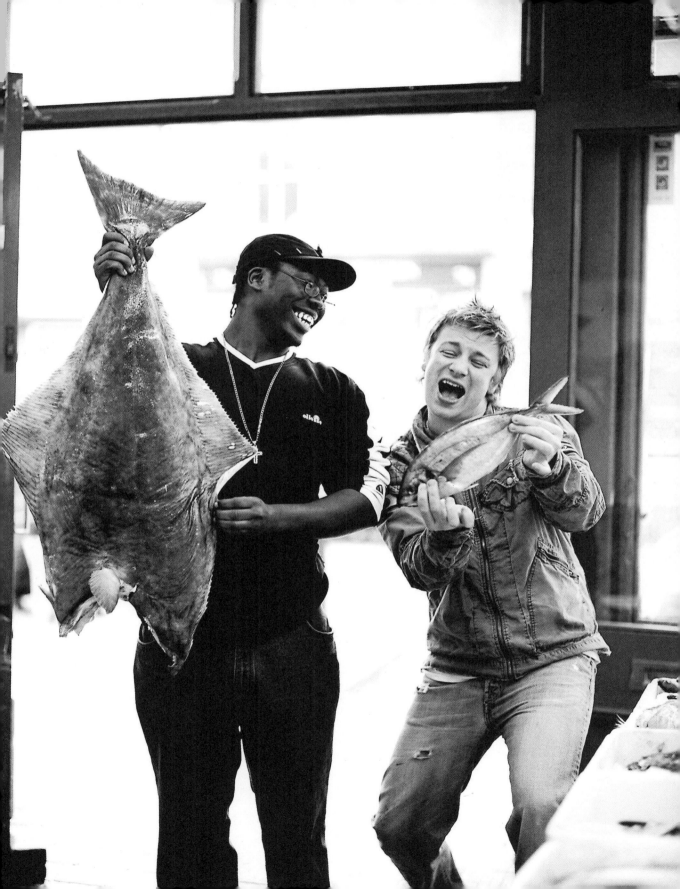

LAKSA-STYLE SCALLOPS WITH SWEET CHILLI SAUCE

A laksa is a cross between a stew and a curry but it uses fragrant flavourings like ginger and lemongrass as opposed to heavy spices, and it's traditionally served with noodles. Instead of scallops you can use cheaper fish like salmon or cod, sliced up – I'd suggest that you need about 400g/14oz. You can even use finely sliced chicken – just simmer it a little more slowly and a bit longer. This recipe really is open to any type of fish or budget – my version is great with prawns in the base and scallops on the top.

SERVES 4
3 limes, zested and halved
300g/11oz peeled prawns, roughly
   chopped
2 tablespoons fish sauce
2–3 fresh red chillies, deseeded
3 cloves of garlic
a large thumb-sized piece of fresh
   ginger, peeled
a large handful of fresh coriander,
   leaves picked, stalks reserved
1 tablespoon sesame oil

a small handful of kaffir lime leaves
olive oil
1 teaspoon tamarind paste
2 x 400ml tins of unsweetened
   coconut milk
140ml/¼ pint chicken stock
sea salt and freshly ground
   black pepper
200g/7oz noodles or rice
12 scallops
optional: 4 finely sliced spring onions
   or 1 punnet of cress, chopped

Put the lime zest into a bowl with your prawns. Squeeze over the juice of 2 of the limes and add your fish sauce. Mix well, and leave to marinate for about 10 minutes. In a pestle and mortar or a food processor, pound or blitz the chillies, garlic, ginger, coriander stalks, sesame oil and lime leaves until you have a paste. Heat a large casserole or wok, pour in a couple of tablespoons of olive oil and add the paste, stirring quickly. Cook for about a minute before adding your prawns and all the flavoursome juices from the bowl. Allow to cook for another minute, stirring. Then add the tamarind paste, coconut milk and chicken stock. Turn the heat down and simmer slowly for about 15 minutes. Taste – you may need to add salt and pepper or more fish sauce, and just enough lime juice to give it a good twang, as Asian food should be hot, salty, sweet and sour.

Get a pot of water boiling for your noodles or rice. Now lightly score the scallops with a criss-cross pattern on one side so that when they cook they will open out to look like flowers. Get a large non-stick frying pan hot and pour in a little olive oil. Put your lightly seasoned scallops into the pan and cook for a couple of minutes on each side until golden. Halfway through, add the noodles or rice to the boiling water and cook according to the packet instructions.

Remove the scallops from the heat. Drain the noodles or rice and divide between four serving bowls, spooning the laksa stew over the top. Sprinkle with the coriander leaves – or you can try some finely sliced spring onions or some cress to give a bit of a crunch. Then lay two or three scallops on top of each bowl. Lovely served with a dollop of sweet chilli jam, which you can buy just about everywhere these days.

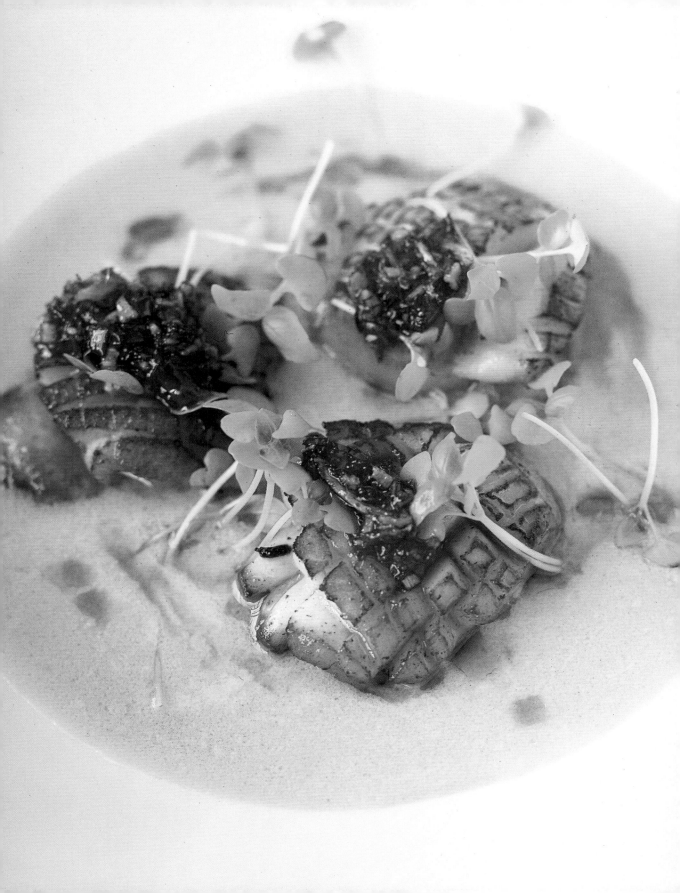

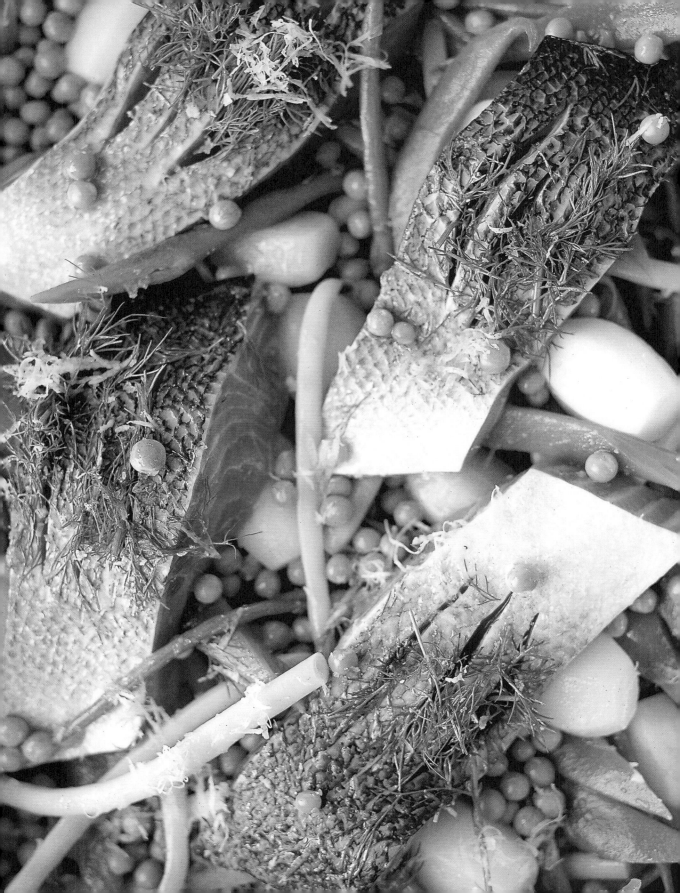

SUMMER TRAY-BAKED SALMON

This is one of those great dishes that you can really make your own by using whatever vegetables are in season – it's particularly nice with broad beans, asparagus or little halved cherry tomatoes. The fish doesn't take long to cook, so you can blanch your veg accordingly and then finish them off in the tray with the fish. It makes life a lot easier if you're cooking for the family or a large group of friends.

SERVES 4
700g/1½lb new potatoes, scrubbed
sea salt and freshly ground black pepper
a large handful of runner beans, sliced into 5cm/2 inch pieces
a large handful of green beans, tops trimmed
optional: a large handful of yellow French beans, tops trimmed
2 handfuls of podded peas
55g/2oz butter
extra virgin olive oil
2 lemons, zested and halved
a handful of fresh basil
a handful of fresh fennel tops or dill
4 x 200g/7oz fillets of salmon, scaled, filleted and pinboned

Preheat the oven to 230°C/495°F/gas 8. Bring a large pan of salted water to the boil, add your new potatoes and cook for 10 to 12 minutes until they are nearly done. Add all your beans to the pan and cook for another 4 minutes. Then drain the potatoes and beans in a colander. Put them into an appropriately sized roasting tray and add your peas, the butter, a little drizzle of olive oil and the zest and juice of the lemons. Season lightly with salt and freshly ground black pepper and toss together while still warm so the flavours are absorbed.

Chop up half the herbs and add to the tray. Score your salmon fillets lightly on the skin side. Rub each fillet with salt, freshly ground black pepper and a little olive oil, and stuff the scores with the remaining herbs. Put into the preheated oven and cook for about 10 to 15 minutes until the salmon is just cooked (don't overcook it) and the veggies are soft. Serve at the table, giving everyone some veggies and potatoes, a nice piece of salmon steak and some of the lovely cooking juices from the bottom of the tray which are like a ready-made sauce. Great with some garlic mayonnaise.

ITALIAN-STYLE UPSIDE-DOWN FISH PIE

This was one of the big revelations of last year for me. Don't think you're going to get your traditional fish pie – with this you'll get something more stylish and subtle. And the great thing about it is that it can be flexible on the budget – you can make it cheaply with things like mussels and haddock, or you can spend a bit more on things like lobster. As long as the fish is sliced around the same thickness it really doesn't matter what you use. But what you will have to do is ask your fishmonger to fillet all the fish for you, and it will also have to be pinboned. If using clams and mussels, make sure they are cleaned and debearded. Throw away any that are open and after cooking chuck away any that remain closed.

SERVES 4
sea salt and freshly ground
    black pepper
150g/5½oz polenta
115g/4oz freshly grated
    Parmesan cheese
150g/5½oz butter
extra virgin olive oil
200g/7oz mixed mushrooms,
    left whole or torn up
2 cloves of garlic, peeled and
    finely chopped

1 x 500g/1lb 2oz bag of spinach
½ a nutmeg
2 lemons, zested and halved
800g/1¾lb mixed fish (red mullet,
    monkfish, bream, prawns, mussels or
    clams), filleted, pinboned and sliced
2 handfuls of red or yellow cherry
    tomatoes, halved
1 red chilli, deseeded and finely
    chopped
a large handful of fresh thyme,
    leaves picked

In a high-sided, thick-bottomed pan cook your polenta according to the packet instructions – it will make a very soft 'blup blup blup' noise! Add the Parmesan and 100g/3½oz of the butter, and season to taste with salt and freshly ground black pepper, otherwise it will be too bland. Once this is done, put a lid on top and keep the polenta warm.

Preheat the oven to 230°C/450°F/gas 8. Put a large ovenproof frying pan or roasting tray on a medium heat on the hob, then add the rest of the butter, a little olive oil, the mushrooms and the garlic. Fry for 2 or 3 minutes, then add the spinach. Continue to cook until the spinach wilts and goes dark green and any liquid has cooked away. Grate over your nutmeg and season very carefully to taste with salt, freshly ground black pepper and a tiny squeeze of lemon juice from one of the lemon halves. At this point you can turn the heat off, shake the pan so the mushrooms lie flat, and pour the wet polenta over the top to give you a nice layer.

In a bowl put the fish, tomatoes, a couple of tablespoons of good olive oil and the zest and juice of the lemons. Season with salt and freshly ground black pepper, add the chilli and thyme, then toss everything together. Sprinkle the fish mixture over the top of the polenta, pouring over any juices from the bowl as well. Cook in the preheated oven for around 10 to 15 minutes. (The fish shouldn't need any longer than this.) Then take straight to the table and serve.

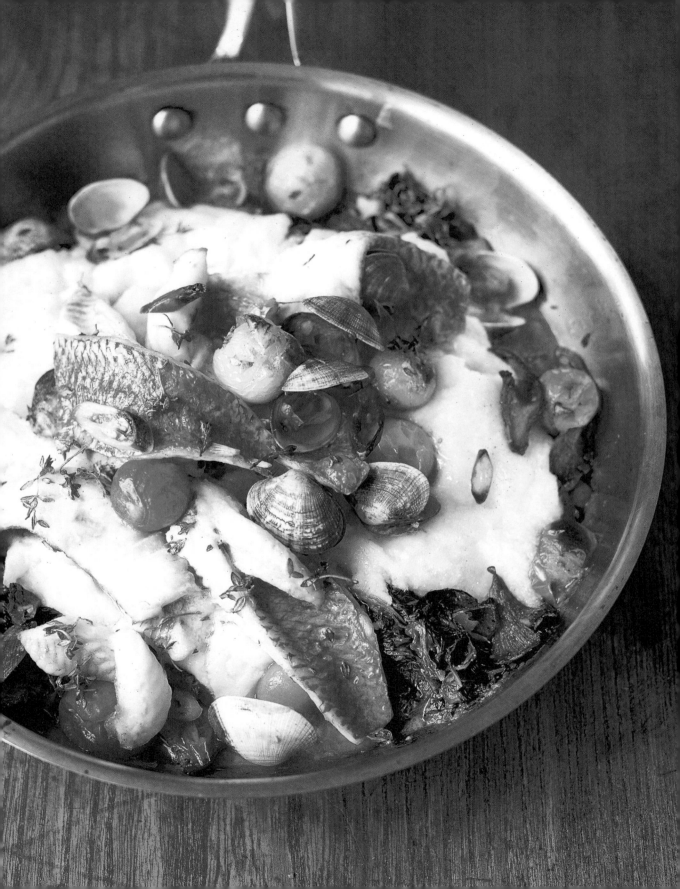

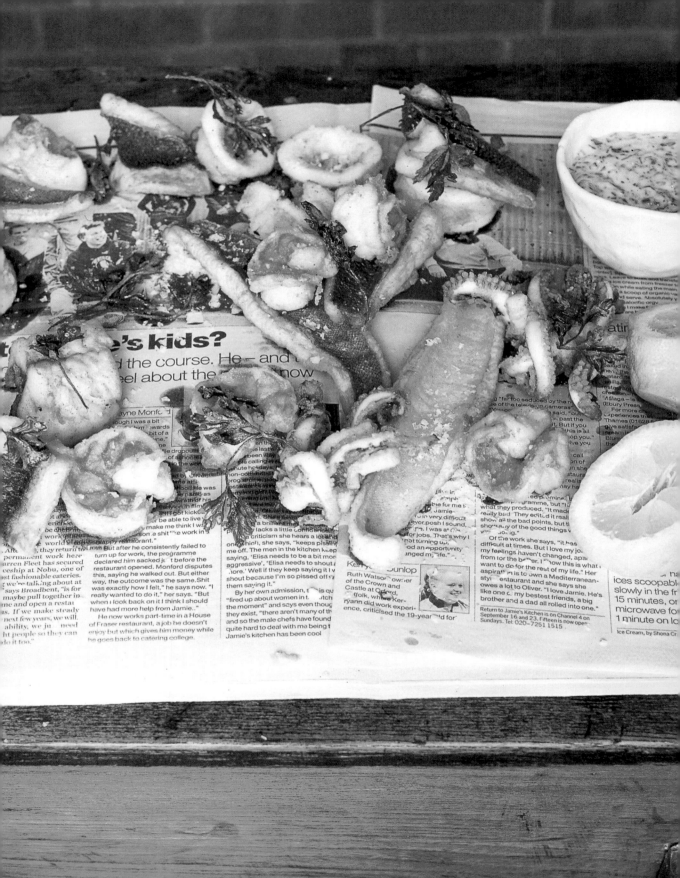

SPICED FRIED FISH WITH A SPEEDY TARTARE SAUCE

I've had lots of fun serving this as an appetizer at dinner parties, or even for a starter at the restaurant. This way you don't need to have a massive pot and loads of oil heating up. And you can get it all done in one or two batches. You can pretty much deep-fry any fish, and they'll all cook together very happily provided they're sliced to the same thickness or size. All you need to do is make sure that the fish have been scaled, filleted and pinboned. In the case of prawns you will need to peel, devein and butterfly them, and if you're using squid it should be skinned and gutted. Ask your fishmonger to give you a selection of fish that will take the same length of time to cook – I particularly love using squid, sole, bass, bream, prawns and mullet. Once you've been to the fishmonger's, let's be honest, most of the work's done for you, so all your love and attention can go on the cooking, which is the key here.

SERVES 4
sea salt and freshly ground
    black pepper
sunflower oil
a small piece of potato
a handful of fennel seeds
75g/2¾oz flour
600g/1lb 6oz mixed fish,
    scaled, filleted, pinboned
    and prepared (see above)
3 dried red chillies

FOR THE TARTARE SAUCE
4 heaped tablespoons mayonnaise
a handful of capers, finely chopped
a handful of gherkins, finely chopped
zest and juice of 1 lemon
a splash of white wine vinegar

Make your tartare sauce by mixing all the ingredients together in a bowl. Season to taste and put to one side. Now get yourself a large, wide casserole pot with reasonably high sides. I wouldn't recommend a wok for this recipe, as they're not all that stable or safe for deep-frying. Fill your pot with an inch and a half of sunflower oil and place a small piece of potato in it. Turn the heat on – by the time the potato is golden and frying you'll know you're at the right frying temperature. It normally takes about 10 minutes to heat up, but as usual you need to be around and be vigilant, so don't leave the pan unattended. If the oil starts to smoke it is too hot, so turn it down.

Meanwhile, in a coffee grinder or a pestle and mortar, whizz or bash your fennel seeds and chillies to a powder. Mix well with the flour. Now, if you've got a big pan you may be able to do all your fish at the same time, but if not then you need to cook them in two batches. Toss all the fish in the spiced flour and gently shake off any excess. Place the fish carefully in the oil, one piece at a time to avoid splashing the oil, making sure the heat is on full whack as the fish will reduce the temperature of the oil and you need it as hot as possible. Using a slotted spoon, slowly move the fish around. Cook for a couple of minutes until golden and crisp, then remove to kitchen paper to soak up any excess oil. Serve at the table on a platter, a plate or even some newspaper! Give it a good sprinkling of sea salt and serve with the tartare sauce. Simple but great.

GRILLED AND TRAY-BAKED RATATOUILLE WITH WHITE FISH

This recipe for delicate white fish baked on top of a sweet and easy ratatouille is just lovely. Again, in the typical tray-baked way, the ratatouille benefits from being flavoured by the fish juices and at the same time it will steam its flavour into the fish. Ratatouille is a kind of vegetable stew which originates from Nice in the South of France. I've made my own version of this dish using a slightly different technique. I think the end result looks great and tastes fantastic, so I hope you enjoy it.

SERVES 4

3 red peppers
1 bulb of fennel, trimmed
1 red onion, peeled
olive oil
3 firm aubergines
4 firm green courgettes, trimmed and chopped into 1cm/½ inch pieces
2 cloves of garlic, peeled and chopped
a handful of fresh basil, leaves picked and stalks chopped

2 x 400g tins of good-quality plum tomatoes, chopped
2 handfuls of black and green olives, destoned
2 bay leaves
1 tablespoon red wine vinegar
sea salt and freshly ground black pepper
900g/2lb white fish, filleted and pinboned, cut into similar-sized pieces (try using lemon or Dover sole, sea bass, monkfish, haddock, or even squid and prawns)
juice of ½ a lemon

Preheat the oven to 190°C/375°F/gas 5. Using a pair of tongs, hold the peppers over a naked flame on a gas hob or place on your barbecue. When the skins have blackened, put the peppers into a plastic bag and secure it. This will allow them to steam – leave them for half an hour before peeling and deseeding. Chop the fennel and onion into rough 1cm/½ inch pieces and put them straight into a large casserole-type pan or roasting tray with a little olive oil. Toss together, then cook over a medium heat while you prepare the rest of the vegetables.

Cut the aubergines in quarters lengthwise and then trim off the fluffy central core and discard it. Then chop the aubergines into 1cm/½ inch pieces, leaving the skin on. When the fennel and onion have had 5 or 6 minutes and have softened nicely, remove them to a plate. Then turn the heat up to full whack, pour in a small amount of olive oil, and add the aubergines, courgettes, garlic and basil stalks. Continue to cook for another 6 minutes, stirring regularly to mix everything together. Add your tomatoes to the vegetables, along with the fennel and onion, olives, bay leaves and red wine vinegar. Season lightly and give it a good stir. Pop the tray into the oven for 40 minutes to allow the sauce to thicken – you can loosely cover the tray with tinfoil or wet greaseproof paper.

Dress your fish with a little olive oil, a squeeze of lemon juice and some salt and freshly ground black pepper. Remove the ratatouille from the oven, taste it and correct the seasoning, then add all the basil leaves, either whole or torn, and give it a good stir. Lay the fish over the top and pop the tray back in the oven. If the fish pieces are reasonably thin they should only need 5 minutes, but give them slightly longer if you prefer. When they're done, remove the tray from the oven and take it straight to the table. Serve with really nice crusty bread and a good glass of wine.

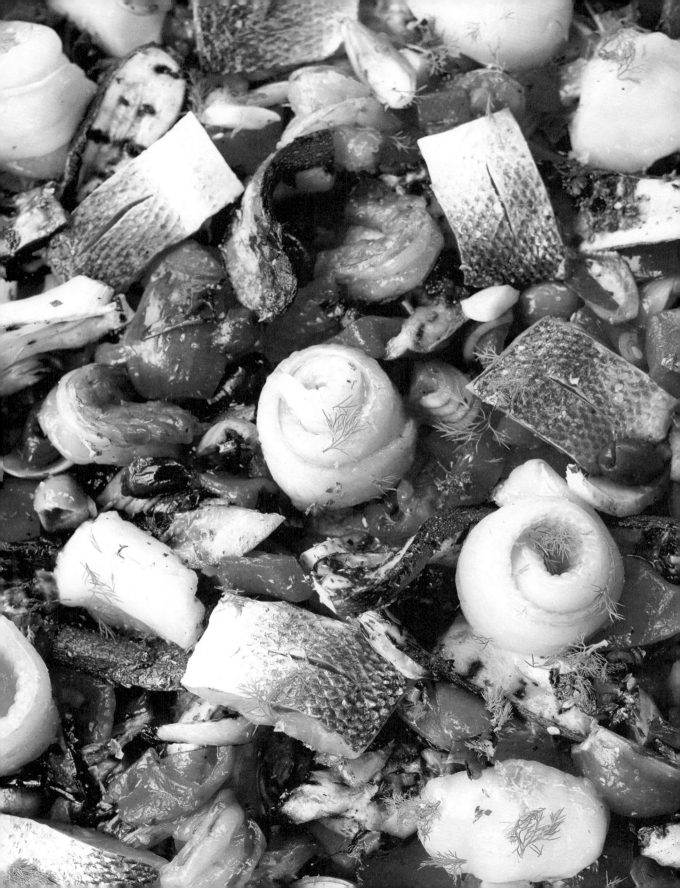

TRAY-BAKED SEA BASS WITH CRISPY ROASTED ASPARAGUS BUNDLES WRAPPED IN BACON

This is another of my favourite tray-baked dishes. I like to serve it in the tray at the table, so that people can help themselves to the bits that they like best. It's a really great way to cook for your family, and your bambinos should love it. What you're going to get from this is some tremendous veg, some wonderfully cooked fish, some crispy smoky bacon and a lovely wine sauce at the bottom of the tray. If you want to have some new potatoes on the side, or a green salad, feel free. You can always swap the mint for basil if you prefer.

SERVES 4
4 x 225g/8oz thin sea bass fillets, scaled, pinboned and trimmed
olive oil
zest and juice of 2 lemons, plus juice of ½ a lemon
a handful of runner beans, tops trimmed
a handful of green or yellow French beans, tops trimmed
a handful of white or green asparagus
a large handful of fresh mint
8 rashers of smoked streaky bacon
2 wineglasses of Chardonnay
sea salt and freshly ground black pepper
85g/3oz butter, diced

Preheat the oven to 250°C/495°F/gas 8, or as high as it will go. Score your sea bass fillets and then get yourself a large clean plastic bag, sandwich bag or dish. Put the fillets into your chosen bag or dish with a little swig of olive oil and the zest and juice of the 2 lemons and leave to marinate for 10 minutes. Meanwhile, parboil all your beans and asparagus for 2–3 minutes until they are softened and tender.

While the veg is cooking, smash up most of the mint in a pestle and mortar (or use a metal bowl with a rolling pin) until you have a pulp. Add a little olive oil to loosen, and the juice from the extra lemon half. Drain the half-cooked beans and asparagus into a colander, then pour them into a large roasting tray and toss them around with the mint oil.

Divide the beans and asparagus into bundles and wrap them snugly with some strips of bacon to secure. Put these bundles into the roasting tray, then remove the fish fillets from the bag and inter-mingle them with the bundles. Pour the wine into the tray, season with salt and freshly ground black pepper and cook in the preheated oven for around 10 minutes or until the fish and bacon are both golden. Remove from the oven, add your small pieces of butter, and allow to rest for a few minutes. Give the tray a shake then take to the table. Serve the fish drizzled with some of the white wine sauce from the tray, and sprinkled with the rest of the mint.

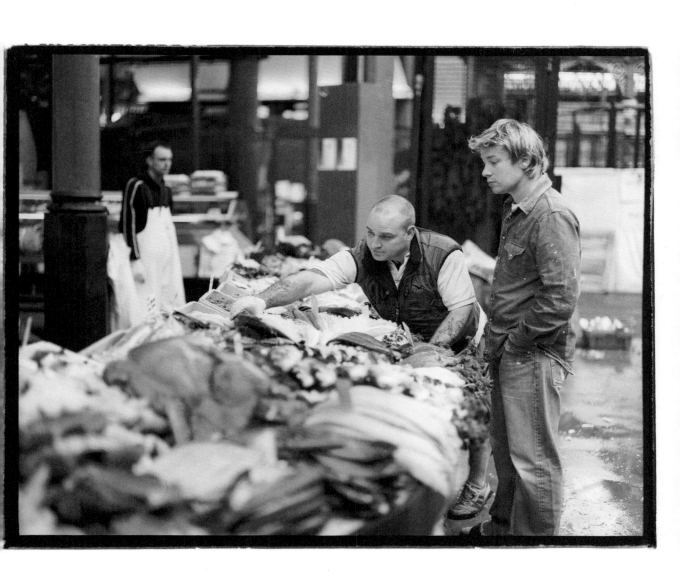

TASTY FISH BAKE

Although I've eaten dishes similar to this in the past, this particular fish bake was brought to my attention recently by one of my students. It's essentially some slow-cooked 'jammified' sweet onions and fennel, layered with lovely, flaky fish, crunchy potatoes and breadcrumbs with a little cream and cheese, and baked in the oven. When you eat it, make sure to get a bit of every layer on your fork! The dish makes wonderful use of trout (as I've used here), sardines, salmon or mackerel – any fish really, but oily ones are great to use, especially for kids. Try to get hold of the freshest fish you can, and ask your fishmonger to prepare it and get rid of the bones for you.

SERVES 4
400g/14oz potatoes, scrubbed and finely sliced
4 tablespoons olive oil
1 clove of garlic, peeled and chopped
1 onion, peeled and sliced
1 bulb of fennel, trimmed and sliced
1 teaspoon fennel seeds
4 medium or 8 small fillets of trout, scaled and pinboned
285ml/½ pint single cream
2 handfuls of freshly grated Parmesan cheese, plus extra for sprinkling
2 anchovy fillets, chopped
sea salt and freshly ground black pepper
2 handfuls of fresh breadcrumbs
2 lemons, halved

Preheat the oven to 200°C/400°F/gas 6. First of all, parboil the sliced potatoes in salted boiling water for a few minutes until softened and then drain in a colander. Place a 20cm/8 inch casserole-type pan on a low heat, and add the oil, garlic, onion, fennel and fennel seeds. Cook slowly for 10 minutes with the lid on, stirring every so often.

Take the pan off the heat. Lay your trout fillets skin-side up over the onion and fennel. Mix together your cream, Parmesan and anchovies, season with salt and freshly ground black pepper, and pour over the fish. Toss the potato slices in a little olive oil, salt and pepper and layer these over the top. Place in the oven for 20 minutes, sprinkling with the breadcrumbs and a little grated Parmesan 5 minutes before the end. Serve with lemon halves, a green salad and cold beers!

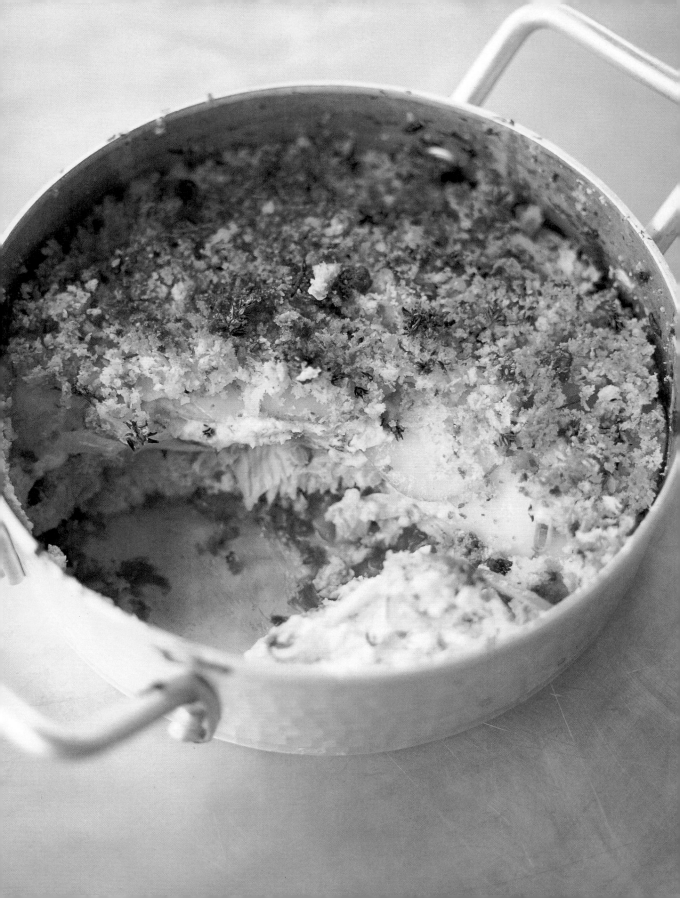

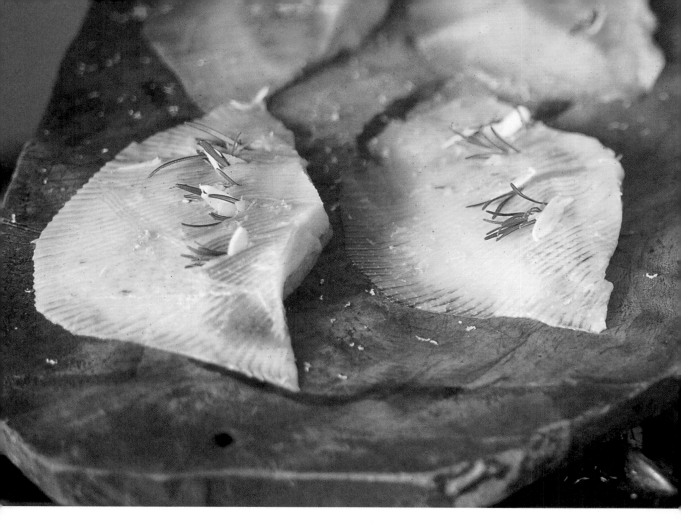

SKATE SIMMERED IN A SWEET TOMATO SAUCE

I got the idea for this skate dish when I was in Sicily and was served a large loin of tuna (the length of my arm!) poached in a fragrant tomato sauce. The results were fantastic – the fish and sauce had each flavoured the other and both had become the better for it. A bit like a good marriage! As large pieces of fresh tuna are reasonably hard to get hold of, I tried it with skate. The results were just as good, as skate has a fantastic meaty texture too, so feel free to use either fish in this recipe.

SERVES 4

4 x 255g/9oz skate wings
1 red onion, peeled and
    finely chopped
4 cloves of garlic, peeled and
    finely chopped
1 teaspoon coriander seeds,
    bashed up
olive oil

3 x 400g tins of good-quality plum
    tomatoes, finely chopped or puréed
zest and juice of 2 lemons
sea salt and freshly ground
    black pepper
12 anchovy fillets, halved
1 small handful of rosemary tips

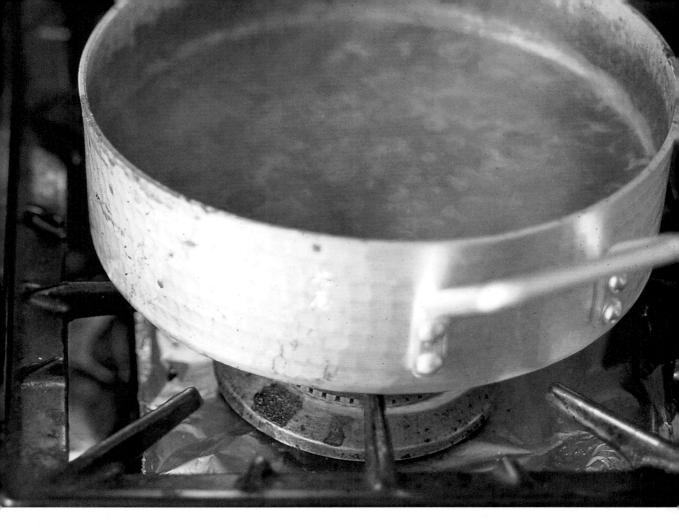

Preheat your oven to 180°C/350°F/gas 4 then find yourself a casserole-type pan or deep roasting tray that will fit all the skate wings in. (The skate needs to be totally covered by the sauce when it cooks, so make sure the fish fits in nice and snugly. You can slightly overlap the thinner ends of the wings.) In this pan or tray, slowly fry the onion, garlic and coriander seeds in a couple of lugs of olive oil until softened but not coloured. Then add your tomatoes, lemon zest and juice and season lightly with the salt and freshly ground black pepper. Bring the sauce to a simmer.

Meanwhile, using the tip of a small, sharp knife, make small incisions in the fatter central part of the fish. Push half an anchovy fillet into each incision and then spike with a small piece of rosemary. Do this three times on both sides of each fish. Now carefully submerge the fish in the tomato sauce, making sure that every part is covered. Put the pan or tray into the oven and cook slowly for around 15 minutes, depending on how thick the skate wings are (if the flesh pulls off the bone you know it's cooked beautifully). Correct the seasoning and take to the table straight away.

This can be served as it is, with just the sauce for company like they do in Italy, or you can have it with things like mashed potato or polenta, salad or garden greens. If you have any left over, you can even flake the fish off the bone and toss it with pasta. But my favourite way is just with some really fresh ciabatta to mop up the tomato sauce.

PAN-COOKED GIANT PRAWNS WITH MANGETOUTS, PEAS AND BUTTER BEANS

This recipe was great fun to make up. I was shopping at Borough Market and decided to buy some fantastic giant prawns, then a jar of butter beans and a handful of mangetouts and peas. Next I bought a paella pan and went along to see my friend Maria, who works at the Borough Market Café. She let me use one of the rings on her gas hob and I got cooking . . . Don't be put off by thinking that large prawns are expensive, because they're actually quite good value. However, this recipe works with all sorts of different prawns.

SERVES 4
olive oil
12 large prawns, peeled and butterflied
1–2 fresh red chillies, finely sliced
a bunch of spring onions, trimmed and finely sliced
4 large handfuls of mangetouts
2 large handfuls of podded peas
2 x 410g tins of butter beans or cannellini beans
500g/1lb 2oz ripe mixed tomatoes, chopped
sea salt and freshly ground black pepper
a large handful of fresh flat-leaf parsley
juice of 1–2 lemons

Get yourself a large paella or casserole pan, wok or sturdy roasting tin. Put it on the hob and get it nice and hot. Pour in 3 or 4 tablespoons of olive oil, let it heat up and immediately add your prawns. Allow them to colour on one side and then turn them over, sprinkling them first with the chilli, then with the spring onions. Add the mangetouts and peas to the pan, give it a shake, then add a splash of water, put a lid (or some tinfoil) on top and let everything steam for a minute.

Remove the lid (or tinfoil) and add the butter beans and tomatoes. Give it all a stir, simmer for a couple of minutes until softened, then correct the seasoning, throw in your chopped parsley and add lemon juice to taste. Serve in the middle of the table – wonderful with rice, couscous or simply on bits of grilled bread.

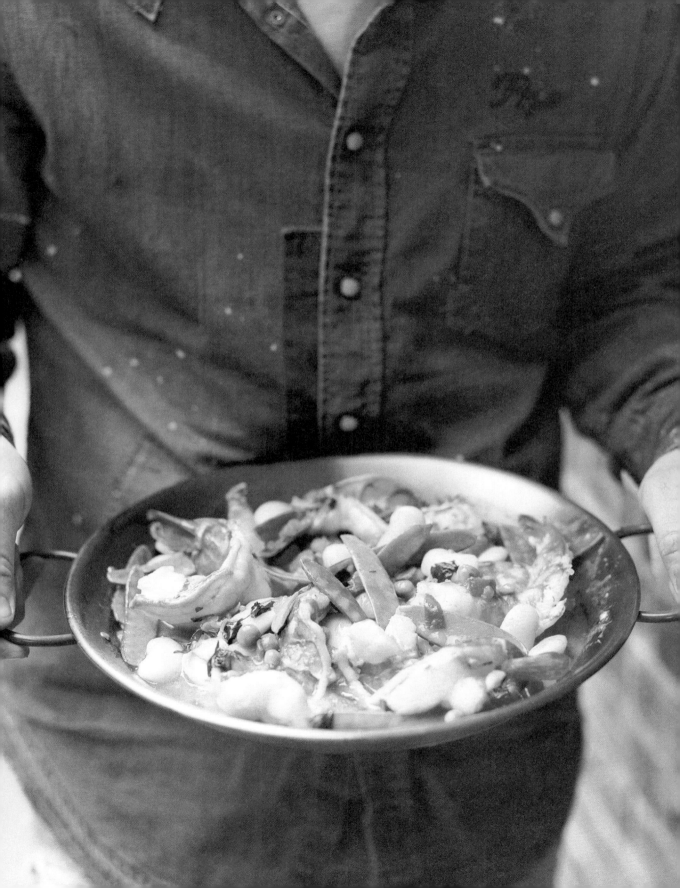

OMEGA 3 AND COUSCOUS

Silly name, but what a great dish! Omega 3 refers to all the lovely goodness that you get from oily fish like red mullet, sardines and fresh anchovies, so do feel free to use any one of these, or a mixture of them. This is also great served with linguine pasta instead of couscous.

SERVES 4

700g/1½lb red mullet and/or sardines, scaled, filleted and bones removed
olive oil
2 red onions, peeled and finely chopped
1 bulb of fennel, herby tops removed and reserved and bulb finely chopped
1 fresh red chilli, finely chopped

1 teaspoon fennel seeds
1 bay leaf
400g/14oz couscous
500g/1lb 2oz mixed ripe tomatoes
2 anchovy fillets, chopped
sea salt and freshly ground black pepper
2 lemons, zested and halved
8 tablespoons natural yoghurt
a small handful of fresh mint, torn

First of all, lay your fish out in one layer on your worktop to give you an idea of how much you are dealing with. Next get yourself a pan with a lid – ideally one that's the right size for the fish to be spread out in one layer. This is so that it can all cook at the same time. Put your pan on the heat, add 4 or 5 tablespoons of olive oil, and slowly fry your onions, fennel, chilli, fennel seeds and bay leaf with the lid on until nice and softened. This should take about 10 minutes.

Meanwhile put your couscous in a bowl and just cover it with salted, boiling water. Put to one side to soak for about 5 minutes. When the onions are sweet and soft, add the tomatoes and anchovies, stir together and carefully season to taste. Shake the pan so that the onions and tomatoes cover the bottom of the pan evenly. Dress the couscous lightly with a little olive oil and the juice and zest of one of the lemons. Sprinkle the couscous over the top of the onions and tomatoes in one even layer. Then place the fish over the top of that and finish off with a drizzle of olive oil. Place the lid on top and simmer slowly on the hob for about 12 minutes.

Meanwhile, season the yoghurt with salt, pepper and the remaining lemon juice and sprinkle over the reserved fennel tops and mint. Serve the pan of fish in the middle of the table with a bowl of yoghurt and let everyone help themselves. Lightly stir the fish up, check the seasoning and eat straight away.

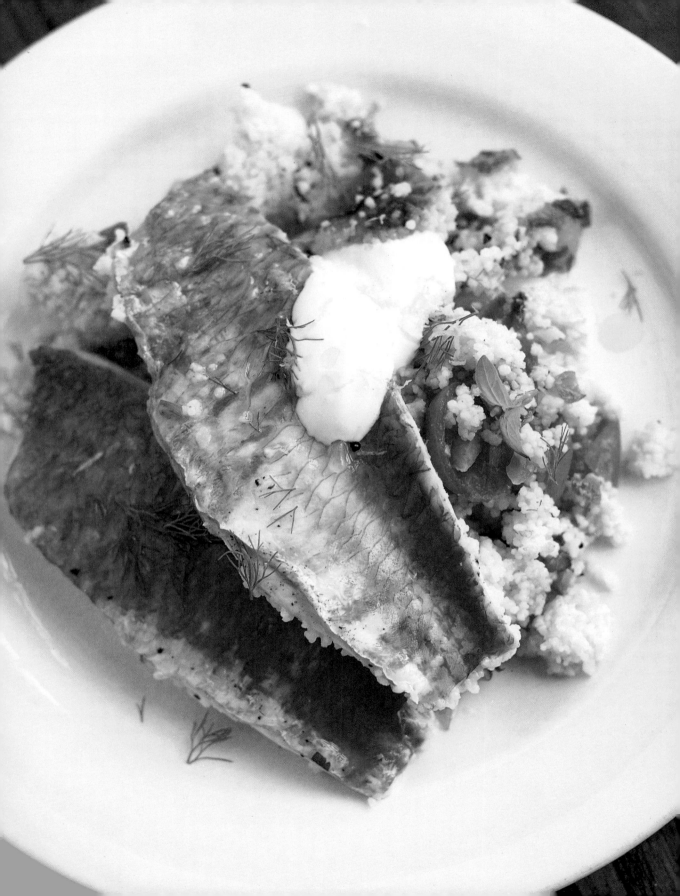

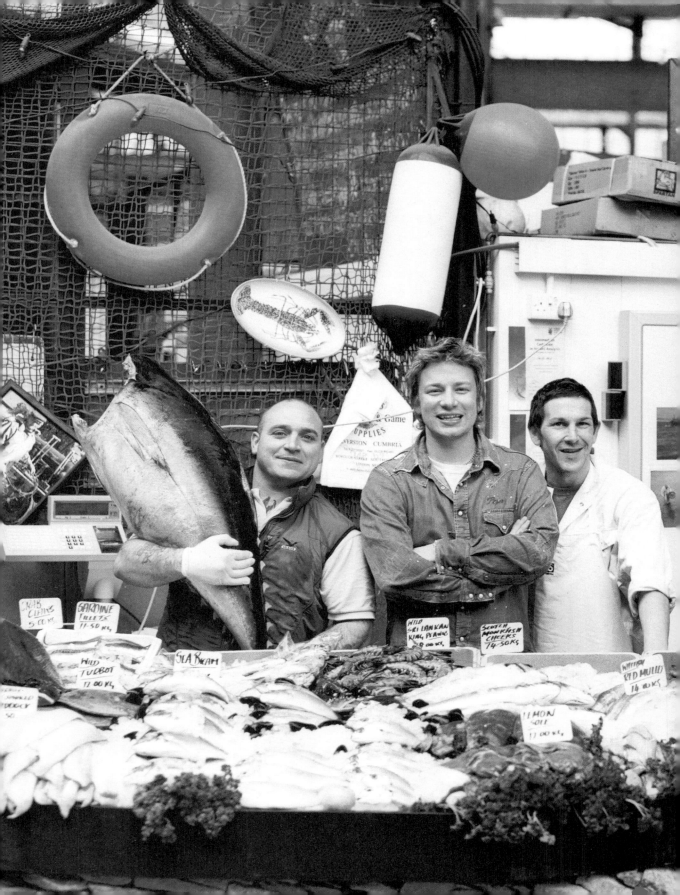

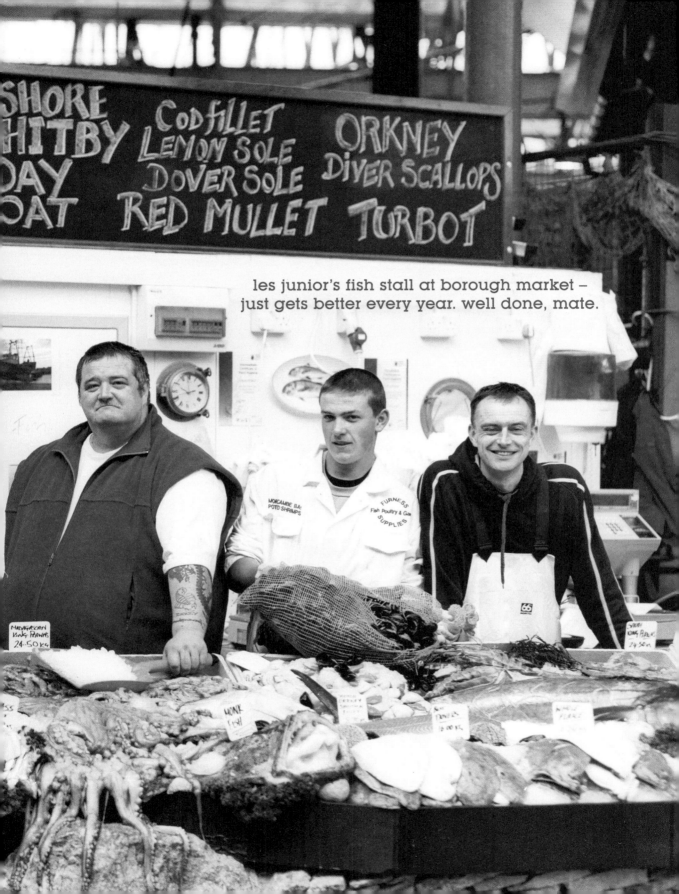

les junior's fish stall at borough market –
just gets better every year. well done, mate.

THE NICEST TRAY-BAKED LEMON SOLE

This recipe can be applied to any size of flat fish. Out of all the soles, lemon sole is the most widely available and generally good value for money. This method of cooking is really simple. Not only does it give you a really clean-tasting fish but it also gives you a juicy, chunky sauce with the added benefit of all the natural fish juices and olive oil. It's really quick and easy and I would recommend serving the whole tray at the table with a big bowl of new potatoes, a mixed salad and some crisp white wine.

SERVES 4
4 whole lemon soles
2 handfuls of red and yellow cherry tomatoes, halved
4 cloves of garlic, peeled and finely sliced
a handful of fresh oregano or basil, leaves picked
a bunch of spring onions, trimmed and finely sliced
1 tablespoon balsamic vinegar
sea salt and freshly ground black pepper
2 lemons, zested and halved
extra virgin olive oil
a handful of black olives, destoned and chopped
a handful of fresh flat-leaf parsley, finely chopped

This is really simple. First of all give your fish a wash, then with a sharp knife score across each fish down to the bone at 2.5cm/1 inch intervals on both sides. This allows flavour to penetrate the fish and lets the fish's juices come out.

Preheat the oven to 200°C/400°F/gas 6. Get yourself a bowl and add the tomatoes, garlic, oregano or basil, spring onions, balsamic vinegar, a pinch of salt and pepper and the zest and juice of 1 lemon to it. Loosen with a couple of good tablespoons of extra virgin olive oil and mix well, then spread over the bottom of a large roasting tray. Use one that will fit all 4 fish quite snugly (or you can use two smaller trays). Place the fish on top – top to tail.

Now add the olives, parsley, juice and zest of the second lemon to the bowl that the tomatoes were in. Loosen with a little olive oil and then divide this mixture between the fish, placing an equal amount on the centre of each. Cook in the preheated oven for 12 to 15 minutes, depending on the size of the fish. To check whether they're done, take the tip of a knife and push it into the thickest part of the fish. When done, the flesh will easily pull away from the bone.

Once cooked, remove the fish from the oven and allow them to rest for 3 or 4 minutes while you get your guests round the table, serve them some wine and dress your salad. Then you can come back to the fish. Divide them up at the table on to 4 plates, making sure that everyone gets some tomatoes and juice spooned over the top of the fish. Lovely!

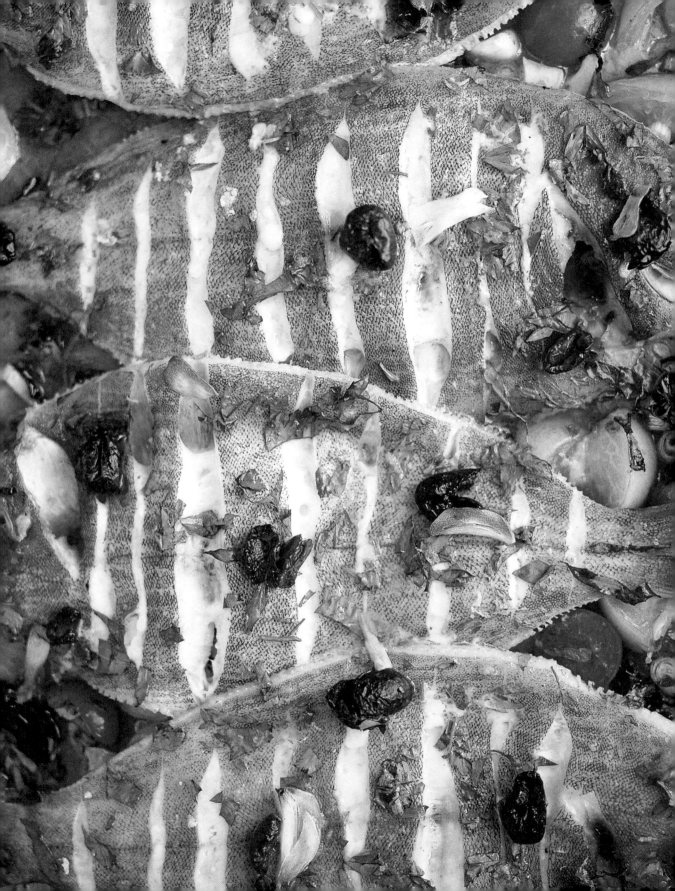

CONCERTINA SQUID

This is a really cool way of prepping squid. It makes the squid look great and allows it to take on flavours and seasoning in a really interesting way. You can see from the picture why I've called it 'concertina squid' as it reminds me of a concertina, or accordion, when it opens out. It can be served hot or cold as a main dish or a salad. Simple but totally scrumptious.

SERVES 4

1kg/2lb 3oz new potatoes, scrubbed
sea salt and freshly ground black pepper
a handful of fresh mint, leaves picked and chopped, stalks tied together
2 knobs of butter
extra virgin olive oil
1kg/2lb 3oz medium-sized squid, skinned and gutted

1–2 fresh red chillies, deseeded and finely sliced
1 red onion, peeled and finely sliced
a large handful of fresh flat-leaf parsley, stalks finely chopped, leaves roughly chopped
1 tablespoon finely ground white pepper
2 cloves of garlic, peeled and finely grated or chopped
juice of 2 lemons

First of all, boil your new potatoes in salted, boiling water with the bundle of mint stalks for 20–25 minutes until slightly overcooked. When done, drain and allow to steam dry while you heat up a large frying pan. Put a knob of butter and a couple of tablespoons of extra virgin olive oil into the pan, add the potatoes and then, using a pair of tongs or a spoon, lightly crush them and toss them around for about 5 minutes until lightly golden. While these are cooking, you are going to prepare your squid – I've given you some step-by-step photographs to help you out (see pages 278–9).

Take a squid and place a large cook's knife, palette knife or wooden spatula into its tube. Using another cook's knife, slice the squid along its length at 1cm/½ inch intervals. As the second knife cuts down on to the first knife, a fantastic effect is achieved whereby the squid retains its overall shape but also opens up a bit like a concertina. Do the same to the remaining squid.

When the potatoes have taken on a little colour, add the sliced onion and parsley stalks and give the pan a good shake. Toss the scored squid in a bowl with the white pepper and a tiny pinch of salt. When the onions are golden, turn them and the potatoes out on to a plate, put the pan back on the heat, add a little olive oil and fry the squid for about 2 minutes on each side. When nicely golden, add the remaining butter, the grated garlic, the chilli and the parsley leaves. Give the squid a really good shake to take on all these beautiful flavours and then put the potatoes and onions back into the pan. Toss together, have a little taste and correct the seasoning. Squeeze over the lemon juice – this will give it all a nice twang – and divide on to 4 plates, sprinkled with the mint leaves.

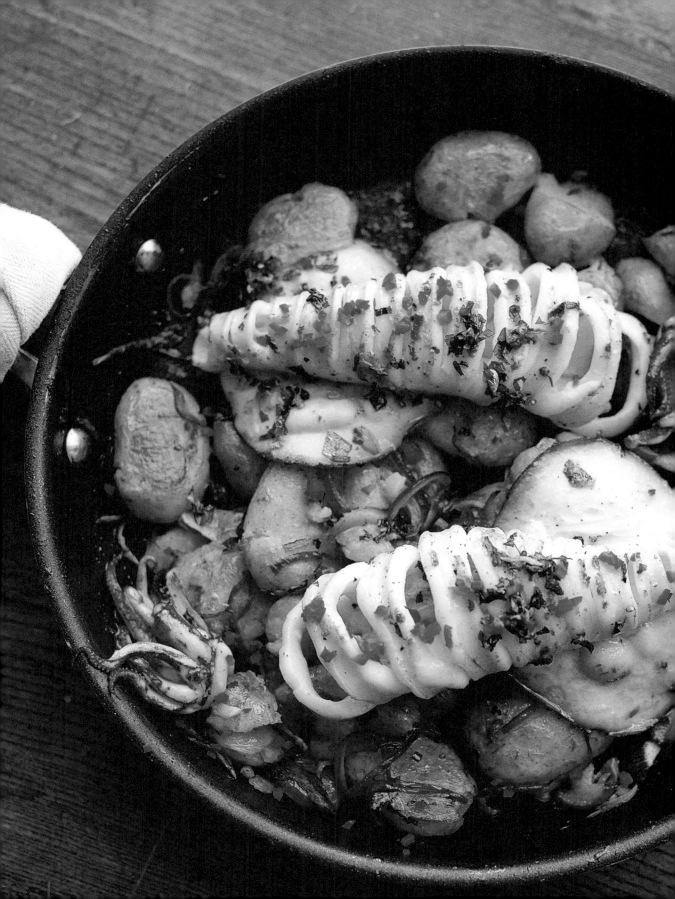

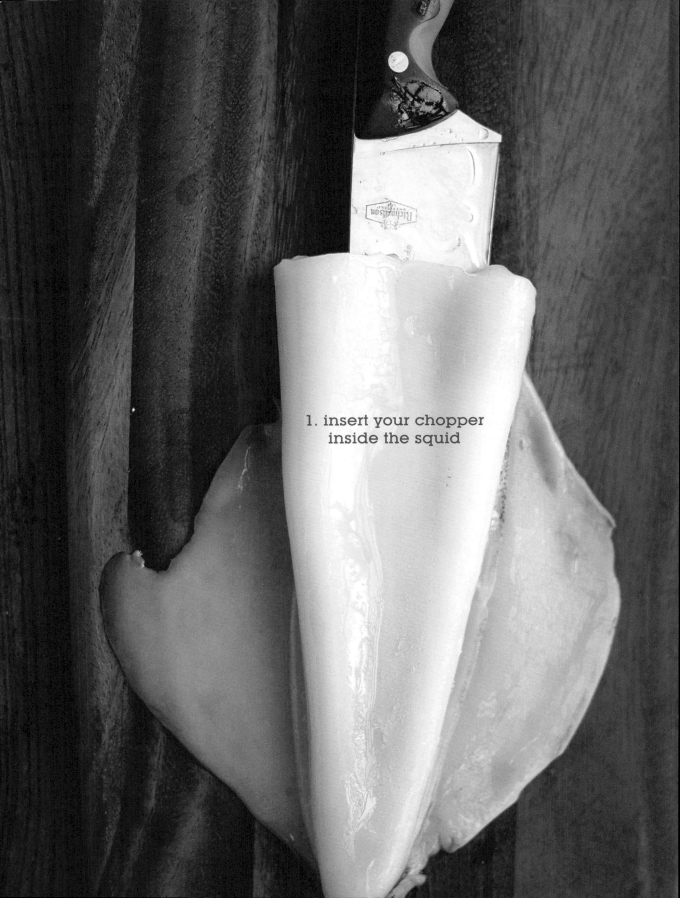

1. insert your chopper
inside the squid

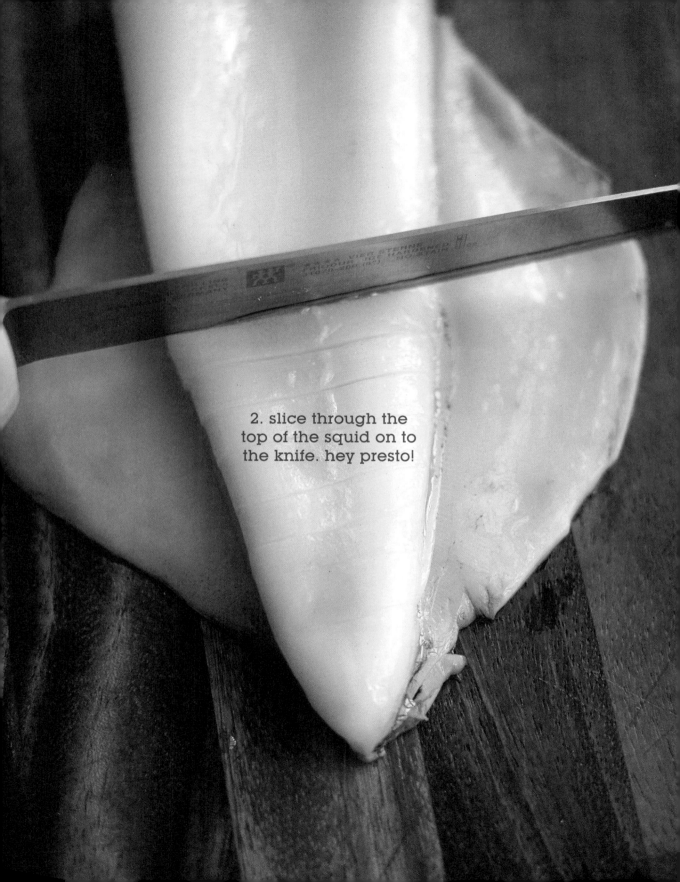

2. slice through the top of the squid on to the knife. hey presto!

SOUTH AMERICAN FISHCAKES

I learnt this recipe from my friend Santos, who comes from Brazil where they make little fritters of this recipe and deep-fry them – more like glorified canapés than fishcakes really. I've adapted his recipe slightly to make actual fishcakes – probably the nicest I've tasted! In Brazil they're called 'bolinho de bacalhau' and are made with salt cod, which is a wonderful fish to use if you can get hold of it. However, for this recipe I've simply used flaked white fish. Quite a few cookbooks have recipes for fishcakes these days, but they all seem to be Thai-influenced, with overly clever and complicated seasonings or dips. The nice thing about this one is that you can taste the potatoes and fish alongside the heat of the chilli and the zing of the lemons and limes. It works a treat.

PS My sister wanted to know if these fishcakes could be pan-fried instead of deep-fried. The answer is yes they can be but you will need to control the temperature. For fishcakes that are ¾ inch thick they will need about 2½ minutes on each side.

MAKES LOTS!

1kg/2lb 3oz haddock fillets, skin on, scaled and pinboned
140ml/¼ pint milk
2 bay leaves
1kg/2lb 3oz potatoes, peeled and diced
a big bunch of fresh flat-leaf parsley, finely chopped
a handful of fresh mint, finely chopped

zest of 2 lemons and 2 limes
1 teaspoon fennel seeds, bashed
2 eggs
1 fresh red chilli, finely chopped
sea salt and freshly ground black pepper
115g/4oz plain flour
sunflower oil, for deep-frying
lemons, to serve

Preheat the oven to 190°C/375°F/gas 5. Place the haddock in a deep baking tray with the milk and bay leaves, then cover the tray with foil and cook for 15 minutes. Meanwhile, cook the potatoes in salted boiling water for about 15 minutes, until soft. Drain them in a colander to get rid of any excess water, then return to the pan on a low heat and mash.

Flake the cooked fish into a large bowl, picking out any bones and removing the skin. Add the mashed potato, parsley, mint, lemon and lime zest, fennel seeds, eggs and chilli and season with salt and freshly ground black pepper. Mix well, taste and add more salt if necessary.

Flour your work surface, then take 1 tablespoon of the mix in your hands with a little flour and pat it into a flattened circle, rolling it in the flour. Rough and ready is good, so don't worry about having them all exactly the same!

Pour enough oil into a large heavy-bottomed saucepan to fill the pan about a third of the way up. Heat over a medium heat until a deep-frying thermometer inserted into the oil reaches 185°C/360°F. (If you don't have a thermometer, heat the oil until a cube of bread will brown in about 3 minutes.) Deep-fry the fishcakes for about 5 minutes until brown and crispy. Drain on kitchen paper, sprinkle with sea salt and serve on a large plate with lots of lemon halves.

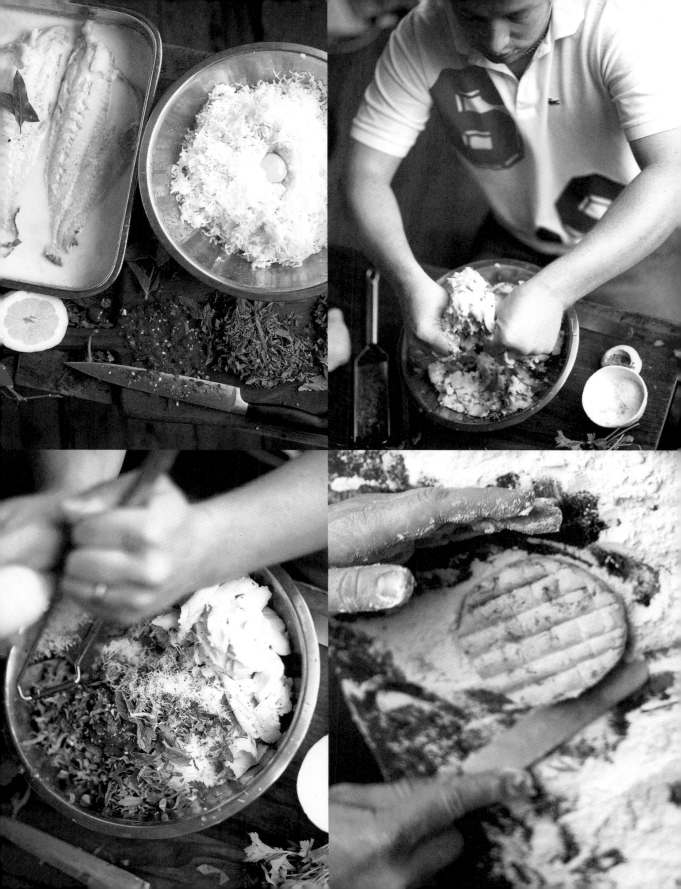

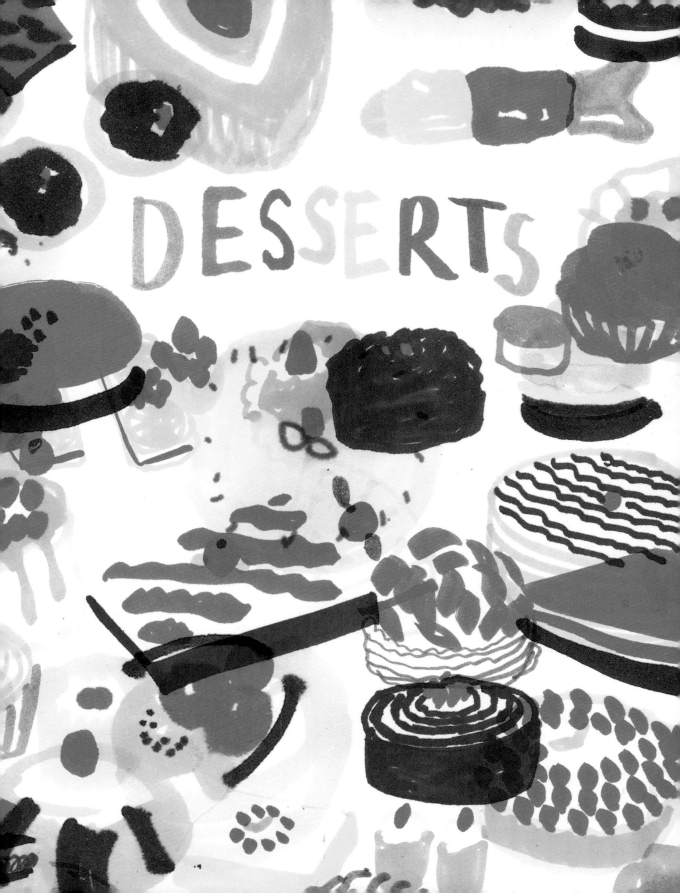

For all of you who like your desserts, there's no major theme for this chapter apart from it's a great collection of really solid recipes that are just perfect for making at home. I've used fruit in most of the recipes, as I think it's always a treat when you're working with rich desserts or sugar. I've also included a few of the great British classics like jam roly poly, sticky toffee pudding or a lovely Bakewell tart, and you must try the scented English creams – perfect for a summer's day as a light dessert. The tarts in particular are great with an afternoon cup of tea or even in your lunchbox as a treat. Mmmmm! Quite a lot of people think they shouldn't eat desserts, but I don't think there's anything wrong with a little – just don't eat the whole lot!

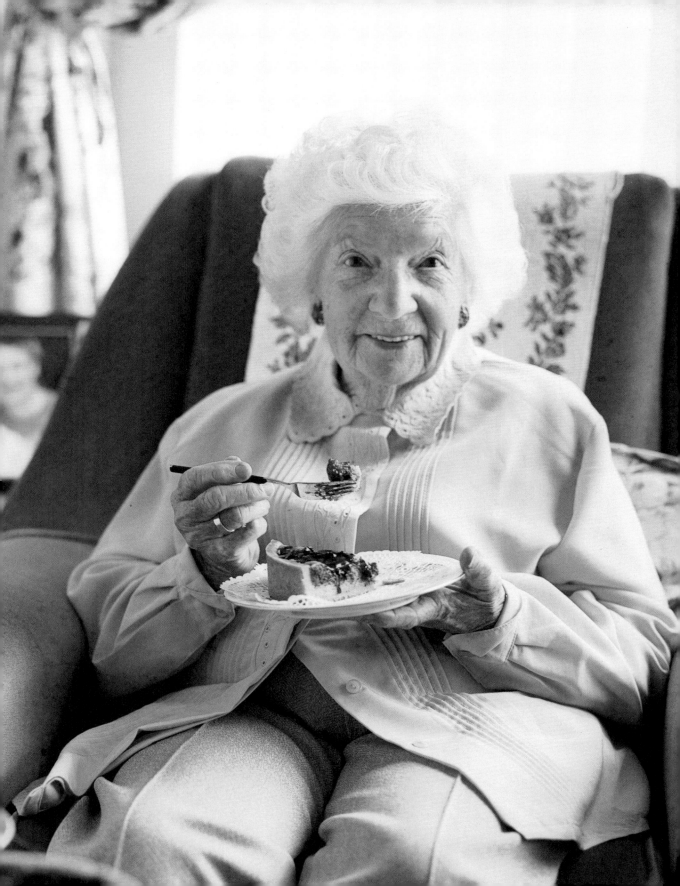

BAKED PEARS WITH WINE AND A SCRUMPTIOUS WALNUT CREAM

When I worked in France I would visit a lovely little bakery once a week to buy a tart filled with a really amazing walnut cream, with poached glazed pears on top. It was such a joy to eat that I wanted to give you a recipe based on these flavours – the combination is fantastic. At Christmas time it's nice to use chestnuts instead of walnuts, or you could even bash up or grate some good-quality chocolate to sprinkle over the pears as well.

SERVES 4
1 vanilla pod
4 good-quality seasonal pears, peeled
125g/4½oz dark muscovado sugar, plus a little extra
2 large wineglasses of red or white wine
2 oranges
200g/7oz peeled walnuts
255g/9oz mascarpone

Preheat the oven to 220°C/425°F/gas 7. Score down the length of the vanilla pod and remove the seeds by scraping a knife down the inside of each half. Put the pears into a tight-fitting ovenproof pot or pan, add the 125g of sugar, wine, vanilla pod and seeds, and the peel and juice of 1 orange and bring to the boil. Sprinkle over half the walnuts and then put in the oven to bake. Every so often, baste the pears with the syrup they are cooking in, as this will give them a nice glaze. Cook for around 20 to 30 minutes, depending on the ripeness, until the pears are tender but still holding their shape, then remove from the oven and allow to cool while you roast the remaining walnuts on a baking tray in the oven for 5 minutes – make sure you keep an eye on them as they can quickly go from golden to black and you don't want burnt walnuts!

Remove the vanilla pod from the syrup. When the walnuts are done, either whizz them in a Magimix or bash them up with a pestle and mortar until you have a paste. Whip up the mascarpone with the walnut paste, the zest and juice of the other orange and enough sugar to sweeten, and serve this cream with the baked pears, the nuts, some orange peel and some of the cooking syrup.

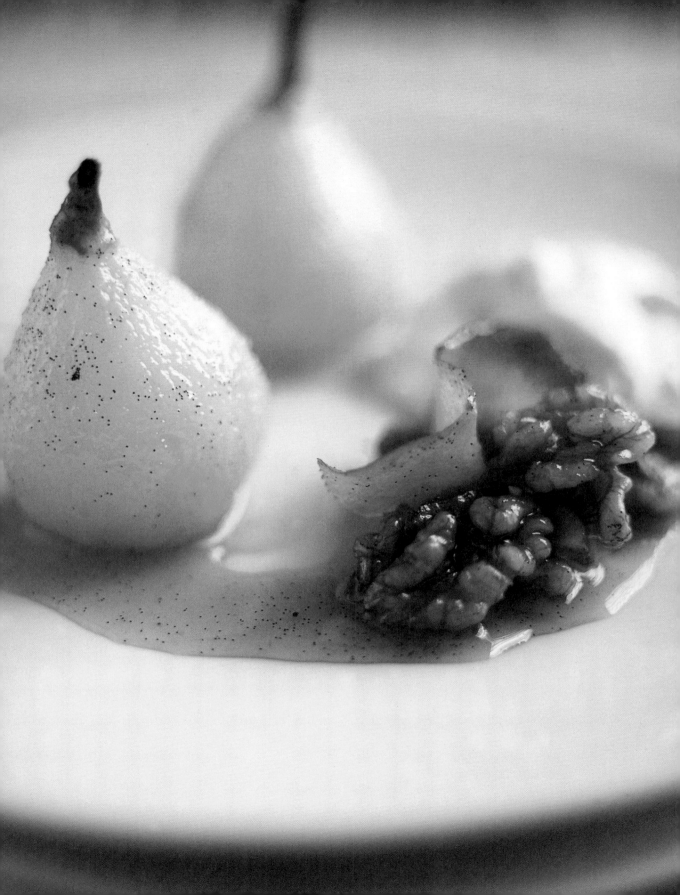

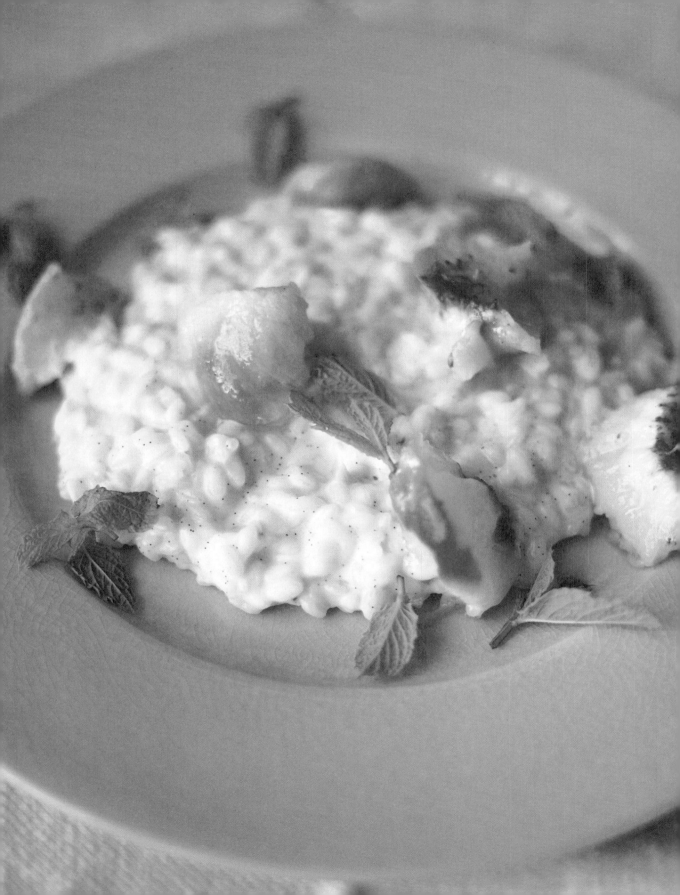

SWEET VANILLA RISOTTO WITH POACHED PEACHES AND CHOCOLATE

People in Britain have always had a bit of a soft spot in their hearts for rice pudding. However, the convenience and relative quality of tinned Ambrosia rice pudding has stopped a lot of people cooking the real thing. I thought it would be good to get you making this lovely old British dessert, but with a northern Italian twist – in the style of a risotto. Pudding rice and risotto rice are both plump, short-grain and starchy, so I thought it would be a good test to see if risotto rice would make great rice pudding – and it did. It has to be one of the best rice puddings I've ever made! It's lovely served with the peaches, but you could also use apricots, strawberries or rhubarb.

SERVES 6

6 ripe peaches, halved
6 tablespoons caster sugar
½ a cinnamon stick
zest and juice of 1 orange
85g/3oz butter
2 vanilla pods
325g/11½oz risotto rice

1 wineglass of white wine
1 litre/1¾ pints full fat milk, preferably organic
100g/3¾oz best white chocolate, grated
100g/3¾oz best-quality dark chocolate (70% cocoa solids)
a handful of fresh mint, leaves picked

When you halve the peaches, leave the stones in – they will come away a lot more easily after they have been cooked. Put them into a small pan with 4 tablespoons of the sugar, the cinnamon stick and the zest and juice of the orange. Put a lid on top and slowly simmer for about 10 to 15 minutes, until the peach skin and stones can be easily removed. You don't want to cook them to pulp – they should be soft but should still hold their shape. Remove from the heat and put to one side.

In an appropriately sized high-sided, thick-bottomed pan with a lid, slowly melt two-thirds of the butter. Score down the length of the vanilla pods and remove the seeds by scraping a knife down the inside of each half. Add the seeds to the butter and stir. Continue to cook for 1 minute before adding your rice with the remaining sugar. Turn the heat up to medium, stir the rice, and add the wine, continuing to stir until it has almost cooked away. Now add the milk little by little. Keep the rice on a slow but constant simmer for about 16 or 17 minutes and stir it as often as you can. In this way you can massage the starch out of the rice and this will give you a silky, oozy end product, much like the classic Italian risotto. When the rice has cooked through it should be soft yet still holding its shape. You may need to add a little more milk or water just to adjust the consistency. Remove from the heat, add the grated white chocolate and the rest of the butter, then stir, place a lid on top and leave for a few minutes.

Remove the skin and stones from the peaches, discard them along with the cinnamon stick, and take the peaches to the table with your block of dark chocolate, snapped into small pieces. Spoon the risotto on to plates, then push a couple of pieces of dark chocolate into the middle of each one. Just so you know, a perfect risotto should slowly creep and ooze to the side of your plate, so don't worry if it starts to spread out! Gently tear the peaches and place some on each plate, then drizzle over some of the lovely juice and sprinkle over a few mint leaves. By the time you go to eat it, the dark chocolate will have melted. Joy joy joy!

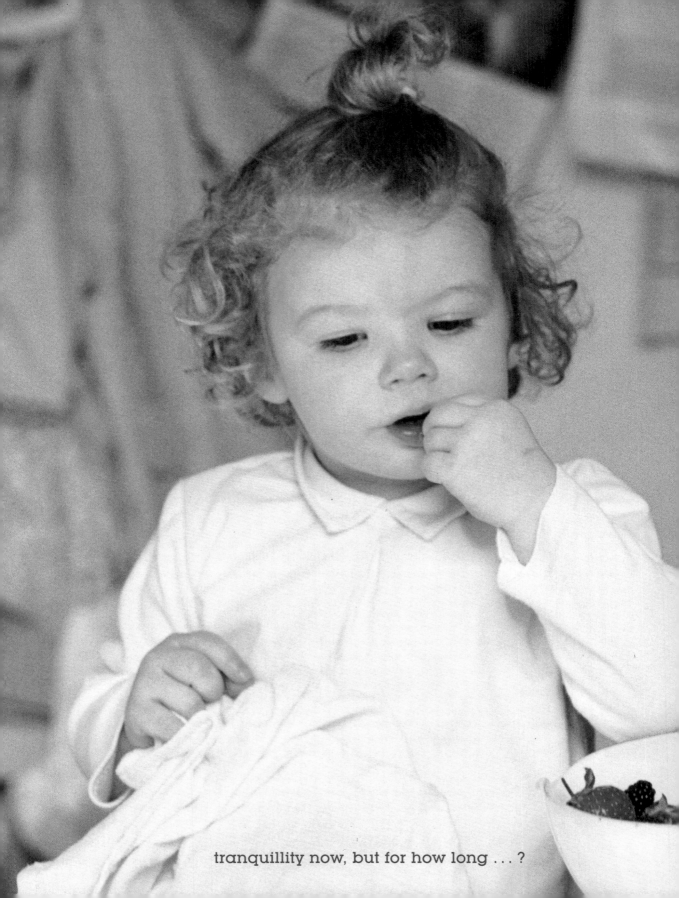

tranquillity now, but for how long . . . ?

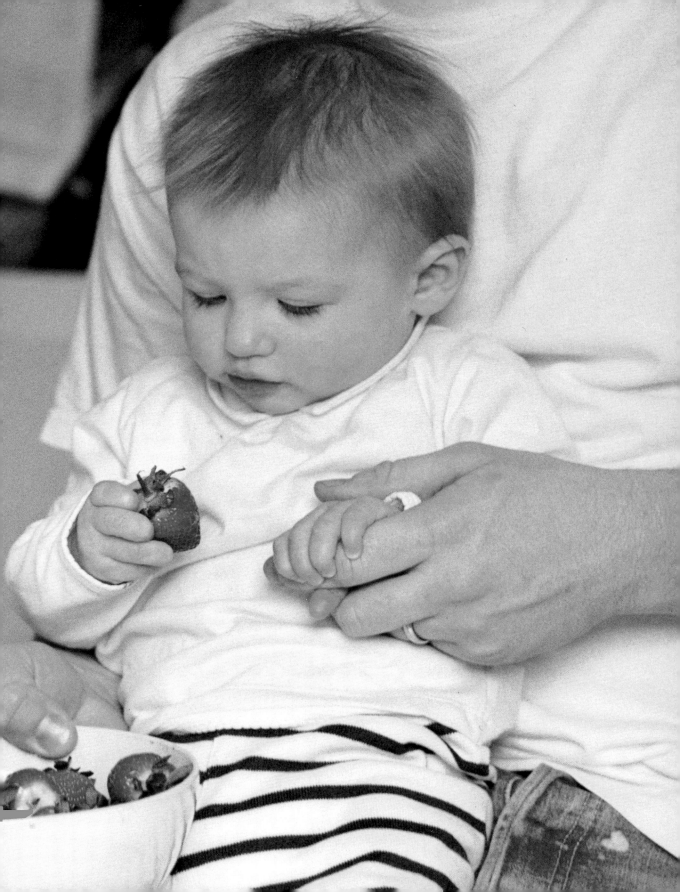

TOFFEE APPLE TART

This is a fantastic dessert that I love to make for friends as they can't get enough of it. The combination of toffee and apples is a fairground classic but feel free to try it with pears, bananas, even strawberries.

SERVES 6–8

FOR THE SHORTCRUST PASTRY
optional: 1 vanilla pod
125g/4½oz butter
100g/3¾oz icing sugar
a small pinch of salt
255g/9oz flour
zest of ½ a lemon
2 egg yolks
2 tablespoons cold milk or water

FOR THE FILLING
2 x 397g tins of condensed milk or
  2 jars of Merchant Gourmet Dulce de
  Leche toffee
4 medium-sized cooking apples
2 heaped tablespoons icing sugar

Put your unopened tins of condensed milk in a high-sided pan, covered with water. Bring to the boil, then reduce the heat and simmer constantly for about 3 hours with a lid on top. It's very important to remember to keep checking the pan, as you don't want it to boil dry – otherwise the tins will explode. It will give you the most amazing toffee. Put the tins to one side and allow to cool.

First of all you need to make your pastry. Score down the length of the vanilla pod, if using, and remove the seeds by scraping a knife down the inside of each half (keep the pod for making vanilla sugar). Cream together the butter, icing sugar and salt and then rub in the flour, vanilla seeds, lemon zest and egg yolks – you can do all this by hand or in a food processor. When the mixture looks like coarse breadcrumbs, add the cold milk or water. Pat and gently work the mixture together until you have a ball of dough, then flour it lightly and roll it into a large sausage shape – don't work the pastry too much otherwise it will become too elastic and chewy, not flaky and short as you want it to be. Wrap the dough in clingfilm and place in the fridge to rest for at least an hour. Remove it from the fridge, slice it up and line a 28cm/11 inch tart mould with the slivers. Push them together, then tidy up the sides by trimming off any excess. Place the tart mould into the freezer for an hour. Preheat the oven to 180°C/350°F/gas 4, then take the pastry case out of the freezer and bake for around 15 minutes or until lightly golden. Remove from the oven and place to one side. Peel and quarter the apples and remove the cores, then slice finely and toss in the icing sugar. Smear the caramel from both tins of condensed milk over the pastry. Place the apples on top and pour any remaining juices over. Cook at the bottom of the preheated oven for about 40 minutes, to give you a crispy base and bubbling toffee over the apples. Serve with vanilla ice cream. Beautiful!

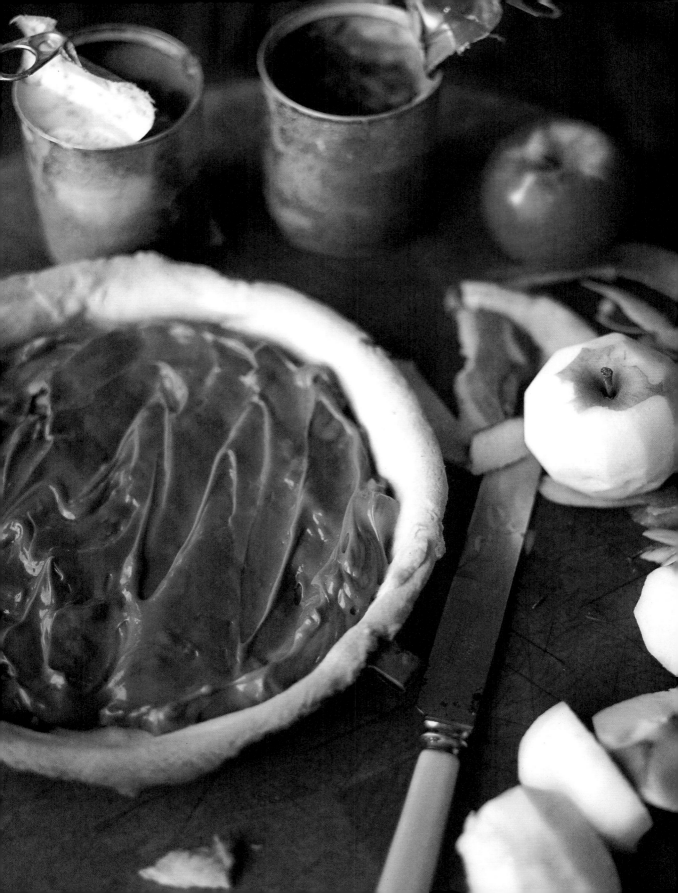

CHOCOLATE CLAFOUTIS WITH CARAMELIZED ORANGES

The nice thing about this recipe is that the fruit accompanying it can be varied – certain things work really well with chocolate, like oranges, clementines, apricots or cherries, so give them a try.

SERVES 6-8

5 oranges
100g/3¾oz best-quality dark
    chocolate (70% cocoa solids)
80g/2¾oz unsalted butter
115g/4oz self-raising flour
115g/4oz ground almonds
115g/4oz sugar

a pinch of salt
2 large eggs
3 egg yolks
180ml/6½fl oz full cream milk
100g/3¾oz best-quality white chocolate,
    broken up
1 x 500ml tub of crème fraîche

Preheat your oven to 200°C/400°F/gas 6. Firstly zest 3 of your oranges, then carefully remove the outer peel and slice them across into wheel-shaped pieces just under 1cm/½ inch thick. Break the dark chocolate up, place in a small bowl and slowly melt it over some simmering water, giving it a stir once in a while with a spatula.

You will need a deep 20cm/8 inch metal tin or earthenware dish to cook the clafoutis in. Rub the inside of it with a little of the butter. To make the clafoutis, sift the flour into a separate bowl, add the almonds, half the sugar, the salt, eggs, yolks, orange zest and milk. Whisk up until smooth and then add the rest of the butter to the melting chocolate. Scrape all the melted chocolate and butter into the batter mix and pour into your tin. Poke little pieces of white chocolate into the batter, then place the tin in the oven and bake for around 16 to 20 minutes. It will rise and should be firm around the edges but sticky and gooey in the middle. This doesn't mean it's undercooked . . . it means it's perfect! So be careful not to overcook it or it will just be like a boring sponge.

While it's cooking, bring the other half of your sugar to the boil with about 6 tablespoons of water on a medium heat until you have a golden caramel. Remove from the heat, add the juice from your remaining oranges and stir it in to loosen the caramel syrup slightly. Arrange your oranges nicely on a plate, pour over the caramel and serve with your chocolate clafoutis and a bowl of crème fraîche.

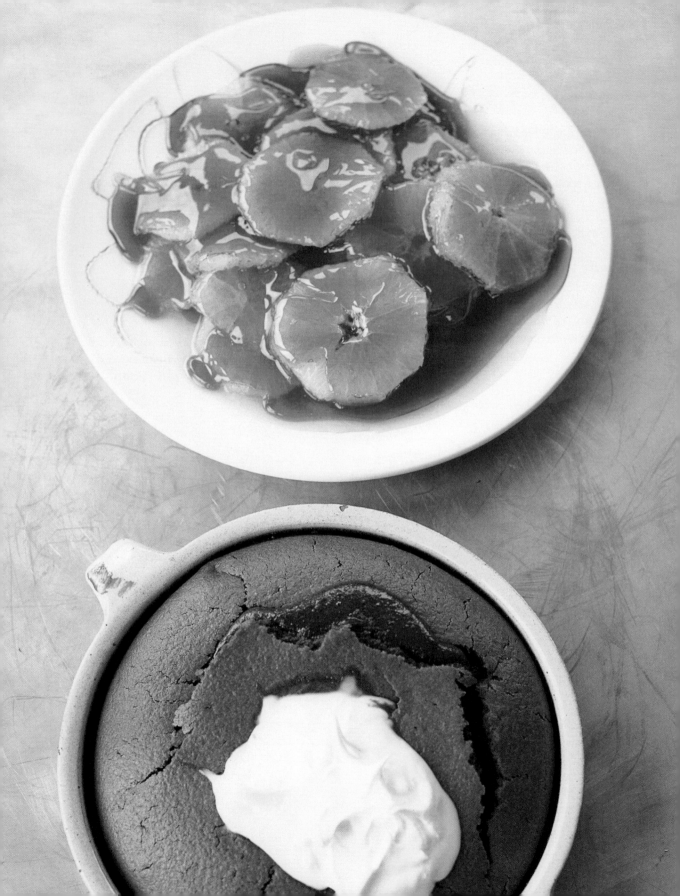

THE ULTIMATE JAM ROLY POLY

This is something I had all the time for school dinner when I was at primary school. My mum also used to make it every now and again and it was always superb. The way the suet – which is completely underrated these days – gives the most fantastic, slightly chewy texture and it's all fluffy in the middle and slightly crisp on the outside … I love it, really really nice. My version of the roly poly is based on the original golden oldie. I don't think it can be improved upon all that much, but what I think is quite nice is to bring some flavour into the batter and also to use some fruit. This works really well with the jam – it gives the whole thing a bit more texture and makes it more luxurious. Feel free to fiddle with different flavours – raspberry and strawberry mixed together is one of my favourites.

SERVES 6
1 vanilla pod
225g/8oz self-raising flour
1 heaped teaspoon baking powder
zest of 1 orange
a pinch of salt
150g/5½oz beef suet, vegetarian
   suet or butter

150ml/5½fl oz milk
175g/6oz strawberry and raspberry jam
3 large handfuls of strawberries and
   raspberries, washed and sliced
1 egg, beaten

Score down the length of the vanilla pod and remove the seeds by scraping a knife down the inside of each half. Sift the flour into a large bowl, then add the baking powder, orange zest and vanilla seeds (keep the pod for making vanilla sugar) with a pinch of salt and the suet or butter. Depending on the flour you're using, you may not need all the milk, so add it slowly until you have a soft but firm dough which isn't sticky. Leave it to rest for half an hour, then lightly dust a surface with flour and roll out the dough so it's about 30 x 30cm/12 x 12 inches. It doesn't have to be too perfect. Leaving a 2.5cm/1 inch rim around the sides of the dough, smear the jam over it and scatter the strawberries on top. Brush the rim with some egg to help give it a nice seal.

The idea of the roly poly is that it's all rolled up so you get lovely layers of jam and sponge, but the jam from the early folds tends to get squeezed out, so what I try to do is put a nice bit of jam in the first bit as I begin to roll it and then, as I fold the dough over, pinch around it so that the jam gets trapped in and can't ooze out. Then I continue to roll and pinch at the ends to keep in all the lovely jam.

When it's all rolled up, lay a piece of buttered greaseproof paper in front of it. Carefully roll the roly poly on to the paper and continue to roll it up so it is covered by the greaseproof. Then get a double-layered sheet of tinfoil and roll the roly poly in this as well, pinching the ends together. Place it on a rack above simmering water in a baking tray and cover it all with tinfoil to allow it to steam in the oven for about 2 hours at 150°C/300°F/gas 2. Top the tray up with boiling water from your kettle every half hour – simply peel back the foil to do this. This is one dessert that just has to be eaten with custard – nothing else will do!

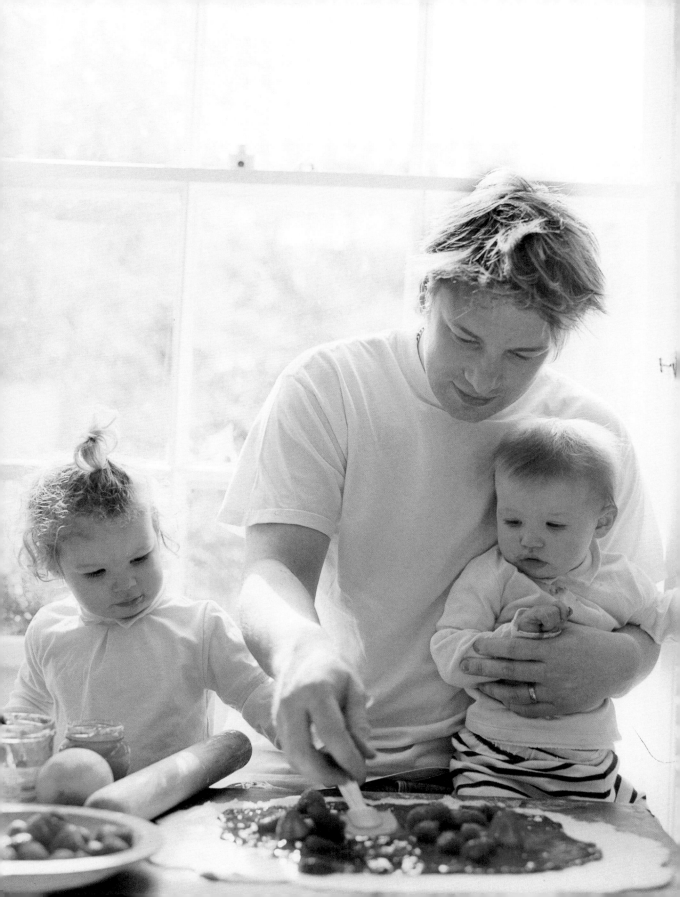

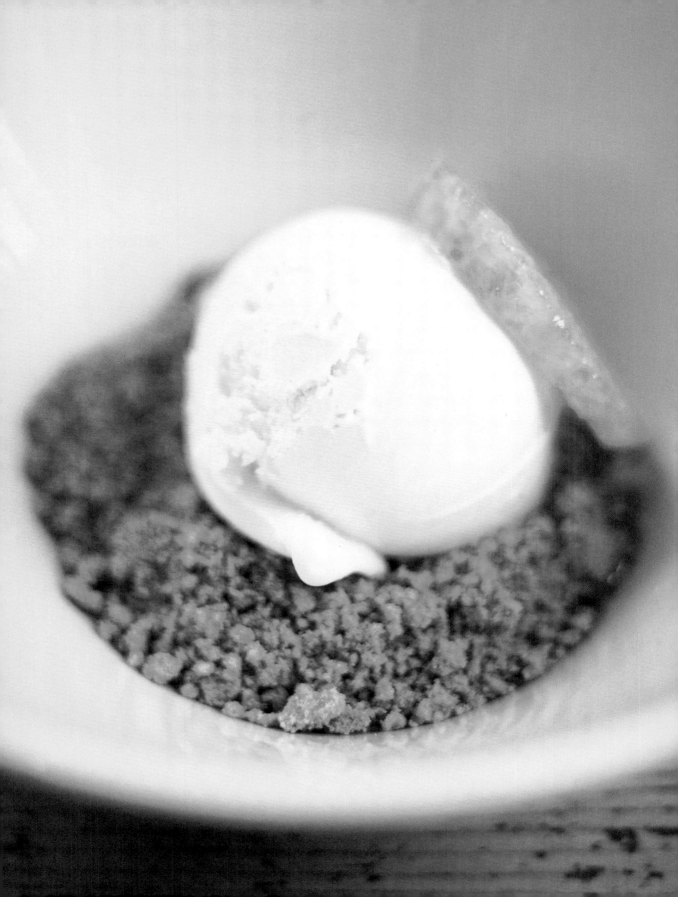

CHEAT'S DESSERT

This is a dessert which is absolutely great for getting you out of trouble at the last minute if you have friends descending on you for dinner.

SERVES 4
4 ginger biscuits
4 blood oranges or clementines, plus the juice of 2 oranges
4 scoops of vanilla ice cream
optional: 55g/2oz caster sugar

Smash the ginger biscuits up into crumbs using a pestle and mortar, or place them in a clean tea towel and bash with a rolling pin. Put them into a dish. Peel and slice the oranges or clementines, making sure you remove any pips. Now all you have to do to serve is put a scoop of ice cream on each plate and either sprinkle with the ginger biscuit crumbs or serve a pile of the crunchy biscuity crumbs under the ice cream, and top with some blood orange slices.

If you want to take this up a notch, bring 55g/2oz of caster sugar to the boil with 6 tablespoons of water on a medium heat until you have a golden caramel. Remove from the heat, add the juice from the extra 2 oranges and stir it in to loosen the caramel syrup slightly. Pour this over your sliced oranges so they marinate in the caramelized juices. Divide the ginger biscuit crumbs between 4 plates and top with a scoop of ice cream and some slices of caramelized orange.

MAPLE SYRUP AND PECAN TART

Maple syrup and pecan nuts are fantastic Canadian flavours. What I've done here is make a traditional English treacle tart, but I've used maple syrup as well as golden syrup and have added nuts.

SERVES 6–8
1 x shortcrust pastry recipe (see page 292)
55g/2oz butter
340g/12oz maple syrup
3 tablespoons golden syrup
170g/6oz breadcrumbs, half fine, half coarse
zest of 2 oranges
2 Cox's apples, grated
a thumb-sized piece of fresh ginger, peeled and finely grated
2 handfuls of shelled pecan nuts
optional: crème fraîche or vanilla ice cream
optional: a handful of thyme flowers

First of all, make your pastry, then line a 28cm/11 inch loose-bottomed tart tin with it and place in the freezer for an hour. Preheat the oven to 180°C/350°F/gas 4. Take the pastry case out of the freezer and bake in the oven for around 15 minutes, until lightly golden. Remove from the oven and allow to cool slightly. Heat the butter, maple syrup and golden syrup together in a pan, then mix in the breadcrumbs, orange zest, apples, ginger and half the pecan nuts. Spoon into the pastry case and sprinkle over the remaining pecans. Put back in the oven and bake for around 20 minutes. Lovely served with some crème fraîche or vanilla ice cream and sprinkled with thyme flowers.

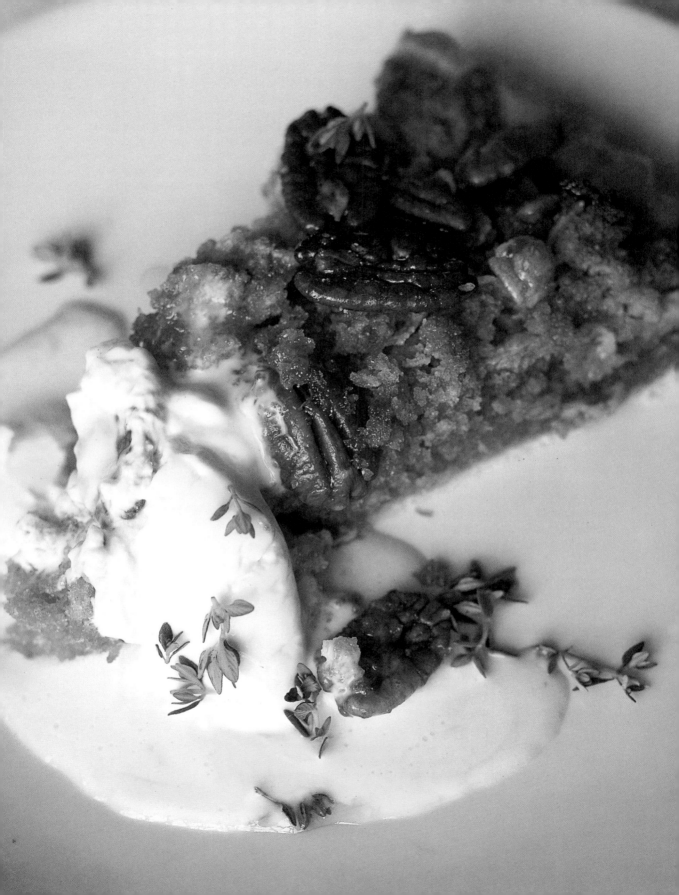

BAKEWELL TART

This is pretty easy because all you need to put it together is a pastry recipe and a frangipane recipe. Bakewell tart is a classic English tea cake which, if made with a bit of love and some quality jam, well deserves to be a dessert in its own right.

SERVES 8
1 x shortcrust pastry recipe (see page 292)

FOR THE FRANGIPANE
350g/12oz blanched whole almonds
300g/11oz unsalted butter
300g/11oz caster sugar
3 free-range eggs
6 tablespoons good-quality strawberry jam
a handful of sliced blanched almonds
1 x 500ml tub of crème fraîche

First of all, make your pastry, then line a 28cm/11 inch loose-bottomed tart tin with it and place in the freezer for an hour. Preheat the oven to 180°C/350°F/gas 4, then take the pastry case out of the freezer and bake for around 15 minutes or until lightly golden. Remove from the oven, place to one side, and turn the heat down to 170°C/325°F/gas 3.

To make the frangipane, blitz the whole almonds in a food processor until you have a fine powder and put this into a bowl. Now blitz the butter and sugar until light and creamy. Add this to the almonds with the lightly beaten eggs and fold in until completely mixed and smooth. Place in the fridge to firm up slightly.

Smear the jam over the bottom of the pastry case, pour the chilled frangipane mixture on top, and sprinkle with some sliced blanched almonds. Bake the tart for about 40 minutes, or until the almond mixture has become firm and golden on the outside but is still soft in the middle. Allow to cool for about 30 minutes and serve with crème fraîche or custard.

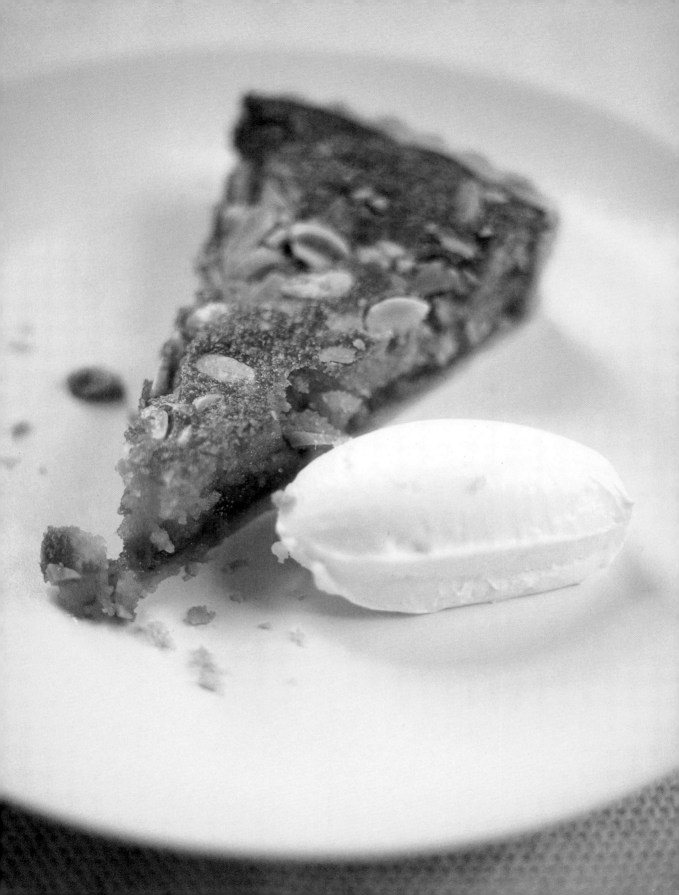

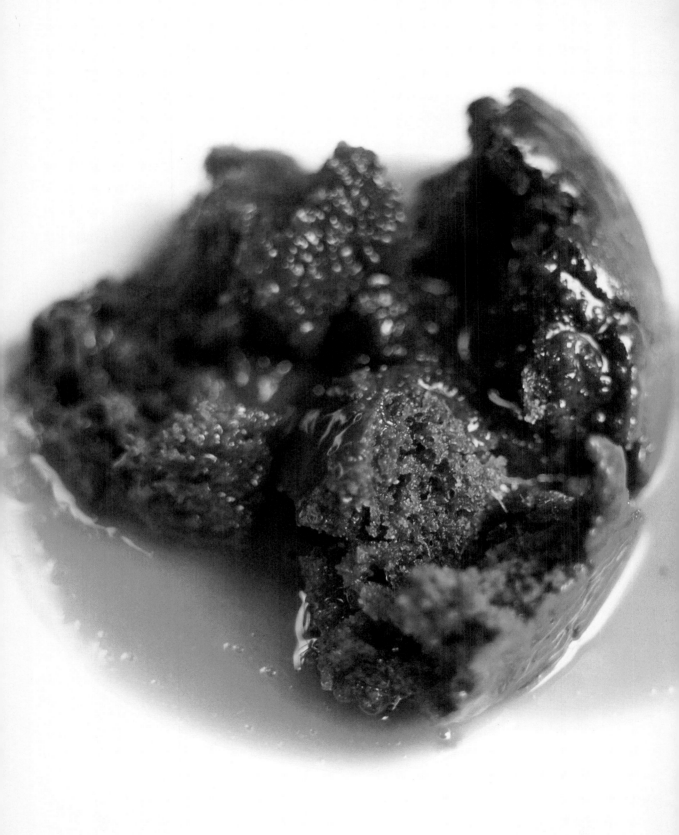

STICKY TOFFEE PUDDING

You are going to love this pudding – it has a rich, fantastic flavour and the sauce is amazing. Fresh Medjool dates are best to use, but dried ones work well too.

SERVES 8
225g/8oz fresh dates, stoned
1 teaspoon bicarbonate of soda
85g/3oz unsalted softened butter
170g/6oz caster sugar
2 large free-range eggs
170g/6oz self-raising flour
¼ teaspoon ground mixed spice

¼ teaspoon ground cinnamon
2 tablespoons Ovaltine
2 tablespoons natural yoghurt

FOR THE TOFFEE SAUCE
115g/4oz unsalted butter
115g/4oz light muscovado sugar
140ml/5fl oz double cream

Preheat your oven to 180°C/350°F/gas 4. Put the dates in a bowl with the bicarbonate of soda and cover with 200ml/7fl oz of boiling water. Leave to stand for a couple of minutes to soften, then drain. Whizz the dates in a food processor until you have a purée. Meanwhile, cream your butter and sugar until pale using a wooden spoon, and add the eggs, flour, mixed spice, cinnamon and Ovaltine. Mix together well, then fold in the yoghurt and your puréed dates. Pour into a buttered, ovenproof dish and bake in the preheated oven for 35 minutes.

While the pudding is cooking, make the toffee sauce by putting the butter, sugar and cream in a pan over a low heat until the sugar has dissolved and the sauce has thickened and darkened in colour. To serve, spoon out the pudding at the table and pour over the toffee sauce.

SCENTED ENGLISH CREAMS

This is a kind of cross between an old-fashioned blancmange milk jelly and a pannacotta and was traditionally made in England as a variation on fruit jelly. It can be spiked with booze, flavoured with things like vanilla, lemon zest, cinnamon, coffee or orange and, like a good pannacotta, wants to be set so that it just holds together and isn't too bouncy or rubbery. I'm giving you a basic recipe to follow, with three different flavours, or scents, to add to it. Each of them uses 2½ leaves of gelatine and this is ideal if you want to make them the day before you need them. If making on the same day as eating, then you'll need an extra ½ a leaf.

MAKES 10
600ml/21fl oz full cream milk
200ml/7fl oz double cream
150g/5½oz caster sugar
2½ leaves of gelatine

FOR AN ORANGE AND
CARDAMOM CREAM
zest of 4 oranges
10 cardamom pods, roasted in a hot
   oven for 5 minutes then bashed up

FOR A BASIL CREAM
a very small bunch of basil, leaves
   picked, stalks reserved and bashed up
optional: 10ml/1 dessertspoon grappa

FOR A STRAWBERRY AND
STAR ANISE CREAM
200g/7oz strawberry jam
   (with strawberry bits!)
5 star anise

Put the milk, cream and sugar into a large pot and place on the heat. For the orange cream, add the zest and cardamom pods to the pot; for the basil cream, add the basil stalks and grappa; and for the strawberry cream just add the star anise. Bring the mixture to a gentle simmer, then remove from the heat and place to one side for the flavours to infuse. While this is happening, soak the gelatine leaves in enough ice-cold water to cover and leave to soak for 10 minutes until they have softened.

Place the pan of milk back on the heat and bring to the boil. Whisk in the softened gelatine leaves until they have dissolved, then strain the liquid into a bowl. If making the orange cream, discard the orange zest and cardamom pods and pour the liquid into little moulds. For the basil cream, bash up the basil leaves and add these to the pan. Give it a good stir and then strain the liquid, discarding the basil leaves and stalks, before pouring into moulds. If making the strawberry version, remove it from the heat and leave to cool to room temperature. While it is cooling, break the jam up with a fork until you have a nice loose consistency but with little bits of strawberry. Whisk the cooled milk liquid, then strain it and discard the star anise before pouring it into the jam. Stir together well and pour into your moulds. Put the moulds into the fridge and leave to set for at least 4 hours, but preferably overnight.

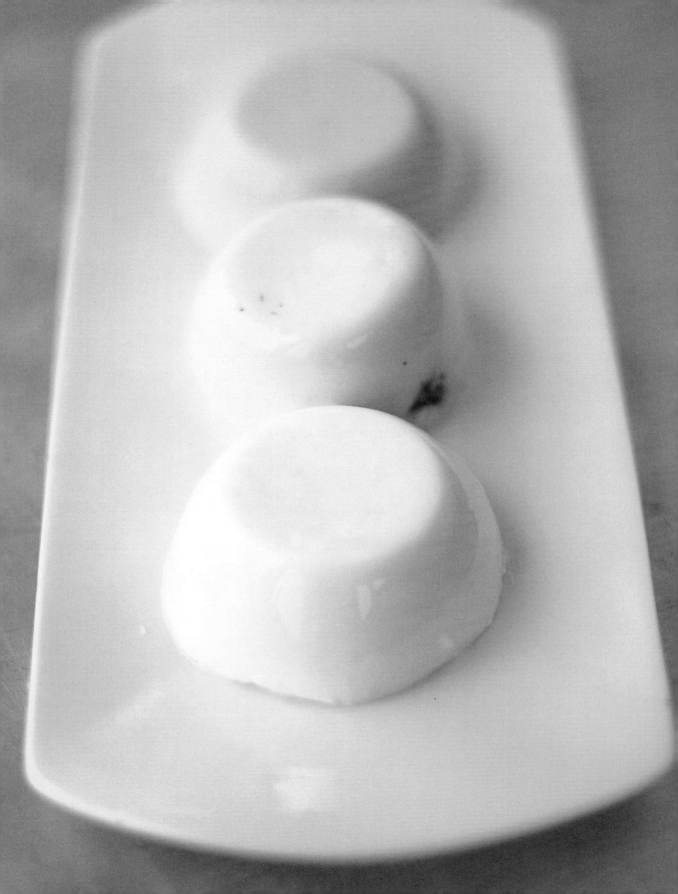

KITCHENS THAT WORK

Loads of friends and people that I meet say, 'Oh, you always make cooking look so easy,' and add, 'I've only got a little kitchen,' as if that means that they can't do the same. The truth is that I don't have a big commercial kitchen that I produce it all from. To this day all my kitchens at home have been really small. The one that was featured on *The Naked Chef* was the most spacious, but it was cheaply made. However, a lot of commonsense to the layout made it work well. So here's a few points to help you get your kitchen organized which will give you more space and hopefully make you feel able to achieve more from it.

Most chefs and architects will agree that very rarely do you have the perfect shell to put a kitchen in – there will always be extraction problems or pillars or plumbing restrictions that make you compromise on the perfect design. If you're lucky enough to be designing a kitchen from scratch or are redoing a kitchen, here are some things to bear in mind. We all want a kitchen that looks good, but functionality is really important. Cupboards are always an issue because space is usually at a premium, especially as things like dishwashers are now built into what would have been extra cupboard space. Following on from here are some basic little hints and tips that will make life less stressful, easier, and which will put on display the most important things that you are going to need access to, making your food tastier! You'll be moving with some form of elegance if every-thing flows well in the kitchen – no more scraping about in the back of dark drawers for forgotten implements.

KITCHEN TIPS

- So, tip number one, get an old laundry rack or pan rack to hang from the ceiling. These are really cheap, easy to install, look really nice and quaint, and if you want to make one look funky, just give it a lick of paint. Straight away you resolve the problem of where to put your pans, your colanders and sieves, and things like cheese graters. It will look like cool clutter. One of the biggest problems to muck up dinner parties is lack of room to cook in and serve from, so on the day have a look at your kitchen surfaces and move all your quaint and homely family memorabilia, your old jars with coins in, funny little juicers that only get used once a year, bills, etc., and put them in a cupboard under the stairs. You'll be surprised at how much room you've gained.

- If you can, it's always nice to have your sink near or in front of a window for good light and a bit of a view whilst doing the washing-up.

- For your work surface I would suggest getting a reasonably thick wooden one. You can do it economically or you can get some flashy hardwood but, most importantly, this allows you to chop straight on to the surface. Now, when my carpenter saw me doing this he nearly cried, but that's because he's never cooked a meal in his life! I think there's nothing more boring than having chopping boards all over the place. All you really need are two: one for fish and one for chicken. Anything else can be chopped straight on to your wooden surfaces and as time goes by they will look better and better. Just squirt with disinfectant after each use – it couldn't be easier! Every month or so drizzle some cheap olive oil over the wood to feed it and stop it cracking. It's always good to have your knives, bottle openers, peelers and cutlery in a drawer near your central prep area (knives can be in a block).

- Always have your larder stocked up with non-perishables like oils, vinegars, spices, herbs, salts, jams, pasta, rice, mustards and tinned items. I like to keep them in those cheap recycled kilner jars that are easy to get hold of. It's good to get all sorts of different sizes and shapes. One of the cheapest shelf-saving solutions is this: every time you finish with a jar of jam or chutney, give it a wash, soak the label off and then put two screws through the lid of each jar and attach them to the bottom of a shelf. To store, just screw the jar into the lid and it will hang under the shelf – dead easy to grab. I think it looks great to have them all on display. That way you can immediately see what you've got or are running out of.

- Bins have always been an afterthought for me, and they've driven me mad for years now. The best thing if you can is to build a bin into your kitchen work surface. It's very simple: get an extra large plastic bin and either have it in a cupboard so you can pull it out, or cut a hole into your work surface so you can put all your rubbish down through it.

- If you're not going to get a ceiling unit for your pans, try using a free-standing metal or wooden shelf unit on which to stack your bowls, whisks, pans and food processors.

- The final test to find out if you've got a kitchen that's working well is to draw an aerial view showing your fridge, your spices on their shelf, your knives in their drawer or block and so on. Think of a dish that you regularly cook. Then, using a red pen, draw the 'journey' of the meal, from going to the fridge, to cutting up food, to seasoning it, to getting commodities from the cupboard, and by the time you've finished the meal and got it in the oven, if there are loads of lines crossing all over the place you kind of know it's not a brilliant design layout! The two main focal points are your chopping area and sink, so try to position them next to each other. As you stand at your sink, the oven should be behind you. You will become more economical in your movements and will be able to work faster.

KITCHEN EQUIPMENT

- **Pans**

  It's really important that you get yourself some sturdy pans. For home use it's best to always go with non-stick if you can – it's definitely the way forward! I've worked with Tefal and can say that their Professional Series would be my first choice. They're widely available, so try to get yourself a few from the range.

- **Cookers**

  With regard to stove-tops/hobs, I think gas ones are far superior to electric and I would go for gas every time. They are more robust, more visual and give you more physical control over temperature. The ideal scenario would be a gas hob and an electric oven. You generally get what you pay for, but when using medium to cheaper ovens I would most definitely advise going for the larger, better-known companies like AEG, Amana, Hotpoint or Aga which have very good warranties, spare parts and servicing departments, as opposed to some of the design-over-content pretentious makes.

- **Knives**

  When it comes to knives, you really do get what you pay for. What I don't want you to do is go out and buy a large, cheap set, because they won't last very long. There are three brands which are great – Victorinox, Global and Sabatier. You won't go far wrong if you buy a large and small chopping knife, a paring knife and a serrated knife from one of these brands.

- **Dishwashers**

  I find it strange that a lot of people still don't have dishwashers even though they have space for one. They were once considered expensive, but you can get hold of them cheaply and second-hand these days. They are great for washing all your stuff – especially glassware – and because of the high temperatures they sterilize everything and are therefore more hygienic, plus they are easy to plumb in (I've always done my own).

- **Freezers and microwaves**

  There seems to be some idea that these are a bit naff, probably because prepacked frozen meals have been associated with them. The truth is that microwaves are great for reheating things for parties, wonderful for steaming, getting your butter soft, boiling things like veg quickly, and the freezer is a brilliant method of preserving food, so I think both of these are essential for the modern household.

- **Barbecues**

  The only ones to go for are charcoal or wood barbecues as opposed to gas ones, which can impart a negative flavour and certainly don't give you the authentic smoky flavour that makes barbecuing what it should be. Sometimes it's easy to burn things on the outside and not cook them through on the inside. But with barbecues you can organize your charcoal high on one side (hot end) and low on the other – this way you can get fast, hot, direct heat to achieve good colour and on the other side your food will cook slowly and remain tasty and moist. I've bought myself the most amazing hand-made barbecue off a bloke in Oxford. It was about two or three times the price of a really good barbecue, but it should last years because it's stainless steel and incredibly thick. So if you're interested in the best barbecue in the world go to www.caribbeancookers.com.

Thanks...

To My darling wife Jools and my girls Poppy and Daisy for making me excited to wake up every morning — thanks to you both

MUM AND DAD FOR READING THROUGH MY BOOK WITH A FINE-TOOTHED COMB

TO MY MANAGEMENT TEAM: FROSTY the perv, Louise 'the Theydon Tongue' HOLLAND, Tessa 'The Tongue' Graham and Tara 'Leather Matrix Outfit' Donovan

TO LORD LOFTUS WHO CONTINUES TO BE THE BEST FOOD PHOTOGRAPHER IN THE WORLD — thanks bro for pulling out the stops — and to his assistant Annabel who has taken EXCEEDINGLY amazing reportage photos — thanks for being supportive over the past year, To CHRIS TERRY incredibly enthusiastic and to his WIERD but lovely assistant DANNY! THANKS TO YOU ALL FOR THE MOST incredible PICTURES.

sexy Annabel

TO THE ENTIRE GANG AT THE OFFICE. I love you all — THANKS FOR DOING A GREAT JOB, FOR SUPPORTING ME AND PUTTING UP WITH ME!

AND A MASSIVE THANKS DANNY McCUBBIN MY NEW PA, FOR SORTING OUT MY C... DIARY AND KEEPING M... LIFE IN ORDER — YOU K... ME LOOKING BEAUTIFU... BRO. WORK MOR... HOURS PLE...

HOWEVER I WOULD LIKE TO THANK THE FOLLOWING PEOPLE FOR WORKING SO HARD ON THE BOOK: GINNY "Cat's Bum!" ROLFE, PETE 'the gorgeous Scotsman'... BEGG, BOBBY THOMSON and EDDIE "The streaker" SEISUN. ALSO THANKS TO KELLY, TOMMY, SUE, CARLY, JENNY, BETH AND NIC FOR HIS 'CARE NOTES'

LUSCIOUS LINDA P.S

Does Anyone "KNOW" WHO TANYA ROBINSON IS? ? ? ? ? see page one 1 ?

I'VE HAD THE HONOUR AND PLEASURE OF WORKING WITH SOME OF THE MOST TALENTED AND DEDICATED PEOPLE IN ON THIS PROJECT. IN NO PARTICULAR ORDER: ZOE COLLINS, ANDREW CONRAD, ROBERT THIRKELL, DOMINIQUE WALKER, LAIA SALAH, GUY GILBERT, TRACEY GARRETT & VANYA BARWELL. THANKS TO YOU ALL.

+ chris & freddie rT

TO JEANETTE ORREY AND HER KITCHEN STAFF AT ST PETERS PRIMARY SCHOOL IN EAST BRIDGFORD, NOTTINGHAMSHIRE. AND TO NORA SANDS AND ALL THE DINNER-LADIES AT KIDBROOKE SCHOOL IN GREENWICH, LONDON.

TO THE TEAM WHO RUN THE CHEEKY CHOPS CHARITY FOR ME — PARTICULARLY TONY, EAMON AND SHARON. AND OF COURSE, TO ALL OF YOU WHO HAVE DONATED TO CHEEKY CHOPS, — PLEASE GIVE US SOME MORE!

AND EVEN THOUGH THIS DOESN'T REALLY HAVE ANYTHING TO DO WITH THE BOOK, I'D LIKE TO THANK NICK AND LISA LYONS HENSON, CORPORATE ENTERTAINMENT FOR TAKING THE STUDENTS AWAY TO WALES FOR 2 DAYS TO HELP US CHOOSE OUR FINAL FIFTEEN EVERY YEAR. I JUST WANTED TO SAY THAT I APPRECIATE IT.

IF YOU EVER NEED A WEEKEND OF TEAM BUILDING FOR YOUR COMPANY they phone these guys on 01443 228565

TO THE STREAKING SLEEPWALKER 'WELDON' - thanks for being the best, @ most supportive, publisher in town (and fairest)

TOM, 'hardnut' hard, HAMILTON

JOHN 'hasn't got hard'

SOPHIE 'good girl' BREWER and the rest of the rights team, SOPHIE 'great cleavage' CALLARD, CHRIS 'paisley' fronts as I do, for LOVING THIS PROJECT as much WORK THAN HE'S PAID TO DO AND for putting in 4 times more

HEWAT AND CATHERINE 'GRR' 'YOU TIGER' HAMMOND FROM PRODUCTION, ANNIE LEE AND KEITH TAYLOR FOR MAKING MY CHITTER CHATTER LEGIBLE,

THE GORGEOUS TORA ORDE-POWLETT AND THE VERY HANDSOME RDB WILLIAMS IN MARKETING,

THE LOVELY KATY NICHOLSON AND SAUCY JANE OPOKO FROM PUBLICITY AND FINALLY TO ALL THE SALES TEAM FOR THEIR HARD WORK.

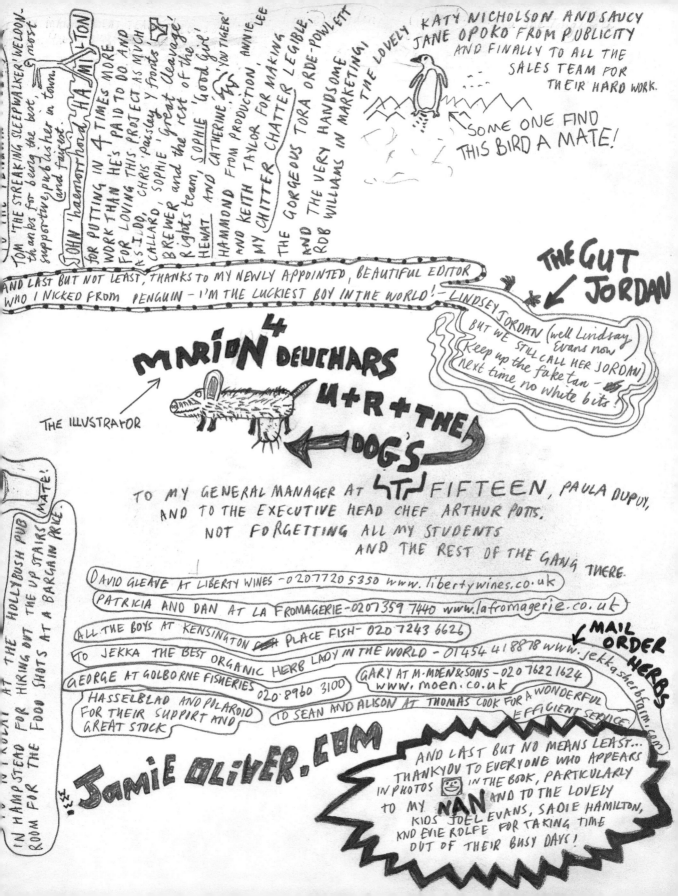

SOME ONE FIND THIS BIRD A MATE!

AND LAST BUT NOT LEAST, THANKS TO MY NEWLY APPOINTED, BEAUTIFUL EDITOR WHO I NICKED FROM PENGUIN - I'M THE LUCKIEST BOY IN THE WORLD! - LINDSEY JORDAN

THE GUT JORDAN

LINDSAY JORDAN (well Lindsay Evans now) but we still call her JORDAN keep up the fake tan - next time, no white bits!

MARION⁴ DEUCHARS

THE ILLUSTRATOR

U + R + THE DOG'S

TO MY GENERAL MANAGER AT FIFTEEN, PAULA DUPUY, AND TO THE EXECUTIVE HEAD CHEF ARTHUR POTTS. NOT FORGETTING ALL MY STUDENTS AND THE REST OF THE GANG THERE.

DAVID GLEAVE AT LIBERTY WINES - 0207 720 5350 www.libertywines.co.uk

PATRICIA AND DAN AT LA FROMAGERIE - 0207 359 7440 www.lafromagerie.co.uk

ALL THE BOYS AT KENSINGTON PLACE FISH - 020 7243 6626

TO JEKKA THE BEST ORGANIC HERB LADY IN THE WORLD - 01454 418878 www.jekkasherbfarm.com

MAIL ORDER HERBS

GEORGE AT GOLBORNE FISHERIES 020 8960 3100

GARY AT M·MOEN & SONS - 020 7622 1624 www.moen.co.uk

HASSELBLAD AND POLAROID FOR THEIR SUPPORT AND GREAT STOCK

TO SEAN AND ALISON AT THOMAS COOK FOR A WONDERFUL EFFICIENT SERVICE

IN HAMPSTEAD AT THE HOLLYBUSH PUB FOR HIRING OUT THE UPSTAIRS ROOM FOR THE FOOD SHOTS AT A BARGAIN PRICE. MATE!

JAMIE OLIVER.COM

AND LAST BUT NO MEANS LEAST... THANKYOU TO EVERYONE WHO APPEARS IN PHOTOS IN THE BOOK, PARTICULARLY TO MY NAN AND TO THE LOVELY KIDS JOEL EVANS, SADIE HAMILTON, AND EVIE ROLFE FOR TAKING TIME OUT OF THEIR BUSY DAYS!

INDEX

v indicates a vegetarian recipe
Page references in **bold** denote an illustration

c

p

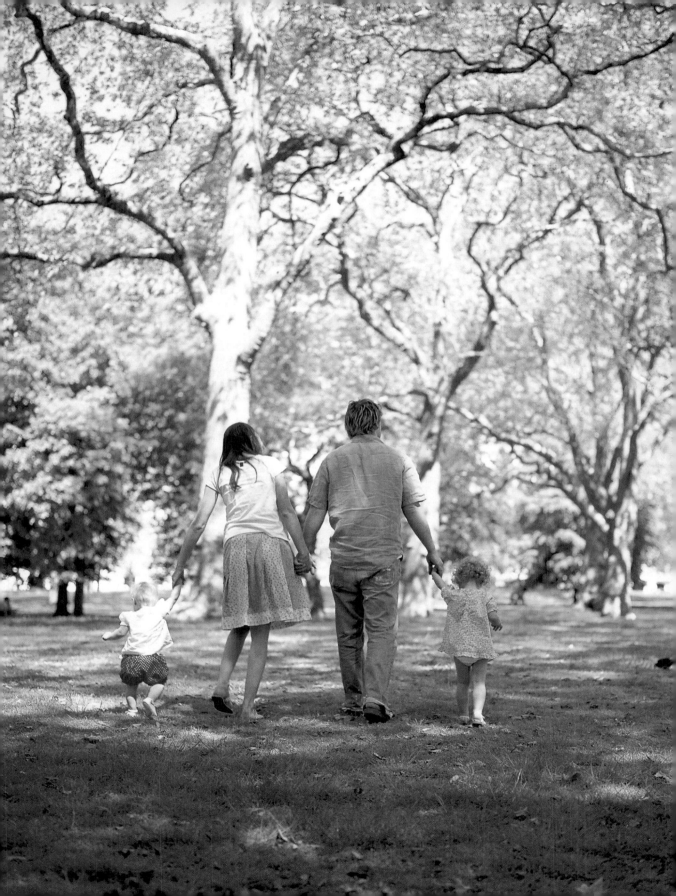